The Limbic System
SECOND EDITION

Robert L. Isaacson

State University of New York at Binghamton
Binghamton, New York

Plenum Press • New York and London

Library of Congress Cataloging in Publication Data

Isacson, Robert Lee, 1928–
  The limbic system.

  Bibliography: p.
  Includes index.
  1. Limbic system. I. Title. [DNLM: 1. Limbic system. WL 307 I73L]
QP383.2.I82 1982   599.01′88   82-9077
ISBN 0-306-40874-0   AACR2

© 1982 Plenum Press, New York
A Division of Plenum Publishing Corporation
233 Spring Street, New York, N.Y. 10013

Printed in the United States of America

Preface to Second Edition

Like the first edition of *The Limbic System*, this book was written as an introduction to the neurobehavioral study of the limbic system; it is intended for students of brain–behavior relationships in psychobiology, neurosciences, physiology, and anatomy, as well as those with clinical interests in the brain and its actions. Also, like the first edition, the book is flavored with my own orientation to the field based on some 22 years of active research.

My own perspective on the limbic system is described in the final chapter. It is an overview of how the different portions of the brain may work in concert to produce mental and behavioral actions. I do not hold to the ideas presented there with strong commitment. This chapter is only an overview and I am sure that other and better comprehensive approaches will be generated. Nevertheless, it helps to have some perspective to integrate diverse facts and information.

In regard to other biases, I still believe that the greatest gains in understanding brain organization will come from studies using the rat, the cat, and the rabbit. Research using nonhuman primates takes even more time and expense now than it did in 1974, and the generation of useful information with such species must therefore proceed slowly. Research using humans which is directed toward understanding brain function must depend on examination of the effects of disease or accidents. Because of this limitation, the study of individuals with similar damage can occur only rarely—if at all. Furthermore, as emphasized throughout this edition, the observable consequences of brain damage depend on genetic endowment, pre- and postdamage experiences, and other factors, as well as on the nature of the damage. Therefore, I doubt that much fundamental knowledge of brain damage will come from studies with the human. As I mentioned in the preface to the first edition, I am convinced that the use of the lesion technique will provide the mainstay of future research, although the goals and methods of lesion studies will be different in the next 10 to 20 years. Despite its difficulties, which are really similar to those using brain stimulation or other approaches,[1] there is no other method that offers a better way to determine just how large portions of the central nervous system interact with each other. In the future such studies will use new neurochemical techniques that offer the promise of distinguishing cellular from axonal damage and more biochemical and pharmacological methods to determine the lesion-induced effects.

In 1974 I admitted that the book could not be considered comprehensive. Only some 500 references were cited at that time, and it was clear that many more could have been included. I tried to concentrate on the ones that seemed most important for current research and theory. In this second edition there are almost 1,400 references and, once again, I am sure that they are not comprehensive. The large increase in the number of references that needed to be noted is a sign of the scientific information explosion in general and an increased interest in limbic system structure and function.

In the original preface I expressed my appreciation to the graduate students who were then in the laboratory. Their thoughts, ideas, and energies about our research were always exciting. Now, another group of students is in the laboratory, helping to unravel the secrets of the brain and behavior. These are John Hannigan, Jr., Joe E. Springer, and Jeanne Ryan. Daniel K. Reinstein, now at the Massachusetts Institute of Technology, was with me for most of the period I was rewriting the book and has helped shape my ideas about the limbic system. To them, my thanks. They keep me young, at least in spirit. In the last year or so, I have also had the benefits of collaboration of two more senior associates, David Hertzler (SUNY–Oswego) and Alex Poplawsky (Bloomsburg State College), who visited the laboratory for extended periods.

---

[1] Isaacson, R. L. Brain stimulation effects related to those of lesions. In M. M. Patterson & R. P. Kesner (Eds.), *Electrical stimulation research techniques.* New York: Academic Press, 1981, pp. 205–220.

When starting this second edition, I wrote to several friends who are recognized authorities in different areas of limbic system research to solicit their ideas about what should be emphasized. They all responded with their ideas and I have tried to follow their suggestions. However, it has taken so long to finish this second edition that I am sure they would make additional or different suggestions now if asked. I appreciate their help in orienting me to their perspectives. Those to whom I wrote originally were Graham Goddard, Sebastian P. Grossman, and Gary W. Van Hoesen. While writing the book I benefited from discussions of the content and ideas with a number of people, especially Peter Donovick, Linda Spear, Paul MacLean, Per Andersen, Larry Swanson, Daniel P. Kimble, and György Buzsaki. It may be hard to recognize the specific contributions made by any of these people to the book itself but they produced strong influences on my thinking and my writing.

No book can be prepared without excellent secretarial assistance. In the first edition it was Mrs. Virginia Walker, at the University of Florida, who was indispensable. This time it was Mrs. JoAnn Kovalich at SUNY–Binghamton. Without her help, the book would not have been finished. Thanks.

ROBERT L. ISAACSON

Binghamton, New York

Preface to First Edition

While this book is intended to be an introduction to the neuroanatomy of the limbic system and to studies of the behavior of animals in which the limbic system is stimulated or damaged, it is primarily intended for advanced students of brain–behavior relationships. I have assumed the reader to have some understanding of the structure of the brain, of basic neurophysiology, and of modern behavioral techniques. It has been written for students in graduate programs in psychobiology, physiological psychology, and the neurosciences, but it also should be of interest to some medical students and to others with catholic interests in the biology of behavior.

In the first chapter, I review the structure of the limbic system and in subsequent chapters consider the behavioral effects of lesions and stimulation of components of the limbic system. Supplemental information derived from recording the electrical signals of the brain is included where it seems appropriate. The final chapter presents a perspective of the limbic system related to brain stem mechanisms and the neocortex. Understanding the behavioral contributions of the limbic system presupposes understanding how the limbic system interacts with other systems of the brain.

Even though there is only one chapter overtly devoted to theoretical issues, various biases of mine influence all chapters. Anyone reading the book with a critical attitude will soon be aware of them. I would like to alert the reader to some of them ahead of time.

Simply put: the book is flavored by my own orientation to research and reading. For the past 15 years, I have been involved in research programs which were directed at elucidating the effects of limbic system destruction on behavior in the rat, cat, and rabbit.

Therefore, studies using these species and using lesion techniques probably are overly represented. Other biases of mine will be apparent.

In many later chapters, consideration is given to the behavioral correlates of electrical rhythms recorded from various limbic structures. In these chapters, the effects of electrical stimulation of various limbic structures on behavior are also discussed. Yet, while these topics are discussed, much less emphasis is placed on them and on studies using other species with which I am less well acquainted.

My biases, the topics and areas given emphasis, come in part from my own research. This research is based on beliefs pertaining to research strategies. I believe that the most substantial knowledge available about the limbic system comes from the use of stimulation and lesion techniques in rats and cats. There is far less useful information available today arising from work using other techniques and other species. Since a great deal more information is needed before an adequate conceptualization can be achieved, this information must come from careful studies using species like the cat and the rat. These animals are amenable to laboratory experimentation and can be used in sufficient numbers so as to provide this information relatively quickly. If we had to rely on studies using nonhuman primates, our understanding of the behavioral contributions made by the limbic system could be greatly delayed. The rat is a necessary laboratory tool, both for neuroanatomists and for those interested in the behavioral contributions of the limbic system. The cat makes its greatest contribution to neurophysiological research.

The other obvious orientation of the book is the emphasis placed on understanding the functions of the limbic system as revealed by destruction of its parts. For 30 years and more, investigations have been underway of the behavior of animals which have had some portion of the limbic system destroyed by aspirative or by electrolytic lesions. Seeking to understand a structure by destroying it is a useful technique for the behaviorally oriented neuroscientist, although it has many faults, dangers, and traps for the unwary experimenter. Nevertheless, equally dangerous are the faults and traps awaiting those using other techniques in the neurobehavioral sciences. In reality, the lesion technique is no better or worse than any other, such as recording electrical rhythms or recording from single units. Satisfactory understanding of the limbic system will not come from the studies of animals with lesions of this or that part of the limbic system or from the analysis of single cell activity but from theoretical contributions derived from the use of all available techniques. Theories must be evaluated on the basis of whether they make sense of the facts to be explained. A theory must provide a meaningful and useful synthesis of information derived from any and all techniques.

Even though the book has a large number of references to published work on the limbic system, it is not a truly comprehensive review of the literature. I doubt that a totally comprehensive review of the experimental literature can be done by anyone. Still, I have tried to represent fairly most of the important studies which have influenced present research directions. Nevertheless, some of my colleagues will be offended by not finding their favorite studies in the book. To them I apologize for the oversight. On the other hand, some studies were omitted because I felt that they had not added a great deal to our understanding of the limbic system. I have tried to select articles from the literature which highlight information of the greatest importance for the understanding of the limbic system.

Theories of limbic function have not been emphasized in this book, since I do not think there are any adequate theories of limbic system function. My theory, presented in the last chapter, is offered in an apologetic fashion. At best, it offers only the broadest outlines for a schema of limbic system function. In almost a playful spirit, it is offered as a potential stimulant to others. In a lecture given at the University of Florida in the spring of 1973, Paul MacLean suggested that scientists did not belong in the laboratory if their work and the generation of ideas were not fun. All of my days in the laboratory have been rewarding. I cannot imagine a more fascinating or more interesting life than struggling to find out how the brain works. Therefore, I hope the reader will evaluate the last chapter with understanding.

But my research and study of the limbic system is motivated by far more than the joy it provides. It is motivated by the belief that learning at least some of the secrets of the nervous system will be of value to mankind. This is not an intangible or abstract motive. Retarded children are very real, as are people with other brain disorders. While much of my present work is directed toward problems of general interest rather than toward retardation specifically, the ultimate goal is to better understand the human condition and to help provide information on which effective therapies and treatments for the brain-damaged can be based.

Accordingly, this is the appropriate time to acknowledge the fact that much of the research summarized in this book, my own included, would not have been possible without the financial support provided by two agencies of the government: the National Institute of Mental Health and the National Science Foundation. The administrators in these agencies who have been advocates and supporters of the peer-review system for the support of biobehavioral sciences have made a real contribution.

Part of the joy which comes from the academic life and the laboratory is the association with young, powerful minds coming to grips with the challenge of science. One of the most pleasant features, therefore, of my academic life has been the opportunity to watch students become accomplished neurobehavioral scientists. I feel that I have been very lucky to count among my former students so many who have made substantial contributions to man's knowledge of brain and behavior. Therefore, if this book has any group to whom it should be dedicated, it would be to my graduate students, both those who have left the laboratory and those who are presently struggling through the ordeals of graduate education. The present group of students has helped me in the preparation of this book by their thoughts and criticisms. These include Michael L. Woodruff, Ron Baisden, Barbara Schneiderman, Linda Lanier, Ted Petit, and Tom Lanthorn.

In addition, in the preparation of this book I have benefited from the advice of friends, well known in neurobehavioral fields, who have read portions of the manuscript. These include Dr. Paul MacLean, Dr. Graham Goddard, Dr. Charles Votaw, Dr. Elliot Valenstein, Dr. Joel Lubar, and Dr. Frederick A. King. Most especially, I would like to acknowledge the comments made by my colleagues Drs. Carol Van Hartesveldt and Peter Molnar. Their ideas and research in the area of the limbic system function always have been top flight.

At last, I would like to thank Mrs. Virginia Walker for her help in preparing the manuscript in all of its various revisions. She has tolerated the almost endless changes of the text I have made and without her assistance the book just could not have been completed.

ROBERT L. ISAACSON

Gainesville, Florida

Contents

1

The Structure of the Limbic System

The term *limbic system* derives from the concept of a *limbic lobe* presented by the French anatomist Broca, in 1878. The word *limbic* refers to a border, fringe, or hem. Broca used the term *limbic lobe* to designate the brain tissue that surrounds the brain stem and that lies beneath the neocortical mantle. In a gross fashion, this term includes the cingulate and hippocampal gyri, as well as the isthmus that connects the two. It also includes the various gyri that surround the olfactory fibers running back from the olfactory bulb and stalk. Within this inner lobe of the brain, the structures are presumed to be organized into two layers. The tissue thought to be phyletically the oldest (the allocortex) makes up the inner ring. The outer limbic ring does not resemble either neocortex or allocortex based on study of its cellular structure. It is therefore called *transitional cortex*, or *juxtallocortex* ("next to the allocortex"). This approach is of some value as a general conceptual scheme, but it fails to recognize that the inner ring is not a uniform band of tissue. In fact, it is a discrete set of structures, which can be identified more or less readily by gross dissection, and it is these structural subunits of the inner ring of the limbic lobe on which our attention will be centered during the remainder of this book.

Broca emphasized two aspects of the limbic lobe: (1) its strong relationships with the olfactory apparatus and (2) its presence as a common denominator among the brains of mammals. The first of these principles is based on the observation that most of the structures of the limbic lobe receive plentiful projections from the olfactory system in the brains of simple animals (e.g., amphibians and reptiles). As a result, the limbic lobe has been considered the rhinencephalon, the "smell brain," presumably responsible for analysis of the olfactory environment.

The structures of the inner portions of the limbic lobe are surrounded by transitional cortical tissue. In different regions of the brain, the transitional cortices are given different names (e.g., entorhinal cortex, retrosplenial cortex, periamygdaloid cortex). Understanding of the limbic system must include understanding the activities of both the inner ring of the limbic structures and the outer ring of transitional cortex (juxtallocortex). Most of the information available today is about the inner ring structures of the limbic lobe. Much less is known about the transitional cortex.

Historically, there have been various debates about the particular anatomical structures of the inner brain that "should be" regarded as belonging to the limbic system. The nervous system is not easily distributed into categories on the basis of hard-and-fast rules. It is possible, in fact, to call a collection of structures a system on some arbitrary basis. The value of a categorizing scheme must be the extent to which it helps us to understand the activities of the brain and its relationship to behavior. For the purposes of this book, I am going to emphasize the role of certain inner core limbic structures and refer to them as the *limbic system*. The structures include the hypothalamus, the amygdala, the hippocampus, and the septal area. Some consideration will be given to the cingulate cortex–anterior thalamus relationships.

The justification for this grouping is based on the fact that the hypothalamus has strong interconnections with all of the other regions. From a functional point of view, this classification can be justified by the fact that many, if not all, of the effects produced by stimulation and lesions of the extrahypothalamic limbic structures can be replicated by stimulation or lesions of the hypothalamus.

THE LIMBIC SYSTEM IN NONMAMMALS

Knowledge of the structure of the limbic system in the amphibian brain can help us to understand the basic organizational plan of the limbic system in mammals. Many of the connections among brain structures in mammalian brain exist in a simpler, more direct form in the salamander. The interrelationships among limbic structures are more difficult to trace in more advanced brains owing in part to the extensive development of the neocortex and the corpus callosum. Their development is correlated with distortions of the fiber pathways of the limbic system.

Probably the most prominent portions of the forebrain of the salamander are the olfactory bulb and the rudimentary cerebral hemispheres. These cerebral hemispheres are made up of cells arranged in a more-or-less laminated fashion, although only a small portion of the hemispheres is considered "general cortex"—the precursor of neocortex. The hemispheres surround the diencephalon and the basal ganglia. These internal structures were considered by Elliot Smith (1910) the heart of a protomammalian brain, and it was around them that higher neural systems are thought to have developed in evolution.

The actual structure of the brains of forerunners to mammals can, of course, only be guessed, since there is no way to determine the brain structures of nonexistent animals. Theories of their structures have to be based on inferences drawn from living species available for study. These species are only the recent progeny of earlier animals and are considerably different from their ancestors. Existing animals in all species are the current products of the forces of natural selection acting over thousands of years on genetic materials that have changed through mutations and selective matings.

Therefore, it is surprising that there seems to be considerable uniformity in the interconnections among the structures of the limbic system in all living vertebrates. It is on this basis that many investigators believe that study of the brains of lower animals can provide help in understanding the patterns of neural organization of all vertebrates.

Figure 1 shows some figures from Herrick's classic book, *The Brain of the Tiger Salamander* (1948). Large pyramidal cells in the area identified as the hippocampus (P. Hip.) project into the area immediately beneath it, labeled as the septal area (Nuc. L.S. and Nuc. M.S.). Some of these fibers project past these septal areas into regions situated along the base of the brain. This is an area containing fibers of the medial forebrain bundle (f. Med.). Its location can be considered approximately that of the lateral hypothalamus. The fibers of hippocampal origin extending into the hypothalamus can be thought of as precursors of the fornix system as it is found in animals with more complex brains. The fornix system connects these three areas, which happen to be close to each other in the salamander. These same relationships are found in the more complex brains, even though the hippocampus, the septal area, and the hypothalamus have become physically separated from each other to a much greater extent.

A conceptual division of the simple salamander forebrain into a mesial division, dealing with the regulation of the internal organs and the autonomic nervous system, and a lateral division, involved with the coordination of somatic activities, has often been proposed. The

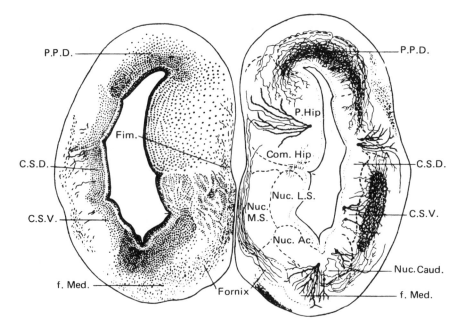

Figure 1. Diagrams of cross sections through brain of tiger salamander. Most anterior section is at top, most posterior at bottom. Drawings have been simplified to emphasize limbic structures and tracts. Abbreviations: P.P.D., primordial dorsal pallii dorsalis (general cortex); P. Hip., primordium hippocampi; Com. Hip., hippocampal commissure; C.S.D., dorsal part of corpus striatum; C.S.V., ventral part of corpus striatum; Nuc. Caud., caudate nucleus; f. Med., medial forebrain bundle; Nuc. Ac., nucleus accumbens septi; Nuc. M.S., medial septal nucleus; Nuc. L.S., lateral septal nucleus; Fim., fimbria; D.B., diagonal band of Broca; Nuc. Amg., amygdala; Com. Amg., amygdalar commissures; Nuc. Po. A., anterior preoptic nucleus; Str. t., stria terminalis; Tr. St. t., striotegmental tract. Figures adapted from Herrick (1948).

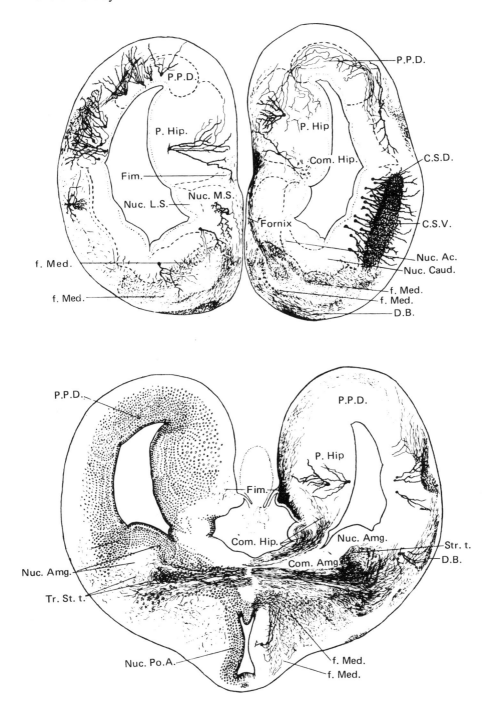

hippocampus and the septal area may be regarded as most closely associated with the mesial division. A substantial portion of the amygdala develops from the lateral systems concerned with somatic activities. Therefore, it could be classified with the basal ganglia, which are related to the lateral forebrain systems. Yet, the amygdala also lies close to the hypothalamus and has rich interconnections with it. The fibers that interconnect the amygdala with the hypothalamus are maintained in the more complex brains of mammals even though the amygdala is much farther away from the hypothalamus than it is in the salamander. In the mammalian brain, the amygdala and the hippocampus lie next to each other in the temporal regions, yet there are very few fibers interconnecting them. Proximity in the more complicated brain does not assure a large number of interconnecting fibers. However, proximity in the relatively simple brain does seem to assure that strong interconnections will be maintained in the more complicated brain.

In Figure 1, some of the commissural systems of the forebrain have been sketched. Commissures connecting the amygdalae and the hippocampi are shown (Com. Amg. and Com. Hip.). The amygdalar commissure is incorporated into the anterior commissure in mammals, whereas the hippocampal commissure maintains itself as a separate system. In more complex brains, such as those of primates, the anterior commissure is mainly a commissural pathway connecting neocortical and limbic structures. The contribution of the fibers of the intermediate olfactory tract that loop from one side of the brain to the other becomes relatively less significant.

The lateral hypothalamic area of the salamander has few, if any, cells in it. It is made up of a dense neuropil consisting of a fine mesh of axons and dendrites. This is the same area through which the fibers of the medial forebrain bundle system pass as they run along the base of the brain. The fibers of the medial forebrain bundle exist in the salamander in the lateral hypothalamic region, just as they do in more complicated brains. The nuclei of the lateral hypothalamus that are found in mammals are thought to be a bed nucleus for the medial forebrain bundle system (Valverde, 1963). Anatomically, the lateral hypothalamic region cannot be dissociated from the medial forebrain bundle. The cells of the lateral hypothalamus live in the midst of a considerable amount of nerve impulse traffic, passing through the medial forebrain bundle.

Many neural systems related to activities of the limbic system are well developed in the salamander. For example, a fiber system running from the habenulae to the ventral tegmentum and the interpeduncular nucleus is very prominent. This fiber system of the habenulae is considered analogous to the habenulopeduncular tract, or tractus retroflexus, found in mammalian brains. The habenulopeduncular tract should be considered a discharge pathway from the limbic system, because the habenulae receive fibers from the septal area, the dorsal hippocampus, and the lateral preoptic area of the anterior hypothalamus, among other areas. A neural tract, the stria medullaris, is the most direct pathway between the septal area and the habenulae, but influences from the septal area and the thalamus may also reach the habenulae by other routes, such as by the inferior thalamic peduncle. Some investigators believe that descending limbic system influences converge on both the hypothalamus and the habenulae. The former is thought to represent a controlling region for the internal organ systems, while the latter may be a controlling region for sensory and somatic systems (e.g., Mok & Mogenson, 1972).

The identification of the habenulopeduncular tract in the salamander brain depends on the identification of regions that can be considered the habenulae and the interpeduncular nucleus. But the "habenulae" and the "interpeduncular nucleus" of the salamander are sometimes identified on the basis of the large fiber tract connecting them. Thus, the identification of both pathways and nuclear areas can be circular. The study of comparative anatomy rests on the criteria used to establish anatomical homologies among various species.

Douglas and Marcellus (1975) have presented evidence that there are two independent evolutionary trends in regard to "higher brains." One of these is the neocortical surface and the subcortical regions closely associated with it. The other is the structures of the limbic system. Some species may be high in one or the other. For example, monkeys have substantial neocortical development but little limbic enlargement. Rabbits are one example of the opposite developmental trend: substantial limbic systems and poor neocortical development. Douglas and Marcellus believe that humans are unique in having substantial advancement on both limbic and neocortical dimensions.

The pathways of the limbic system do not become diminished in brains that have great neocortical development. Even though in the brains of animals with a large neocortical development the relative volume of the limbic system structures has become less, the number of axons in the fiber tracts has become greater, both in absolute number and relative to other fiber systems of the brain. In humans, for example, there are five times the number of fibers in the fornix as in the optic tracts.

THE QUESTION OF HOMOLOGY

At this point, it may be worthwhile to consider some general issues related to "homologous" neural structures. What are the criteria by which a nuclear group or fiber system in the brain of one species can be said to be comparable to a nuclear group or fiber system found in the brain of another species? One example is the habenulopeduncular tract. How can a set of fibers identified in the amphibian be homologous to a set found in a more complex mammalian brain? It depends on the identification of an area in front of the tectum as being "homologous" to the highly organized habenular nuclei of the mammalian brain. This identification is based on the large fiber system coming from it and descending into the ventral portion. Thus, it is impossible to separate the criteria used to identify nuclear and fiber systems. Fiber systems define nuclear areas and nuclear areas define fiber systems—the essence of circular reasoning.

Another possible means of identifying homologous nuclear areas would be similarities of cytological structure. For example, this approach would imply that a nuclear area densely populated with small cells in the brain of one species ought to be populated with small, densely packed cells in all species. In some cases, this criterion may be useful, but it cannot be of general applicability, since many areas of any brain share similar cytoarchitectural characteristics. The two types of criteria can be used together. Nuclear areas could be considered homologous if they had structural similarities *and* shared similar input and output characteristics. The famous anatomist C. J. Herrick used both types of criteria but considered the similarity of structural anatomy the more important. His identification of the hippocampus in the brain of the tiger salamander was based on the fact that this area contains pyramidal cells similar to those found in the hippocampus of mammalian brains. In addition, he found the area identified as the hippocampus to be interconnected with the hypothalamus and an area he identified as the septal area on the basis of cytoarchitecture.

Other anatomists believe that the only appropriate criterion for regarding brain regions of different species as homologous is the origin of the cells in these regions. Two brain areas in different species should be considered homologous only if they arise from similar cell groups during development.

Campbell and Hodos (1970) have discussed the various criteria used to establish homologous areas. They concluded that neither the ontogenetic ("common ancestor") criterion nor the anatomical similarity criterion should be used exclusively. They proposed that many criteria must be used to establish whether two brain areas of different species are homologous. The experimentally determined fiber connections between areas, the topology and topography of the areas involved, the position of reliable sulci, the origin of the areas in embryonic development, the morphology of the nerve cells, the histochemical composition of the areas, the electrophysiological activity of the areas, and finally the comparability of behavioral changes found after lesions or stimulation of the areas all must be taken into consideration. Each of these is a "soft criterion" for the establishment of homologous brain areas. It is only when all, or many, of them converge on a similar conclusion that the areas should be considered "homologous."

Given these considerations, the many similarities that have been described in the organization of limbic areas in salamanders and mammals become less certain. Only a few criteria have been used to identify the septal area, the hippocampus, the amygdala, etc., in the nonmammalian vertebrate brain. Even if the identifications of homologous areas in amphibians have been correct, their interconnections only approximate those found in other species. They provide information only about the general pattern of interconnections among limbic regions and tell nothing about the fine-grain patterns of interconnections that are the hallmark of a particular species. Thus, the evolutionary approach is a vague and uncertain guide to understanding the anatomy of the limbic system. The serious student of comparative anatomy must study the specific patterns of limbic interconnections found in particular species.

At the same time, however, there can be a progression in understanding from the general to the specific. While each species does have its unusual modifications of limbic system anatomy, there is a basic plan that appears in the mammals and that is foreshadowed in the amphibian and reptile brains. In the next sections, the patterns of limbic system organization revealed in the mammalian brain are presented with some comments, where appropriate, on the variations of pattern found in certain species.

THE HYPOTHALAMUS

For many years, the hypothalamus has been known as that region of the forebrain most concerned with the regulation of the internal organs. In fact, it has been called the *head ganglion* of the autonomic nervous system. In addition, the hypothalamus plays an important role in the release of hormones from the anterior pituitary as well as producing hormones of its own, as is discussed later in this chapter. Consequently, the hypothalamus has been a major target of research relating the brain to endocrine activities.

However, it is now well established that the hypothalamus is also concerned with the regulation of somatic activities. In addition, it can alter the level of neural activity in widespread areas of the forebrain. Its effects are exerted both forward into limbic structures and neocortex and backward into midbrain, brain stem, and spinal cord.

The hypothalamus is the most ventral structural "unit" of the diencephalon. Other major diencephalic components are the dorsal thalamus, the ventral thalamus, and the epithalamus.[1] The hypothalamus is a bilaterally symmetrical structure, being divided into left and right halves by the third ventricle. At its rostral extreme, the hypothalamus merges with the preoptic area. It is called *preoptic* because it is rostral to the optic chiasm. There is no clear boundary between these regions, and consequently, the separation is made arbitrarily.[2] The posterior margin of the hypothalamus is usually considered the caudal aspect of the mammillary bodies. Laterally, the

---

[1] This descriptive summary follows the approach proposed by Crosby, Humphrey, and Lauer (1962).

hypothalamus is limited by various nuclei of the ventral thalamus and, in other regions, by various fiber tracts.

In looking at the base of the brain, the following landmarks can be seen: the paired or single protuberance (depending on the species) of the mammillary bodies caudally; a raised, longitudinally oriented middle section called the *tuber cinereum;* a small median eminence leading to the stalk of the pituitary gland; the pituitary gland; and, most rostrally, the optic chiasm.

Throughout the hypothalamus, three zones or regions can be described running from the third ventricle toward the more lateral aspects. These are (1) a periventricular region, (2) a middle or medial zone, and (3) a lateral region. For the most part, cells in the periventricular region are small and lie in rows adjacent to the ventricular lining. The periventricular nucleus is a columnar arrangement of cells in the periventricular gray extending from the infundibular region to an area behind the ventromedial nucleus. It is found along the base of the third ventricle. It is thought not to have a glia cell barrier separating it from the ependymal lining of the ventricle. Fibers of the medial forebrain bundle pass between the medial and the lateral hypothalamic areas, as well as *through* the lateral area, thus producing one obvious anatomical distinction between these regions.

Nuclear Groups

Most of the nuclei of the hypothalamus lie within the medial region of the hypothalamus. The supraoptic and paraventricular nuclei are the most rostral of the medial nuclei. The supraoptic nuclei are found at the lateral margins of the optic tract. The paraventricular nuclei are located along the top of the third ventricle. They extend laterally for a moderate distance from the top of the ventricle. Some fibers from these nuclei extend to the neural lobe of the pituitary gland. The suprachiasmatic nuclei lie above the optic chiasm as a paired bilateral structure. The arcuate nuclei are bilaterally paired nuclear groups along the ventral portion of the third ventricle. In a

---

[2] Some authors consider the preoptic area a component of the hypothalamus, and the term *prothalamus* has been used to include the preoptic area and the anterior hypothalamus.

way, they seem to be symmetrical with the paraventricular nuclei. These nuclei stand out from the top of the third ventricle, while the arcuate nuclei extend from the bottom of the ventricle when viewed in cross sections of the hypothalamus.

The anterior hypothalamic area (AHA) is a region beginning behind the preoptic area and extending past the infundibular and middle regions of the hypothalamus. It has small, relatively evenly distributed cells that are richly interconnected with the forebrain and thalamic areas.

The ventromedial nuclei are found in the ventral parts of the medial hypothalamus. The nucleus contains large cells, although they are not as large as the large cells of the paraventricular nucleus and other nuclear groups thought to have neurosecretory functions. Proceeding caudally from its anterior origin, the nucleus grows rapidly in size and comes to occupy most of the ventral regions of the hypothalamus. Laterally, the AHA merges with the lateral hypothalamic region, and caudally, the area extends until the dorsomedial and ventromedial nuclei appear. Even though there are no well-demarked regions, it is possible to detect several subregions of the area (for further details, see Saper, Swanson, & Cowan, 1978). The dorsomedial nuclei are located above the ventromedial nuclei. In the rat, the ventromedial nuclei are more prominent than the dorsomedial nuclei, but both may be seen without difficulty with usual histological stains. The dorsomedial nuclei are less prominent in primates than in most nonprimate mammals. Above and extending caudally past the dorsomedial nuclei is the posterior hypothalamic area. More anteriorly, this region is continuous with the dorsal hypothalamic area.

In some regions of the hypothalamus, the columns of the fornix are surrounded by cells that are called the *perifornical nucleus*.

Primates have paired mammillary bodies, but the rat has only a single eminence at the posterior aspect of the hypothalamus, although within this prominence there are several nuclei. The medial mammillary nuclei are the largest of the mammillary complex. Fibers from the fornix also richly penetrate the region. The supramammillary commissure contains fibers of the fornix and the medial forebrain bundle that cross from one side to the other, although fibers from the red nuclei and several tegmental nuclei also pass in this commissure.

Behind the medial mammillary nuclei is the most posterior portion of the hypothalamus, sometimes called the *posterior mammillary nucleus*. Just rostral to the mammillary nuclei are the dorsal and ventral premammillary nuclei, which are considered by some investigators "bed nuclei" for the periventricular system. A nuclear group dorsal to the medial mammillary nuclei is called the *supramammillary nucleus*. A simplified schematic drawing of the hypothalamic nuclei is shown in Figure 2.

The pituitary gland is composed of three parts: a posterior, "neural pituitary" connected to the median eminence and the hypothalamus, an anterior portion that does not receive nerve fibers from the hypothalamus or the posterior lobe, and an intermediate lobe or area that does receive some small neural fibers from the hypothalamus. This intermediate area is poorly vascularized, and the release of the hormones from this area is probably not due to chemical influences transported over the portal venous system.

In the rat the suprachiasmatic nuclei are bilateral nuclear groups above, and partly embedded in, the posterior portions of the optic

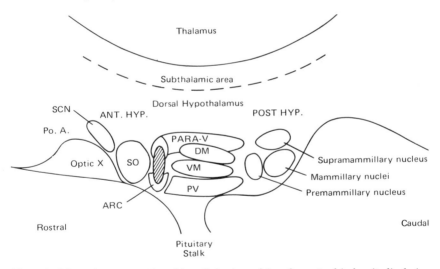

Figure 2. Schematic representation of hypothalamic nuclei as they extend in longitudinal view of the diencephalon. Abbreviations: Po. A., anterior preoptic area; SCN, suprachiasmatic nucleus; SO, supraoptic nuclei; DM, dorsomedial nucleus; VM, ventromedial nucleus; PARA-V, paraventricular nucleus; PV, periventricular nucleus; ARC, arcuate nucleus; ANT HYP, anterior hypothalamic area; POST HYP, posterior hypothalamic area; Optic X, optic chiasm. The shaded eliptic shape surrounded by the PARA-V and ARC regions in the figure represents the ventral extension of the third ventricle.

chiasm. They are divided from each other by the bottom of the third ventricle. They are surrounded laterally by the anterior hypothalamus.

Retinal projections to the paired suprachiasmatic nuclei of the hypothalamus are now well established in the rat (R. Y. Moore, 1973; Moore & Lenn, 1972; Mason & Lincoln, 1976) as well as in many other species, including primates. Fibers from one retina reach nuclei on both sides of the brain and end in their ventrolateral portions. The fibers reaching the suprachiasmatic nucleus seem to be collaterals that arise from axons of various sizes in the optic tract and chiasm (Millhouse, 1977).

Another projection to the suprachiasmatic nuclei arises from the ventral lateral geniculate nucleus (Swanson, Cowan, & Jones, 1974). Catecholamine and cholinergic fibers reach the suprachiasmatic nucleus, and there is an especially heavy serotonin distribution arising from the medial raphe area (Fuxe, 1965; Aghajanian, Bloom, & Sheard, 1969). Information probably related to visual environment reaches cells in the lateral hypothalamus from the superior colliculi. These fibers do not seem to contact the suprachiasmatic nucleus directly, but indirect influences on the nucleus are possible. How the fibers from the superior colliculi contact the cells of the hypothalamus is curious. Apparently, these fibers run forward in the optic chiasm, and nerves do not leave these bundles. Dendrites from the hypothalamic cells grow into the bundles to make synaptic contacts (Fallon & Moore, 1979).

The efferents from the suprachiasmatic nuclei would be anticipated to reach neuroendocrine-related portions of the hypothalamus because of this nucleus's association with rhythmic activities of the individual. Swanson and Cowan (1975c) found that fibers from this nucleus go caudally and dorsally to the periventricular area and make contact with dendrites of cells in the ventromedial, dorsomedial, and arcuate nuclei. Other axons progress caudally in the medial forebrain bundle. Another, smaller group of fibers reaches toward the median eminence of the hypothalamus. The projections are not discretely defined; rather they tend to end in neuropil, which contains a few cells, but is largely made up of cell processes. The axons that project to the median eminence have been reported to contain vasopressin-neurophysin (Vandesande, Dierckx, & DeMey, 1975).

Metabolic activity in this nucleus measured by the uptake of a radioactively labeled glucose analogue seems to be related to both time of day and environmental lighting conditions (Schwartz & Gainer, 1977).

Fiber Systems

Many of the fiber systems related to the hypothalamus have little or no myelin and are difficult to visualize with standard light-microscopic techniques. Only recently have experimental techniques been developed that allow reasonably complete knowledge to be gained concerning hypothalamic fiber connections. These new developments in experimental methods have revealed a great deal of new information about the short fiber pathways of the hypothalamus and have also changed some of the old ideas about the longer pathways.

The major fiber pathways associated with the hypothalamus are shown in Figures 3 and 4. These schematic diagrams represent a composite of results of many studies of hypothalamic fiber connections and interconnections.[3] Despite the complexities of the figures, they should be regarded as simplified representations of reality.

As can be seen from Figure 3, most of the neural input to the hypothalamus from the forebrain arises from areas of the limbic system and the olfactory regions, while most of the ascending fibers from the brain stem come from midbrain regions and the medial periventricular system. The output of the hypothalamus is also restricted in nature. Primary targets include the brain stem sites of origin of the monoamine-containing neurons, the reticular formation, the limbic regions, and the median eminence and posterior pituitary gland. With the exception of limited anterior regions of the prefrontal cortex, there are few connections with the neocortical mantle, the major sensory-thalamic-cortical systems, or the basal ganglia.

The preoptic area has strong connections with the anterior hypothalamus. This could be anticipated from the fact that there is no

---

[3] While the fiber distributions of the hypothalamus have been drawn from many sources, interested readers are especially urged to consult Saper, Swanson, and Cowan (1976, 1978, 1979).

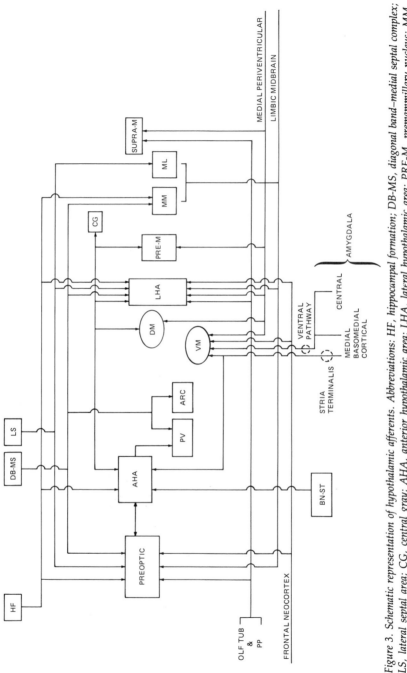

Figure 3. Schematic representation of hypothalamic afferents. Abbreviations: HF, hippocampal formation; DB-MS, diagonal band–medial septal complex; LS, lateral septal area; CG, central gray; AHA, anterior hypothalamic area; LHA, lateral hypothalamic area; PRE-M, premammillary nucleus; MM, medial mammillary nucleus; ML, lateral mammillary nucleus; SUPRA-M, supramammillary nucleus; OLF TUB & PP, olfactory tubercle and prepiriform area; BN-ST, bed nucleus of stria terminalis. Other abbreviations as given in Figure 2.

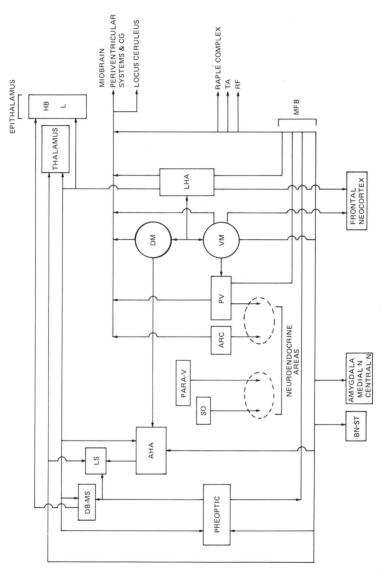

Figure 4. Schematic representation of hypothalamic efferents. Abbreviations: HB L, lateral nucleus of habenula; MFB, medial forebrain bundle; RF, reticular formation; TA, tegmental areas; MEDIAL N, medial nucleus; CENTRAL N, central nucleus. Other abbreviations as given in Figures 2 and 3.

clear boundary between these regions, even though the preoptic area is regarded as being of telencephalic origin, while the anterior hypothalamus is a diencephalic region.

A major afferent source of neural input to the hypothalamus arrives over the mammillary peduncles. Some fibers in this fiber pathway originate in the "dorsal visceral gray" in the primate brain. This region of the midbrain is thought to be concerned with information about taste. Some of these fibers ascend in the medial lemnisci and leave the lemnisci in the midbrain to turn into the mammillary peduncle. However, there are many fiber bundles in the mammillary peduncle. Some come from tegmental nuclei and others from the brain-stem reticular formation. Some fibers of the mammillary peduncle may also arise from the substantia nigra. As the mammillary peduncle approaches the diencephalon, it exchanges fibers with various nuclei in the anterior midbrain region. The fibers of the mammillary peduncle are thought to terminate in the lateral mammillary nucleus and the anterior portions of the medial mammillary nucleus in the cat.

The medial forebrain bundle courses through the lateral hypothalamic area connecting structures of the medial aspects of the hemispheres with preoptic, hypothalamic, and midbrain regions. The terminology describing the hypothalamus is such that some authors prefer to say that the medial forebrain bundle ends in the hypothalamus and that further interconnections with the midbrain are by means of the anterior and posterior hypothalamotegmental tracts.

The anterior hypothalamotegmental tract interconnects the preoptic area and the anterior hypothalamus with the tegmentum, particularly the region ventral to the red nucleus. As this tract travels along the ventromedial aspect of the medial forebrain bundle, it collects fibers from the ventromedial nucleus, the periventricular nucleus, and the posterior hypothalamus. The posterior hypothalamotegmental tract arises mainly from the ventromedial nucleus and reaches to areas above the red nucleus. Thus, the red nucleus is surrounded, top and bottom, by fibers from the posterior and anterior hypothalamotegmental tracts. The point is, however, that the hypothalamus, by means of these components of the medial forebrain bundle, has ample interactions with various tegmental and midbrain

suprachiasmatic nucleus. In addition, Swanson (1977) has reported a tract containing neurophysins (polypeptides binding either to oxytocin or to vasopressin) originating from the paraventricular nucleus with processes that extend to the diagonal band of Broca, the amygdala, the locus ceruleus, and various spinal cord locations, including the dorsal motor nucleus of the vagus.[4] Some fibers from these nuclei join the supraopticohypophyseal tract and terminate on blood vessels along the stalk of the pituitary gland and the posterior lobe of the pituitary.

The best-known route is the oxytocin and vasopressin transport system to the posterior pituitary. These hormones are stored in the nerve endings in the posterior pituitary until their release is triggered by a pulse of neural impulses along the fibers. Then, through exocytosis, the hormones are released into extracellular fluids and from there into the capillary network and the general blood supply of the body.

The anterior pituitary produces and releases a number of hormones with general and specific effects on target organ systems in the body. These include growth hormone, ACTH, thyroid-stimulating hormone, follicle stimulating hormone, luteinizing hormone, prolactin, and a lipid-mobilizing hormone (β-LPH) that may have significance because of its possible cleavage into peptide chains with important behavioral functions (i.e., the endorphins). Because of the neural isolation of the anterior pituitary, the release of the hormones in this area is stimulated chemically by other hormones of posterior pituitary or hypothalamic origin that reach it over the portal blood complex. These substances are called *releasing* or *inhibiting hormones* (formerly referred to as *factors*). These hormones are released in the area of the hypothalamus known as the *median eminence*, a relatively cell-free area where nerve endings come close to capillary loops of the portal complex. There probably is considerable localization of the cells in the hypothalamus that contain the various releasing and inhibiting hormones as well as the locations of their processes in the median eminence. Recent methods of analysis have shown that both luteinizing hormone-releasing hormone (LH-RH) and thyrotropin-re-

---

[4] More detailed reviews of neurosecretory functions of the hypothalamus should be consulted for additional details (e.g., Defendini & Zimmerman, 1978; Knigge, Joseph, & Hoffman, 1978; Hökfelt, 1978).

leasing hormone (TRH) are localized in the ventromedial nucleus (VM), although their concentrations are not homogenous within the nucleus. The VM also has been shown to contain substantial amounts of somatostatin. It is surprising that there are few, if any, projections from this nucleus to the median eminence (Saper, Swanson, & Cowan, 1976). It is possible that the hormones are located not in cells of the VM but in fibers reaching the nucleus from other hypothalamic sites. However, it is also possible that hormones released in the VM are transported to the portal venous system or into the third ventricle. The intermediate lobe of the pituitary gland is the site of production of melanocyte-stimulating hormone (MSH). The role of MSH in mammals is unclear, but subtle behavioral effects can be induced by the administration of this hormone. Both stimulating and inhibiting hormones for MSH release have been discovered.

The hypothalamus, or at least certain portions of it, must be regarded as one of the principal regulators of endocrine responses to the environment. Both long-term (e.g., number of daylight hours) and short-term (e.g., stressors) changes in the environment can affect the endocrine-dominated functions of the organism. For many of these responses, the hypothalamus represents the final pathway of neural control. However, many portions of the limbic system are involved in the regulation of endocrine activities and are sensitive to hormones in the blood or in the brain itself.

The study of the binding of radioactive hormones or their metabolites to cell membranes or to intracellular sites provides further insight into the interactions of the hypothalamus and regions of the limbic system with neuroendocrine activities. In general, the binding of the estrogens, androgens, and glucocorticoids is not identical. In hypothalamic areas, estradiol- and testosterone-concentrating neurons are found in many similar regions, but differences can also be observed. However, the glucocorticoid-concentrating neurons are chiefly localized outside the hypothalamus, in other areas associated with the limbic system. Cells with the capacity to bind the sex-steroid hormones seem to be located in areas around the third and fourth ventricles but also are found in the brain stem (i.e., the area postrema of the medulla). The medial nucleus of the amygdala is an important binding site for both androgen and estrogen but not the corticosteroids. The corticosteroids seem to have an affinity for the central and basal nuclei of the amygdala as well as the hippocampus. It should also be noted that the sex hormones affect a variety of sites in the lower brain stem.

Some neurons in the arcuate nucleus of the hypothalamus contain the transmitter dopamine, but others contain ACTH and β-endorphin. The neurons that contain dopamine do not also contain the neuropeptides. The neuropeptide-containing hormones seem to be predominantly in the ventral portion of the arcuate nucleus but are also found spread out into the ventromedial nucleus and the area between the arcuate and the ventromedial nuclei. Dopamine-containing neurons are largely in the dorsal regions of the arcuate nucleus (Bugnon, Block, Lenys, Gouget, & Fellman, 1979).

THE AMYGDALA

The *amygdala* is the name of a collection of nuclei found in the anterior portions of the temporal lobes in the brains of primates. Its cellular composition makes the nuclear group "stand out" from surrounding cortical areas when appropriately stained and viewed microscopically. In general shape, the nuclear complex resembles an almond; hence, its name. *Amygdala* is the Greek word for "almond."

The amygdalar nuclei are found in different locations in different animals. In marsupials, they are in the floor of the temporal horn of the lateral ventricles, but in most mammals, the nuclei lie both forward of and ventral to the temporal tip of the lateral ventricles.

Nuclear Groups

Many subdivisions have been made of the amygdalar nuclei. The most prominent of these are those of Gurdjian (1928) and Brodal (1947) for the rat and of Fox (1940) for the cat. The subdivision of the amygdala into nuclear groups has produced counts of from 5 to 22 in various species and by various authors. In the past, two major nuclear divisions were recognized: the corticomedial division and the basolateral division (Johnston, 1923). It should be noted, however, that these descriptions were based, almost entirely, on the appearance of the tissue without regard to afferent or efferent connections. More recently, experimental studies have cast doubt on the usefulness of such broad divisions. Many of the nuclear subgroups within each division have been found to be different in cellular structure and, more important, in regard to their interconnections with other brain regions (e.g., Price, 1973; Scalia & Winans, 1975). The following description of amygdala areas and interconnections follows the descriptions of Krettek and Price (1977a,b,c; 1978a,b) based on extensive experimental studies using modern anatomical techniques. In the amygdala region, the following nuclear groups can be distinguished:

- Basolateral
- Lateral
- Central
- Basomedial

In addition, the following cortical structures are closely associated with the amygdala region:

- The medial nucleus and the posterior cortical nucleus
- The amygdalohippocampal area
- The anterior cortical nucleus and the periamygdaloid cortex
- The nucleus of the lateral olfactory tract
- The endopiriform nucleus and the prepiriform cortex

A brief description of these structures and a summary of their major efferent connections is given below. It should be emphasized that these descriptions are much abbreviated, and the interested reader should consult the original papers for more detail. Sketches of the position of these regions are shown in Figure 5.

The basolateral nucleus contains the largest cells in the amygdala complex; thus, it is distinguishable from the lateral and basomedial nuclei, which lie above and below it in the middle reaches of the complex. Anterior and posterior subdivisions are found in the structure based on subtle differences in cell size. Ben-Ari, Zigmond, Shute, and Lewis (1977) have found this nucleus rich in acetylcholinesterase and acetyltransferase in the rat and the cat.

The lateral nucleus is the largest of the amygdalar complex. It can be found throughout the entire rostral-caudal extent of the complex. A "shell" subdivision lies adjacent to the external capsule. The body of the nucleus can be subdivided into a dorsolateral portion and a ventromedial portion. These three divisions can also be differentiated by methods that selectively stain heavy metals. This selective staining

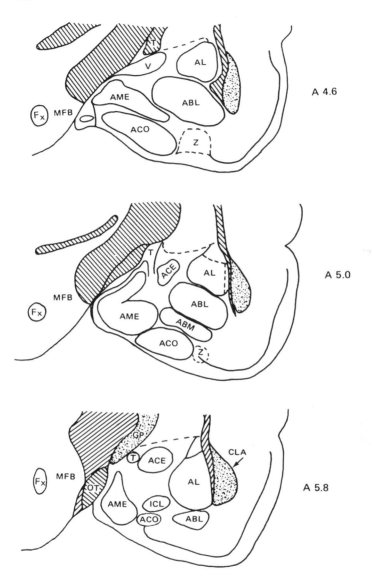

Figure 5. Drawings of major amygdalar nuclei in rat. The letters and numbers to the right of each figure represent the anterior–posterior coordinates of the de Groot atlas from which the drawing was made. Abbreviations of amygdalar nuclei: AL, lateral nucleus; ABL, basal nucleus, lateral part; ABM, basal nucleus, medial part; AME, medial nucleus; ACO, cortical nucleus; ACE, central nucleus; OT, optic tract; T, stria terminalis; V, ventricle; GP, globus pallidus; CLA, claustrum; Z, transitional zone; ICL, intercalated nucleus; Fx, fornix; MFB, medial forebrain bundle. Redrawn from de Groot (1959).

suggests differences in heavy metal content in the regions, probably associated with different enzymatic reactions in them. Anterior and posterior divisions can also be made. In some regions, the distinction between the lateral and the basolateral nuclei is made on the basis of cell size.

The central amygdaloid nucleus lies medial to the lateral and basolateral nuclei. Fibers of stria terminalis separate it from the medial nucleus. At its rostral and caudal extents, it merges into the anterior amygdaloid area and putamen, respectively. Medial and lateral subdivisions are sometimes made within the nucleus.

The cells of the basomedial nucleus are small to medium in size. They are generally smaller than those of the basolateral nucleus. With Nissl stains, they have a lighter appearance as well. The basomedial nucleus is located in the posterior two-thirds of the complex and lies beneath the basolateral nucleus and above (dorsal to) the periamygdaloid cortex.

The medial nucleus lies in the ventromedial edge of the ventral hemispheres in the cat. In the rat, as well, it occupies this position and can be easily distinguished because of the small, tightly packed cells of which it is composed. It is especially prominent in the rostral portions of the complex. Caudally, it merges with the posterior cortical nucleus and the amygdalohippocampal area.

The amygdalohippocampal area is a thick band of darkly staining cells with an indistinct boundary with the subiculum of the hippocampal formation. It appears at the posterior boundary of the medial nucleus. Its connections are similar both to those of amygdala regions and to the hippocampal formation. It also has been called the *posteromedial basal nucleus* (B_3) by Scalia and Winans (1975).

The anterior cortical nucleus begins rostrally immediately lateral to the nucleus of the lateral olfactory tract. It is found in the rostral third of the amygdaloid region. It has three cell layers; the deeper layers form a well-defined oval mass. It receives fibers from the olfactory bulb and from prepiriform cortex, suggesting it may best be considered a cortical region related to olfaction rather than an important component of the amygdaloid complex. It projects to several areas of olfactory cortex, including the prepiriform cortex and the periamygdaloid cortex.

The periamygdaloid cortex lies ventral and medial to the prepiriform cortex, but it is distinguishable from it on the basis of a thinner layer II and a less-well-developed layer III. The prepiriform cortex is not considered part of the amygdala complex, but it lies lateral to the amygdala throughout its extent. The periamygdaloid cortex is distinguishable from the anterior cortical nucleus by its larger and more tightly packed cells in layer II.

The nucleus of the lateral olfactory cortex lies lateral to the amygdala and can be differentiated on the basis of cytoarchitecture. The endopiriform nucleus is a collection of medium-sized cells that lie underneath layer III of the prepiriform cortex and lateral and ventral to the external capsule.

Functional or quasi-functional assumptions about the organization of the amygdala can be made on several bases, although all are highly speculative at this time. It is interesting, however, that the basolateral nucleus projects to areas in the forebrain that also receive the greatest amount of dopamine innervation from brain stem regions, namely, the olfactory tubercle, the nucleus accumbens, and the prelimbic, infralimbic, and insular frontal cortex. All are areas that maintain electrical self-stimulation behavior (Wurtz & Olds, 1963; Routtenberg & Sloan, 1972; Rolls, 1975). The basolateral nucleus is also rich in acetylcholinesterase and acetylcholine transferase (Ben-Ari *et al.*, 1977), presenting another similarity to the ventral-striatal regions. However, the central nucleus and the bed nucleus of stria terminalis are the areas with the greatest amounts of enkephalin (Elde, Hökfeldt, Johansson, & Terenius, 1976; Simantov, Kuhar, Uhl, & Snyder, 1977). The central nucleus also receives a substantial adrenergic innervation (Swanson & Hartman, 1975).

The internal connections of these amygdala regions are summarized in Figure 6, while the major external afferents and efferents are shown in Figure 7. These have been derived from a large variety of sources, especially the work of Krettek and Price (1978a,b), and include information from Wakefield (1979), McBride and Sutin (1977), and others. The relationships shown in these figures have been simplified, and not all of the fine-grain breakdowns have been included. For example, the distinction between the medial and lateral portions of the bed nucleus of stria terminalis have been omitted.

The bed nucleus of the stria terminalis, a major efferent pathway of some amygdalar groups, lies on top of the anterior hypothalamic region to the ventral portion of the lateral septal area. It has both medial and lateral subdivisions. It receives input from many regions

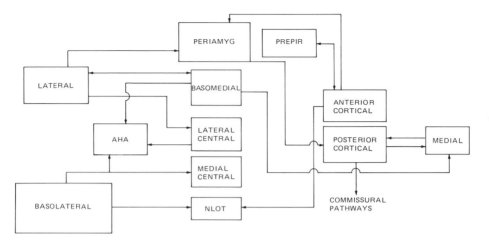

Figure 6. Simplified schematic representation of some of the interconnections among divisions of the amygdala complex. Abbreviations: PERIAMYG, periamygdaloid area; PREPIR, prepiriform cortex; LATERAL, lateral nucleus; BASOMEDIAL, basomedial nucleus; ANTERIOR CORTICAL, anterior cortical nucleus; POSTERIOR CORTICAL, posterior cortical nucleus; MEDIAL, medial nucleus; LATERAL CENTRAL, lateral division of central nucleus; MEDIAL CENTRAL, medial division of central nucleus; NLOT, nucleus of the lateral olfactory tract; AHA, anterior hypothalamic area; BASOLATERAL, basolateral nucleus of amygdala.

of the amygdala and sends axons to a variety of other forebrain regions, acting as if it were a relay station for the amygdala groups with which it is associated. Specifically, its lateral division receives fibers from the basolateral, the basomedial, and the central amygdaloid nuclei. The medial division receives fibers from the medial and posterior nuclei of the amygdala, the amygdalohippocampal area, and the basomedial nucleus. Most fibers traveling in the stria terminalis contribute to those reaching the bed nucleus. The lateral nucleus seems to contribute some fibers to the stria near its origin in the amygdala, but they disappear before reaching the bed nucleus.

The bed nucleus of the stria terminalis receives fibers from most nuclear groups of the amygdala and from the transitional area between the amygdala and the hippocampus. The surprising part is the large number of areas that receive projections from this nucleus (Swanson & Cowan, 1979). These include the entire hypothalamus (except the suprachiasmatic and the ventromedial nucleus), the parataenialis and paraventricular nuclei of the thalamus, the medial habenula, the nucleus accumbens, the substantia innominata (the region between the bed nucleus of the stria terminalis and the nucleus of the diagonal band), the ventral tegmental areas, the central gray of the midbrain, the rostral pole of locus ceruleus, and the anterodorsal and anteroventral nuclei of the thalamus—an impressive distribution list for a rather small nucleus.

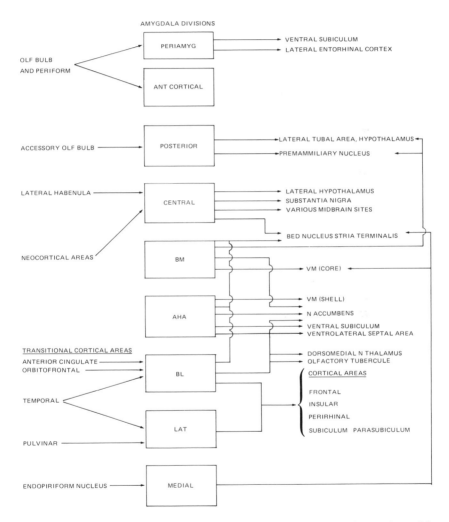

Figure 7. Simplified schematic representation of major afferent and efferent pathways of amygdala complex. Abbreviations: ACCESSORY OLF B, accessory olfactory bulb. Other abbreviations as in preceding figures.

Fiber Systems

The fiber connections of the amygdala are less than perfectly understood, but two main efferent systems are recognized. These are the stria terminalis and the ventrofugal bundles (ventral amygdalofugal pathways). Fibers of amygdalar origin pass to more anterior regions of the forebrain, primarily the preoptic and ventromedial areas of the hypothalamus, over the stria terminalis. The stria terminalis probably arises predominantly from the central and medial nuclei of the amygdala, although the basolateral nucleus also contributes some fibers to it. The ventral amygdalofugal pathways to the hypothalamus are thought to arise from many nuclei, but many fibers in this pathway arise from periamygdaloid cortex rather than from the amygdala itself in many species, including the rat. At least in the rat, and perhaps in other species as well, the stria terminalis and the associated bed nucleus are the major efferent pathways to telencephalic and diencephalic structures.

The fibers in the stria terminalis from the amygdala reach the hypothalamus and preoptic areas, some coursing in front of and others behind the anterior commissure. There are at least three components of the stria terminalis: dorsal, ventral, and commissural. According to DeOlmos (1972), the dorsal component sends fibers to the bed nucleus of the stria terminalis, the basal part of the lateral septal nucleus, the posterior-medial part of nucleus accumbens septi, the olfactory tubercle, portions of the anterior olfactory nucleus, the granular layer of the accessory bulb, the medial preoptic area, the area around the ventromedial nucleus of the hypothalamus, and an area just ahead of the mammillary nuclei. The ventral component distributes to the bed nucleus of the stria terminalis, the junction of the preoptic area and the hypothalamus, the central core of the ventromedial nucleus of the hypothalamus, and the premammillary area. A commissural component connects the amygdalae of the two hemispheres through the anterior commissure, as does a small portion of the dorsal component of the stria terminalis.

An apparent redundancy occurs in the termination of the two major fiber systems, the stria terminalis and the ventral amygdalofugal pathways. For example, fibers from both the stria terminalis and the ventral amygdalofugal fibers end in the lateral preoptic areas.

However, the fact that one component of the limbic system projects to another area over two (or more) different routes does not necessarily imply redundancy in the system. In the case of the amygdala, it is likely that each of the various components has its own special pattern of projections in the hypothalamus. This may imply different routes of regulatory control, and perhaps different types of control, by different cell groups of the amygdala.

The distribution of fibers originating in the amygdala and reaching forebrain sites over the ventral pathways has been difficult to establish owing to the difficulty of producing lesions restricted to the amygdalar nuclei. When lesions are made in the amygdala, there is always incidental damage to periamygdaloid cortex and an interruption of fibers passing through the amygdalar complex. Therefore, it is difficult to establish the contribution of the amygdalar groups *per se* as opposed to fibers originating outside the amygdala. A rostral segment of the ventral fibers forms a more-or-less compact bundle containing axons of cells located in the piriform cortex and in the basolateral group. This tract courses between the central and lateral nuclei and forms a part of the "longitudinal association bundle" of Johnston (1923). At its rostral extreme, the ventral fiber systems turn medially to go toward the substantia innominata, some ending there but most passing through and terminating in the bed nucleus of the stria terminalis. Other fibers in this rostral, compact pathway go to the ventral portions of the ventral striatum and the olfactory tubercle.

In addition to the compact, rostral component of the ventral amygdalofugal fibers, there is a diffuse projection of fibers in this pathway. Some of the small fibers in this group take origin in the nuclei of the amygdala, but other small fibers and most of the large fibers probably originate in the nearly cortical areas.

Projections from the amygdala reach the posterior aspects of the dorsomedial nucleus of the thalamus. This is of significance because of the strong interconnections between the dorsomedial nucleus and the lateral and orbital frontal cortex. In primates, influences from the amygdala can also reach the prefrontal neocortical areas by another route as well, that is, the uncinate fasciculus, which runs between the anterior temporal lobe and the prefrontal areas.

Another area that receives fibers from the stria terminalis system is the ventral portion of the lateral septal area. In addition, some fibers from the amygdala come over the stria terminalis to turn caudally at the level of the septal area to run through stria medullaris to the habenular complex.

There are further complications of the stria terminalis system. These include fibers that leave the stria terminalis at its most rostral extent and turn into the fornix. These fibers terminate in the septal area much as do other fibers in the fornix that arise from the hippocampal formation.

Both the medial forebrain bundle and the system of the habenulopeduncular tract provide means for conveying impulses from amygdala and other limbic areas to the midbrain tegmentum and central gray. Some fibers from these systems also spread out into the region of the mesencephalic reticular formation. There is the possibility of direct connections between the amygdala and the midbrain reticular formation as well, although these have been demonstrated only in electrophysiological studies. Schwaber, Kapp, and Higgins (1980) have reported a direct connection from the central nucleus to the autonomic regulatory nuclei of the brain stem.

THE HIPPOCAMPUS

One of the problems faced by the student of the limbic system anatomy is what is meant by the term *hippocampus*. Those concerned with human anatomy often use the term to mean all of the tissue making up the hippocampal gyrus found on the medial and ventral areas of the temporal lobe. This use of the term is too broad, since it includes too many neural tissues of a diverse nature. It is more useful to use the term *hippocampus* to refer to the structures within the hippocampal formation that have a simple laminar composition. The hippocampus is marked by a dense layer of pyramidal cells and the dentate area by a dense band of small pyramidal or granule cells that result in a distinctive appearance in Nissl-stained histological preparations in most species. The hippocampal pyramidal regions appear to be laid out with "ruling-pen neatness," as described by some investigators. In this book, *hippocampus* is used to designate the unit comprised of the hippocampus and the dentate area, while *hippocampal formation* is used to designate the hippocampus proper, the dentate gyrus, and the transitional cortical areas connected with both the hippocampus and neocortical areas.[5]

A diagram of the hippocampus and the dentate gyrus as they would be seen in a horizontal section of the right hemisphere in a rodent brain is shown in Figure 8. This diagram is oversimplified, of course, and tries to convey only an overview of the principal subdivisions and the general configuration of cells in different regions. As can be seen in this figure, the hippocampus and the dentate gyrus appear to be interlocked gyri. It should also be noted that the outer surface of the neocortex continues around to the hippocampal fissure and around the edge of this fissure until the fornix–fimbria complex is reached. Thus, the leftmost edge of the hippocampus and the dentate gyrus in this figure represents the most medial aspects of the structure. Inside this medial edge is the diencephalon or the brain stem, depending on the height in the brain at which the section is made. The point is that the most medial aspects of the hippocampus and the dentate gyrus are really their "outer surface," and the most lateral aspects are comparable to the deeper layers of neocortex. The deepest major layer of the hippocampus would be the alveus, while the "deepest" layers of the dentate gyrus would be the fiber complex found at the junction of the hippocampus and the dentate gyrus, through which the axons enter and leave the dentate gyrus.

Layers of the Hippocampus

Although the hippocampus and the dentate gyrus are often said to be primitive because they have fewer layers of cells than does the neocortex, a translation of a book on the hippocampus by Ramon y Cajal (1968) indicates that this great anatomist accepted a seven-layered conceptualization of the structures, which reveal marked similarity to other cortical regions of the brain, including the neocortex. The following represents a brief summary of the descriptions provided by Ramon y Cajal of the layers found in the hippocampus.

---

[5] Like other descriptions in this chapter, the description of the anatomy of the hippocampus must be somewhat simplified. The interested reader may wish to consult the chapters by Chronister and White, by Angevine, by Stranghan, by Kuhar, and by Andersen in Isaacson and Pribram (1975).

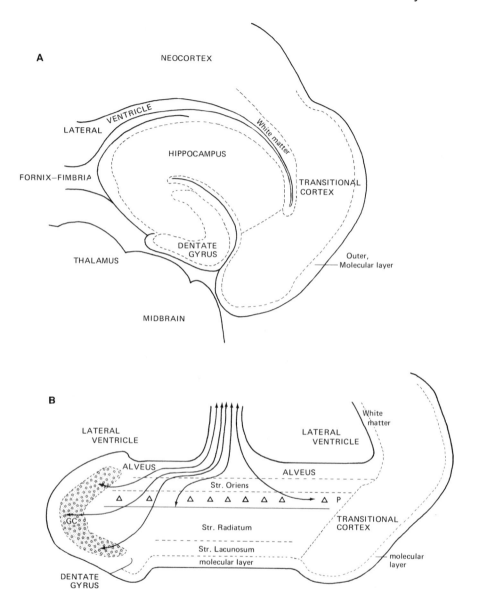

Figure 8. (A) Sketch of hippocampal formation as seen in horizontal section made through right hemisphere of rat brain. (B) Sketch of "unfolded" hippocampal formation. This drawing shows the similarity of the alveus to the deep white matter of the nonlimbic cortex and the continuity of the molecular layer of the hippocampus with the outer molecular layer of hemispheres. The traditional layers of the hippocampus are labeled. Abbreviations: Str., stratum; P, stratum of pyramidal cells; GC, granule cells of dentate gyrus.

1. Stratum Moleculare. The outermost zone of the hippocampus and the dentate gyrus (which are continuous with each other) is called the *stratum moleculare*. It contains many nerve fibers but relatively few cells. At least some fibers run horizontally in the molecular zones, and probably these are long dendritic processes of the pyramidal cells. Other fibers in this zone are probably axons entering the hippocampus from the subiculum. The few cells found in this zone give rise to fibers running parallel to the direction of the molecular layer for short distances.

2. Stratum Lacunosum. The stratum lacunosum consists of many irregularly spaced cells and rather a large number of fibers. Large bundles of parallel fibers run through the stratum lacunosum. Some arise from the "inferior" region of the hippocampus and reach to the subiculum. Some of these fibers are collaterals from pyramidal cells. Other fibers of unknown origin enter the stratum lacunosum from the white matter (alveus) beneath and send processes both to the cells in the pyramidal layer and to the cells in the stratum lacunosum.

3. Stratum Radiatum. The stratum radiatum lies between the stratum lacunosum and the pyramidal cell layer below. It is less densely populated by cells than the stratum lacunosum and contains many bushy dendritic arborizations of the pyramidal cells beneath it. It also contains many fiber systems coursing through it from various points of origin. Ramon y Cajal believed that the layers designated as stratum moleculare, stratum lacunosum, and stratum radiatum together were comparable to the outermost layer, the molecular layer (layer 1) of the neocortex.

4. Pyramidal Layer. The large pyramidal cells of the hippocampus are found in the pyramidal layer below the stratum radiatum. In many animals, the pyramidal cells are closely packed. There may be three or four tightly packed rows of cells in the pyramidal layer, with the outer cells being somewhat smaller than the inner cells. Ramon y Cajal noted the suggestion made earlier by Schaffer that the large and small pyramidal cells found in the neocortex in different layers (3 and 5) have become collapsed into a single layer in the hippocampus. However, the usefulness of this view is suspect since the pyramidal cells of the hippocampus are markedly different from pyramidal cells of the neocortex. In the hippocampus, the pyramidal cells have tufted dendritic arborizations extending both toward the surface (toward the stratum moleculare) and toward the deeper regions (the alveus). For this reason, the pyramidal cells of the hippocampus are often called *double pyramids*. The pyramidal cells of the neocortex are marked by long dendritic processes directed toward the surface (the apical dendrites) and by bushy processes extending around the base of the cell (basilar dendrites). Herrick (1926) pointed out that double pyramidal cells are characteristic of neurons in the reptilian cortex, and he felt that this indicated that the hippocampal tissue of mammals is probably the neural inheritance from primitive ancestors.

Axons from the pyramidal cells descend toward the alveus, giving off some collaterals along the way. Some fibers reach the alveus and continue forward in the fornix to reach the septal area or other regions. Some axons bifurcate in the alveus. One branch apparently exits through the fornix, while the other goes in a "decidedly different" direction.

There are many types of collateral fibers given off from cells in all layers of the hippocampus. These collaterals ascend and descend to different layers while bifurcating frequently. In the region of the hippocampus adjacent to the dentate gyrus, thick collaterals arise from the axons of pyramidal cells that come off a descending axon in the stratum oriens. The main portion of the axon continues to the alveus, while other collaterals continue for some distance to contact cells of the hippocampal areas farther away from the dentate gyrus, the subicular complex, the entorhinal area, and the lateral septal complex on the same side of the brain (Swanson, Sawchenko, & Cowan, 1980). These large, myelinated fibers were described by Karl Schaffer toward the end of the nineteenth century and have been called *Schaffer collaterals*. The Schaffer collaterals reach the superior region through the stratum radiatum and stratum oriens (Hjorth-Simonsen, 1973).

5. *Stratum Oriens.* The stratum oriens lies below the pyramidal cells and above the white matter of the alveus. Many of the cells appearing in this region resemble cells found in the deeper layers of the neocortex. Cells in the region are predominantly oriented parallel to the underlying fibers of the alveus, although some axons have been traced upward into the pyramidal cell layer. This is also the region into which the deep tufts of the double pyramidal cells are directed. There are some large cells in this zone whose axons turn upward and reach the molecular layer.

6. *Alveus.* For the most part, the alveus is composed of white matter, that is, axons arising from pyramidal cells deeper within the

hippocampus and from other regions. There are some polymorphic cells in it that are thought to be displaced from the stratum oriens.

7. Epithelial Zone. The hippocampus lies inside the lateral ventricle, and separating it from the ventricle is a layer of epithelial cells. Ordinarily, this layer would not be considered a part of the neural organization of the hippocampus and consequently not one of the "layers" of the structure, but Ramon y Cajal found that processes of these cells reached into the hippocampus to terminate in the stratum oriens in very young animals. In older animals, these fibers terminated in the alveus.

The description by Ramon y Cajal of seven layers of the hippocampus is somewhat misleading. When describing the neocortex, the underlying white matter and its epithelial zones (in areas bordering the lateral ventricles) would not be considered cortical "layers." Furthermore, as noted before, layers 1, 2, and 3 should be considered together as being homologous to the molecular layer of the neocortex. Therefore, it may be proper to combine the various layers described by Ramon y Cajal in order to provide a simple summary of the cell layers of the hippocampus.

Ramon y Cajal layers 1, 2, and 3 = Hippocampal layer 1
Ramon y Cajal layer 4 = Hippocampal layer 2 (pyramids)
Ramon y Cajal layer 5 = Hippocampal layer 3

The main differences between this cortical arrangement and that of the neocortex would lie in the fact that the neocortex has two pyramidal cell layers (layers 3 and 5) and a granule cell layer (layer 4) interposed between these two pyramidal cell layers. In addition, the appearance of the pyramidal cells in the neocortex and the hippocampus is quite different, being "single" in the former and "double" in the latter.

Subdivisions of the Hippocampal Formation

The hippocampal formation is larger than the hippocampus proper. The formation includes the dentate gyrus and the cortical areas adjacent to the hippocampus. Indeed, there is some question about just what should be included in the terms *hippocampus* and *hippocampal formation*. Leaving aside these terminological matters for the moment, we first consider the various subdivisions of the hippocampus.

The hippocampal formation exists as a long prominence in the lateral ventricles. A photograph of the hippocampus in the human is shown in Figure 9. The end of the structure closest to the tip of the temporal lobe is called the *temporal end*. The other end is called the *septal termination;* and the imaginary line between these two extremes is called the *septotemporal axis* of the structure. In rodents, the hippocampal septotemporal axis is almost at right angles to the caudal-rostral orientation brain so that the septal end is dorsal, and the temporal end is ventral. Certain subdivisions of the hippocampus and the dentate gyrus can be found along the septotemporal axis. The neural input and output relationships are somewhat different in the rat dorsal and ventral portions. Neurochemical differences are also found between dorsal and ventral regions (Gage, Armstrong, & Thompson, 1980). It is likely that there are functional units existing like chips across the septotemporal axis. These cross-sectional units are called *lamellae* (e.g., Lømo, 1971; Andersen, Bland, & Dudar, 1973).

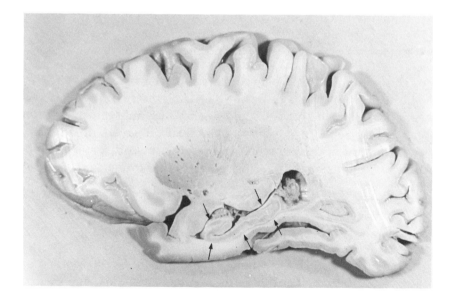

Figure 9. A photograph of longitudinal section of human brain cut through the temporal lobe. The hippocampus lying in the lateral ventricle is indicated by arrows. Photograph of brain section courtesy of Dr. Donald A. Dewsbury.

Based on the genetic analysis of inheritance of cell populations along the septotemporal axis, at least four subdivisions of the hippocampus along this axis should be recognized (Wimer, Wimer, Chernow, & Balvanz, 1980).

The most widely known subdivisions of the hippocampus are based on its structure as represented in sections made at right angles to the septotemporal axes. In such sections, two major subdivisions are found: the superior region and the inferior region.

The superior region is a zone beginning with a compact layer of pyramidal cells and extending to the point where this layer becomes less compact. This is the boundary between the superior and the inferior regions. As can be seen in Figure 10, the inferior part of the

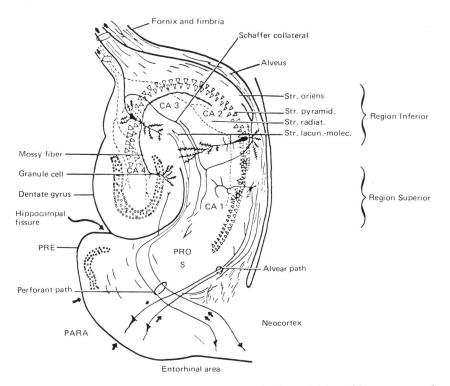

Figure 10. Schematic drawing illustrating superior and inferior divisions of hippocampus and divisions into CA fields. Abbreviations: Str. oriens, stratum oriens; Str. pyramid., stratum pyramidale; Str. radiat., stratum radiatum; Str. lacun.-molec., stratum lacunosum-moleculare; PRO, prosubiculum; S, subiculum; PRE, presubiculum; PARA, parasubiculum. Drawing adapted from Brodal (1969). Reproduced by permission of the author and Oxford University Press.

hippocampus lies "ahead" of (rostral to) the superior region and extends throughout the frontal convexity of the hippocampus. The hippocampus was further subdivided into "fields" by the anatomist Lorente de No. These fields are designated by the letters *CA* (meaning *Cornu Ammonis* or Ammon's horn) and numerals from 1 to 4. The superior part of hippocampus corresponds to CA_1. The inferior region is CA_3. A small region between CA_1 and CA_3 is designated CA_2. Region CA_4 is a small area distinct from CA_3 which appears at the transition of the hippocampus and the dentate gyrus.

Ramon y Cajal considered the fascia dentate, or dentate gyrus, to be a simple three-layered cortex imposed on the end of the molecular layer of the hippocampus proper. It has a molecular zone, a granule cell zone, and a zone of polymorphic cells.

There are only a few neurons with very short processes in the molecular layer. The granule cell layer consists of densely packed cells in several layers. These cells resemble the pyramidal cells of the hippocampus proper but contain little protoplasm and have very few basal dendrites. The axons from the granule cells descend into the polymorphic cell zone of the dentate and into the molecular and pyramidal layers of the hippocampus proper.

The axons of cells in the dentate gyrus have a dense, mossy appearance as they wander above and below the pyramidal cell layer of the hippocampus. As a result, they are sometimes called "mossy fibers." These fibers end abruptly at the transition from the inferior to the superior region of the hippocampus. As a result, the granule cells are thought to communicate primarily with the pyramidal cells of the inferior region of the hippocampus.

Transitional Cortical Areas

The transition between the cortex and the hippocampus begins with the entorhinal cortex.[6] The anatomical designation of the entorhinal cortex is based on a plexus of nerve fibers that are found in layers 2 and 3 of the cortex. This is illustrated in Figure 11. This plexus marks the limits of the entorhinal cortex. At the inner edge of the entorhinal cortex is the parasubiculum. Inside the parasubiculum is

---

[6] The following description is based on anatomical studies of the rat hippocampal complex (e.g., Blackstad, 1956; L. E. White, 1959).

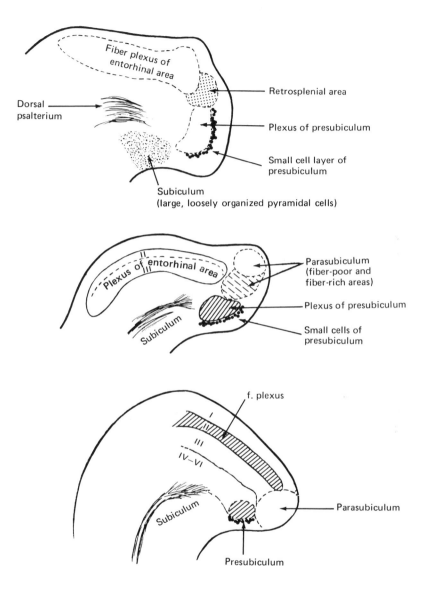

Figure 11. Highly simplified, schematic drawings of transitional regions outside the hippocampus in rat. The three drawings represent sections made through upper, middle, and lower parts of entorhinal and parasubicular areas. Modified from Blackstad (1956, Fig. 5, p. 427).

an area called the *presubiculum*. It is marked by a dense fiber plexus and by a layer of granular cells. The next area leading to the hippocampus is the subiculum itself. The cells in this region do not have a laminated appearance but are scattered in an apparently unsystematic fashion throughout a wide area. The beginning of the hippocampus is marked by the appearance of the densely packed pyramidal cell layer that is the beginning of the region superior. Near the dorsal aspects of the hippocampus, a triangular area is found inserted between the parasubiculum and the presubiculum. This area is called *area entorhinalis e* in the rat. It is practically devoid of fibers. It becomes smaller and finally disappears as the hippocampal formation is followed ventrally.

The main types of fiber input to the hippocampus from the entorhinal region that can be noted are the perforant path, the alveus pathway, and the psalterium. The last of these is a commissural system connecting the hippocampal formations of each hemisphere. Fibers entering the hippocampus from the psalterium mix with fibers in the fimbria before their final termination in the hippocampus. The perforant path enters the hippocampus from the entorhinal region, crosses the hippocampal fissure, and reaches the molecular layer (broadly defined) of the hippocampus and the dentate gyrus. The fibers in the perforant path make contact with the apical arborizations of dendrites of pyramidal cells in all areas of the hippocampus and the dentate (Blackstad, 1958).

The fibers reaching the hippocampus over the psalterium are from the contralateral hippocampus. Such fibers reach the superior sector, making contact with the apical dendrites near the cell body and with the basilar dendrites. In addition, fibers from the contralateral entorhinal cortex reach the granule cells in the fascia dentata. These fibers make contact nearer the cell body than do the ipsilateral afferents from the entorhinal cortex to the same cells, which arrive over the perforant path. Thus, there is a spatial distribution of terminations on the dendrites of cells in the hippocampus and the dentate gyrus based on the ipsilateral or contralateral sources of the fibers. In general, the distal portions of the dendrites receive ipsilateral input over the perforant path, while the proximal portions of the dendrites receive input from commissural, contralateral fibers. The origin of the perforant path seems to lie in the medial and lateral regions of the entorhinal cortex (Hjorth-Simonsen, 1972). There is some question about whether the perforant pathway acts in a homogenous fashion (Harris, Lasher, & Steward, 1979) or whether it should be regarded as comprised of two subdivisions (McNaughton, 1980).

Hjorth-Simonsen and Jeune (1972) have described the termination of the perforant pathway in the rat as being in the middle regions of the molecular layer of the dentate gyrus and the region lacunosum–moleculare, near the stratum radiatum, in the inferior region of the hippocampus. Terminations were not found in the superior region. It is of some interest that Hjorth-Simonsen (1971) has demonstrated fibers from the inferior region to the entorhinal cortex that may be considered reciprocals of the perforant pathway fibers. Cells in the superior region of the hippocampus project to the subiculum, near the boundary with the presubiculum, by means of fibers that travel in the alveus (Hjorth-Simonsen, 1973).

Afferents and Efferents

The neural input to the hippocampus arises over two main pathways: (1) those mediated through the transitional cortical regions and (2) those over the fimbria–fornix system. Parallel efferent systems exist over these systems. Each is discussed separately.

Transitional Cortex Routes. Basically, the major input system to the hippocampal formation is the perforant pathway from the entorhinal cortex. This pathway reaches the dentate and, to some degree, portions of area CA_3. From the dentate, it is distributed to fields CA_4, CA_3, and CA_2 of the hippocampus. The CA_2 and CA_3 regions project to the CA_1 region and to some degree to the subiculum. Field CA_1 projects to the subiculum, the entorhinal cortex, and the perirhinal cortex. Some cells of CA_4 also project back on the dentate gyrus. There is reason to believe that cells in all areas of CA_1, CA_2, and CA_3 project to the subiculum and that cells in some portions of these regions send fibers to the transitional cortical areas and to retrosplenial and cingulate cortices as well (Swanson & Cowan, 1977). It is of special interest that most of the principal outflow of the hippocampal formation to the diencephalon and other regions is from the subiculum.

There are strong parallels between the intrahippocampal association projections and the crossed, commissural projections to the hippocampus and the dentate gyrus on the opposite side of the brain (Swanson, Wyss, & Cowan, 1978).

The output of the hippocampal formation contains large components directed toward the association cortical areas. For example, when radioactively labeled amino acids are injected into the parahippocampal areas in nonhuman primates, considerable label is detected in all neocortical association areas. These include regions of the frontal, the parietal, the temporal, and the occipital lobes. These association areas are the ones usually thought to be of special importance in the performance of intellectual activities (i.e., higher functions). The parahippocampal region receives afferents directly from the hippocampal formation. These fibers arise from the subiculum and reach the association areas without making synapses at other locations. Other fibers project to the amygdala (mediobasal nucleus) and cingulate cortex (Rosene & Van Hoesen, 1977). Projections have been found from the subiculum to the areas of the rhinal sulcus and the inferotemporal cortex. In a way, these connections evidence a reciprocity with hippocampal afferent fibers from the same regions and are supportive of the idea that the subicular region represents a final output pathway of information received by the hippocampus.

These results indicate that the transitional cortical areas of the hippocampal formation represent the critical portion of the structure for the influencing of other cortical regions of the brain. The hippocampal pyramidal zones of the CA_3 area have relatively few projections beyond those that reach the septal area.

Since the entorhinal area provides a massive input to subicular regions, it is of value to know something of its connections. Three main sources of input can be recognized: (1) from the middle portion of the medial aspects of the ventral temporal lobe (area TH of Bonin & Bailey, 1947); (2) from an area just caudal to the entorhinal region, the prepiriform region (Brodmann's area 51), and an area just rostral to the entorhinal area; and (3) from the orbitofrontal cortex. Two anatomical subdivisions of the entorhinal region (medial and lateral) receive different patterns of input from the three areas. The medial zone of the entorhinal region projects to the dentate gyrus. The lateral area projects to the apical dendrites of both the dentate gyrus and the pyramidal cells of the hippocampus (Van Hoesen, Pandya, & Butters, 1972).

The Fornix.   One emphasis in research on the distribution of fibers to and from the hippocampal formation involves those fibers that course through the fimbria and continue into the fornix system. In addition to commissural fibers, which partly follow this course, this system contains fibers that interconnect the hippocampus with the septal area and with lateral preoptic and hypothalamic areas. Fibers to and from the medial forebrain bundle also pass through this system. Between the hippocampus and the hypothalamus, the fornix can be regarded as having two components: (1) postcommissural and (2) precommissural. The postcommissural fornix system is made up of fibers from the hippocampal formation that do not enter the septal area but continue beyond it, passing behind the anterior commissure. Axons of cells of the hippocampus proper are almost entirely confined to the precommissural fornix and terminate in the lateral septal areas. Cells in the subiculum and the adjoining presubiculum and parasubiculum send axons over the postcommissural route to the hypothalamus. Dorsal subicular and nearby transitional cortical areas project to the mammillary body region. Those from the ventral portions reach the area of the arcuate and ventromedial nuclei over the corticohypothalamic tract (Swanson & Cowan, 1975a,b). A comprehensive study of the efferents of the hippocampal formation was made by Swanson and Cowan (1977). In general, their results were similar to those described above. A schematic representation of their results is shown in Figure 12. Fibers that take origin from the ventral subicular regions other than those passing over the corticohypothalamic tract include ones that reach the bed nucleus of stria terminalis, the nucleus accumbens, the anterior olfactory nucleus, and the infralimbic area. The presubiculum and parasubiculum project to the anterior and lateral thalamic nuclei. However, diverging from this general view, Krayniak, Meibach, and Siegel (1981) have found that the projections to the nucleus accumbens may arise only from the entorhinal cortex rather than from the subiculum.

The CA_1 region and the adjacent subiculum project through the fimbria and the precommissural fornix to the lateral septal nucleus on the same side of the brain. The CA_3 region projects bilaterally to the lateral septal nuclei. The hippocampus and the subiculum also project to the posterior septal nuclei, from which cells project to the habenulae and the interpeduncular nuclei.

A dorsal–ventral difference in projections of the CA_1 area should be noted. Projections in the dorsal (septal) portions of the hippocam-

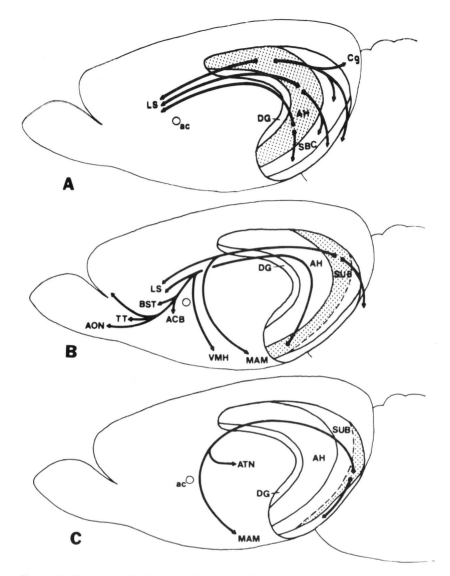

Figure 12. Three schematic drawings of the major efferent connections of the hippocampal formation. In A, the projections of the hippocampus proper to the septal area are noted. In B and C, the more extended projections of the transitional cortical regions are shown. Abbreviations: LS, lateral septal area; ac, anterior commissure; DG, dentate gyrus; AH, Ammon's horn (hippocampus proper); Cg, posterior cingulate cortex; SBC, subicular cortex; AON, anterior olfactory nucleus; TT, Taenia tecta; BST, bed nucleus of stria terminalis; ACB, nucleus accumbens; VMH, ventral medial nucleus; MAM, mammillary bodies; SUB, subiculum; ATN, anterior nucleus of the thalamus. From "An Autoradiographic Study of the Organization of the Efferent Connections of the Hippocampal Formation in the Rat" by L. W. Swanson and W. M. Cowan, Journal of Comparative Neurology, *1977, 172, 49–84. Copyright 1977 by Alan R. Liss, Inc. Reprinted by permission.*

pus reached the perirhinal area. In the ventral (temporal) regions, the projections went only to the subiculum and to the medial and lateral entorhinal cortex (Swanson *et al.*, 1978).

Afferents to the hippocampal formation arise from cells in a large number of subcortical regions. In general, afferents arise from a more-or-less continuous cellular population from the lateral preoptic area along the base of the brain to the ventral tegmental area (Wyss, Swanson, & Cowan, 1979a). In addition, there is evidence of hippocampal afferents arising from the following regions: (1) thalamic nuclear groups: reuniens, parataenialis, paraventricular, anterodorsal, anteromedial, laterodorsal, lateral posterior; (2) hypothalamic nuclei and areas: the lateral preoptic area, the magnocellular preoptic nucleus, the dorsomedial nucleus, the lateral and posterior areas, the ventral premammillary nucleus, the supramammillary region, and various subdivisions of the mammillary nucleus; and (3) the medial septal area and the diagonal band of Broca. The substantia innominata, the anterior amygdala area, and the amygdalohippocampal region also contribute fibers to the hippocampal formation (Wyss, Swanson, & Cowan, 1979b). These connections were found in the rat, and similar ones have been found in the squirrel monkey (DeVito, 1980).

Of special interest are afferents from the monoamine-containing cell groups of the brain stem. The afferents from the locus ceruleus reach the hippocampus through the cingulum bundle and a very dorsal part of the fornix system. They reach the dorsal-posterior hippocampus but not the dentate gyrus. Raphe nuclei project to the hippocampus through the two routes used by the locus ceruleus fibers and also the fimbria to reach both dorsal and ventral hippocampus (Pasquier & Reinoso-Suarez, 1978). These authors suggested that on the basis of the large numbers of neurons projecting to the hippocampus from the hypothalamus, the diagonal band, and the entorhinal area, these regions should be considered the primary origins of extrinsic hippocampal afferents.

In the cat, fornix fibers project to the intralaminar nucleus of the thalamus; fibers projecting to the lateral thalamic nucleus or to the medial hypothalamic areas have not been reported (Siegel & Tassoni, 1971a,b). The cat is perhaps distinctive because of its massive fornix projections to the central gray of the diencephalon. In the monkey, there are some direct projections from the fornix system to the anteroventral nucleus and the intralaminar complex of the thalamus.

The nucleus lateralis dorsalis also receives an abundant supply of fornix fibers, suggesting a strong relationship of the fornix system to the parietal association areas of the neocortex in this animal. In addition, the dorsomedial nucleus of the thalamus receives fibers from the fornix system and from the amygdala, suggesting a dual activation of the dorsomedial nucleus by both the hippocampal and the amygdalar systems, and suggesting that they may help to regulate activities in the dorsolateral prefrontal cortex in primates.

In terms of projections reaching the midbrain, the greatest number is found in the guinea pig, and only a few, if any, in the rat. These projections are essentially absent in cat and monkey as well. In the guinea pig, there are at least three sets of fibers that run past the mammillary bodies. There are the fibers that turn to the central gray just behind the mammillary bodies, a set of fibers that reaches the posterior hypothalamic nucleus (which is a medially located nucleus behind the mammillary bodies), and a ventral tegmental bundle reaching toward the nucleus of Bechterew. This last bundle turns dorsally into central tegmental areas. In addition, there are branches of the fornix into the subthalamic field H of Forel below the medial geniculate nucleus. These fibers are not found in the rat but have been reported in the monkey. At one time, these tegmental pathways were thought to be of septal origin in the rat, but Nauta (1972) believes that these fibers arise from the hippocampal formation and go over the corpus callosum in the dorsal fornix. It is likely that the fibers to the tegmental regions arise from several areas and not only from the hippocampus or the septal area. In the cat, a few fibers of hippocampal origin extend past the mammillary bodies into the midbrain to terminate in the nucleus of Darkschewitsch (Siegel & Tassoni, 1971a).

The hippocampus sends fibers over the fornix system that take a rather extended course. These are the fibers of the dorsal fornix, sometimes called the *fornix superior* or the *fornix longus*. These depart from the main body of the fornix and enter the corpus callosum, penetrate it, and turn rostrally over it to the septal area. Then, they turn downward into the medial septal area. Some of the supracallosal fibers (also known as the *stripes of Lancisi*) do not reach the medial forebrain bundle and the anterior hypothalamus but terminate in the intralaminar nucleus of the thalamus, the anterior nuclei of the thalamus, the habenula, and the mammillary bodies.

THE SEPTAL AREA

The septal area lies in a special position relative to the limbic system and to the rest of the brain. Parts of it stand as unpaired medial structures. All parts receive massive input from a wide variety of limbic regions as well as from the hypothalamus. Its influences on other brain regions are as widespread as its sources of incoming neural traffic. Part of the challenge is to discover the ways in which the septal area acts to integrate and regulate the diverse areas with which it is connected.

The septal area is prominent in nonprimate mammals and is found in an area below the anterior portions of the corpus callosum, bounded in front by the anterior hippocampal rudiment[7] and in back by the hippocampal commissures. The homologous nuclei in primates may be those found in the front of the anterior commissure at the base of the brain. The septum pellucidum in humans is not homologous to the septal area complex of nonprimates. There have been suggestions relating the size of the septal complex to the development of the hippocampus, but this correlation is by no means certain.

Nuclear Divisions

Largely located underneath the anterior and middle regions of the corpus callosum, the septal region is a large midline structure in the rodent and certain other nonprimate species. The largest nuclear mass belongs to the paired lateral septal nuclei that extend from a plane anterior to the optic chiasm to the posterior termination of the structure. The lateral septal area is bounded by the anterior horns of the lateral ventricles, and at or near the posterior boundary, the lateral ventricles fuse with the third ventricle to form the interventricular formation (the foramen of Monro). This posterior region is comprised

---

[7] The anterior hippocampal rudiment, or precommissural hippocampus, is an area marked by vertical columns of darkly staining pyramidal cells at the inner edges of the hemispheres just below the genu of the corpus callosum. These cells seem to be continuous with a very thin band of similar cells that stretch over the top of the corpus callosum, called the *indusium griseum*. Both the anterior hippocampal rudiment and the indusium griseum are thought to represent displaced pyramidal cells of the hippocampus.

almost entirely of fibers of the fornix and hippocampal commissural systems. The lateral septal area is often divided into dorsal, intermediate, and ventral regions, although the cytoarchitectural differentiation of these subregions is not great.

The medial septal division is made up of cells of larger size on the average than those of the lateral division. It is probably wise to regard the cells of the diagonal band of Broca and the cells of the medial septal nucleus as being functionally and anatomically associated as the "medial division" of the septal area. The cells of the nucleus of the diagonal band lie anterior to the medial septal area and curve dorsally before curving back to merge with cells in the medial septal nucleus. Recently, the medial septal nucleus has come to be seen as the most posterior portion of the nucleus of the diagonal band and is not regarded as an independent structure.

In the posterior portion of the septal area, the septofimbrial nucleus and the triangular nucleus are thought to make up a posterior division. The bed nuclei of the stria terminalis lie below and lateral to the lateral septal nuclei, inside the boundary of the caudate, and above the corpus callosum. This nuclear group receives many fibers from the amygdala over the stria terminalis.

The tail of the nucleus accumbens reaches to the septal complex, but this nuclear group is associated with basal forebrain striatal mechanisms rather than with the septal complex.

Fiber Connections

The major fiber connections from the septal complex are described on the basis of the nuclear subgroups.[8]

The efferent fibers from the medial septal nucleus and the diagonal band of Broca are quite similar. Some of the major targets of medial-septal–diagonal-band cells are three systems:

---

[8] The efferent and afferent connections are described following the results reported and summarized by Swanson and Cowan (1979). As mentioned by these investigators, there are problems in describing afferents by the horseradish peroxidase (HRP) technique in the septal area. Even small injections seem to be picked up and transported by fibers of passage. Therefore, an exhaustive description of afferents with this procedure does not seem likely. Most available information comes from anterograde transport of ³H amino acids from selected projection sites.

1. The habenula
2. The hypothalamus
3. The hippocampus

The habenular projection from the medial-septal–diagonal-band complex reaches its targets by passing through the stria medullaris.

The medial septal projections to the hypothalamus reach the medial preoptic region, the lateral hypothalamus, and portions of the mammillary complex, and some continue to the dorsal raphe nucleus and the ventral tegmental area.

The fibers that project to the hippocampus end in the strata radiatum and oriens of CA_3 (but not CA_1), the hilar region of the dentate gyrus, and the subicular and entorhinal transitional cortex regions.

Efferents that travel substantial distances from the lateral septal group arise from the intermediate and ventral subdivisions. Efferents from the dorsal subgroup project primarily to the nucleus of the diagonal band and the medial-septal areas.

Both of the other lateral subgroups have heavy projections to the medial septal nucleus and the diagonal band complex. Both project to areas above the mammillary complex, although there are some differences in the specific areas receiving fibers from the intermediate and ventral regions. Both project to the ventral tegmental area. The intermediate subregion of the lateral septal area projects to the lateral hypothalamus and the dorsomedial nucleus, while the ventral subregion projects to the medial preoptic and the anterior hypothalamic areas. Afferents to the preoptic and the supramammillary regions have also been described (Krayniak, Weiner, & Siegel, 1980).

The main target for fibers from the posterior septal nuclei (septofimbrial and triangular) are the medial and lateral habenula by way of the stria medullaris. The fibers originating in the septal area are joined by fibers from the hippocampus formation, at least in some species. Some of the septal and hippocampal fibers continue through the tractus retroflexus to the interpeduncular nucleus. It is possible to regard the posterior septal nuclei as a link in a neural system connecting with the interpeduncular nucleus via the habenulae.

As described earlier in discussing the hippocampus, a major input to the lateral septal nucleus comes from the hippocampus proper and the subiculum.

The projections reaching the lateral septal area come from areas CA_3 and CA_2 of both sides, with fibers from the contralateral side crossing in the ventral hippocampal commissures. Fibers from area CA_1 and the subiculum are directed only ipsilaterally (Swanson & Cowan, 1979). The projections of the hippocampus onto the lateral septal area are topographically organized, as are the efferents from this nucleus to the hypothalamus. The most rostral (toward the septal area) portions of the hippocampus (and the subiculum) reach the dorsal portions of the lateral septal nucleus, and the most ventral hippocampal and subicular cells project to the ventral septal area and the bed nucleus of the stria terminalis. Dopaminergic and noradrenergic fibers also reach this area from the ventral tegmental area (Moore, Björklund, & Stenevi, 1971) and the locus ceruleus (Swanson & Hartman, 1975; R. Y. Moore, 1978).

Efferents from the dorsal parts of the lateral septal nucleus reach the preoptic and lateral hypothalamic regions, while those from the ventral portions of the lateral septal nucleus reach more posterior areas, like the area of the supramammillary region (Krayniak et al., 1980).

Therefore, a topographical relationship exists encompassing the hippocampal formation and the hypothalamus with a synaptic relay in the lateral septal nucleus—the dorsal hippocampal formation with anterior hypothalamic regions, the ventral with more posterior hypothalamic regions.

Fibers from the amygdala reach the ventral portions of the lateral septal nucleus, although in limited numbers. A much more substantial input reaches the bed nucleus of the stria terminalis (Krettek & Price, 1978b). Other afferents from the olfactory tubercle, the piriform cortex, and possibly the forebrain striatal complex are likely.

Input from the lateral preoptic and lateral hypothalamic regions reach the medial-septal–diagonal-band aggregate (Swanson, 1976). The anterior hypothalamus sends fibers to the ventral portions of the lateral septal area, as does the ventromedial nucleus (Saper, Swanson, & Cowan, 1976).

The vertical limb of the diagonal band projects to the hippocampal formation with cells near the midline projecting to the more dorsal (septal) regions and with more lateral cells projecting to the more ventral regions. Fibers arising from the horizontal limbs are distributed in a rather similar fashion, except that these regions also project to the ventral tegmental area and the interpeduncular nucleus (Krayniak et al., 1980).

A NOTE ON THE HABENULAE

The paired structures at the caudal end of the dorsal thalamus are usually considered a part of the thalamus or the epithalamus. They differ from most thalamic structures by having few fibers projecting rostrally in comparison with the heavy ascending projections of most thalamic nuclear groups. The main habenular output is by the large fiber pathway, the tractus retroflexus (or habenulopeduncular tract), that projects to the interpeduncular nucleus and the midbrain raphe complex. The main input to the habenula is the stria medullaris. It contains fibers originating in the supracommissural septal area, the nucleus of the diagonal-band–medial-septal area, the preoptic and lateral hypothalamic areas, and the globus pallidus. It has been suggested that the habenulae be regarded as having three primary divisions based on their predominant afferent supplies: the medial nucleus, receiving its predominant input from the supracommissural septum; the medial part of the lateral habenular nucleus, receiving its predominant input from the basal forebrain; and the lateral portion of the lateral nucleus, receiving its major input from the entopeduncular nucleus (the nonprimate homologue of the internal segment of the globus pallidus) (Herkenham & Nauta, 1979). Both medial and lateral habenular areas receive cholinergic projections from the diagonal-band–medial-septal complex (Gottesfeld & Jacobowitz, 1979).

Other fibers of significance reach the habenular complex, including ones from the suprachiasmatic nucleus (to the medial portion of the lateral habenular nucleus) and from the ventral tegmental area (to the lateral portion of the lateral habenular nucleus).

Efferents from the three habenular groups also differ. The medial nucleus projects almost entirely to the interpeduncular nucleus. These fibers probably contain acetylcholine and/or substance P. This projection does not seem to be reciprocal in that there is no evidence supporting a projection from the interpeduncular nucleus to the habenula. The medial portion of the lateral habenula projects to the raphe complex, the adjacent central gray, the medial and lateral hypothalamus, the preoptic area, and ventral portions of the septal area. The lateral portion of the lateral habenular nucleus projects to the midbrain reticular formation and to the pontine tegmental areas. Both divisions of the lateral habenular nucleus project to the substantia nigra and the ventral tegmental area.

THE PAPEZ CIRCUIT

The mammillary bodies, the anterior nuclei of the thalamus, and the cingulate cortex were given a prominent place in the theories of the limbic system proposed by Papez (1937). Papez considered the limbic system the anatomical basis of the emotions. The influences of the limbic system converging with those of the cingulate cortex were thought to be the two major governing systems acting on the hypothalamus. Papez assumed, as has often been the case, that the cerebral cortex had to participate in activities in order for the human or the animal to experience emotional phenomena. He did not, however, believe that the cingulate cortex, or any other part of the neocortex, need be involved in the mechanisms responsible for the behavioral expression of emotion. It is worthwhile to note this distinction, which is often found in the literature, between the mechanisms responsible for the overt expression of internal events and the experience of the internal events. It may be that the distinction is justified, at least in some conditions, but certainly emotions can be influenced by bodily actions. The major output of the mammillary bodies is directed to the anterior thalamic nuclei over the mammillothalamic tract (tract of Vicq d'Azyr). From these, fibers arise that project to the cingulate cortex via the thalamocortical radiations. Changes in neural activity arising in the cingulate cortex are thought to pass into the areas bordering the hippocampal formation, and into the hippocampus itself. Papez's circuit is completed when changes in neural activity are sent from the hippocampus to the mammillary bodies by way of the fornix.

In such a system, neural activity representing the emotional processes originating in the neocortex would be passed along into the hippocampus, the fornix, the mammillary bodies, and the anterior nuclei of the thalamus and would finally be projected onto the receptive region of the "emotional cortex" (i.e., the cingulate cortex). From the cingulate cortex, activity representing emotional processes could pass into the other regions of the cerebral cortex and "add emotional coloring to psychic processes occurring elsewhere." Papez thought that emotional experience could arise in one of two ways, either as a result of "psychic activity" (presumably neocortical activity) or as a result of activities originating in the mammillary bodies.

The cingulate cortex borders and lies directly above the corpus callosum on the medial side of the hemispheres. The gyrus cinguli is sometimes called the *gyrus fornicatus*. In more complicated brains, it is separated from adjacent cortex by the cingulate sulcus. At its posterior extent, it broadens out into a transitional area called *precuneatus*, which curves around the splenium of the corpus callosum. This region merges with the hippocampal gyrus. At its anterior end, it merges with the neocortex around the genu of the corpus callosum and continues forward as subgenual cortex. This region is also called the *anterior limbic region* by some authors. A fiber bundle designated the *cingulum bundle* courses through the cingulate cortex.

One of the early approaches to the study of the structure of the cingulate cortex involved the use of strychnine neuronography. In this technique, small amounts of strychnine are applied to neural tissue, and intermittent epileptiform activity is produced at the site of application and later at more remote sites to which the fibers of the cells in the affected area project. In the monkey, Pribram and MacLean (1953) found that the application of strychnine to any part of the cingulate cortex could induce responses in all other areas of the cingulate system. This finding suggests rich interconnections among all regions of the cingulate system. When strychnine was applied to the posterior cingulate regions, evoked activity could be recorded in the precuneate region and in the posterior hippocampal areas as well. The most predominant responses were found in the subicular areas. Strychnine stimulation of the anterior cingulate regions was found to produce activity in the motor cortex and the prefrontal and orbitofrontal regions (Dunsmore & Lennox, 1950). Projections to the centrum medianum nucleus of the thalamus and the reticular formation have also been found by means of stimulation techniques (French, Hernandez-Peon, & Livingston, 1955). These studies, taken together, reveal that the cingulate cortex is richly interconnected with many regions of the brain in some species, and that there is a differentiation of the projection systems found within the cingulate cortex.

Subdivisions of the medial aspects in the rat's hemisphere are shown in Figure 13. These subdivisions of the cingulate cortex are based on cytoarchitectural differences among the areas, extensively examined and reported by M. Rose (1929). There are pronounced anatomical and physiological differences between the anterior and the posterior portions of the medial cortical regions.

Through studies using experimental degeneration techniques, Domesick (1969, 1972) has been able to follow projections from the anterior cingulate areas to the dorsomedial, the anteromedial, and, to a lesser extent, the ventromedial nuclei of the thalamus. Degeneration was not found in these thalamic areas after lesions in the posterior cingulate regions. Posterior cingulate lesions produced degeneration limited to the anteroventral and laterodorsal (lateral) thalamic nuclei. Degeneration could be found in extrathalamic regions after lesions in the anterior and posterior cingulate areas, which included the caudate-putamen region, the zona incerta, the pretectal area, the superior colliculus (lower layers), the tegmentum, the central gray, and the gray matter of the pons. All regions of the cingulate cortex projected to these areas. A similar pattern of degeneration had been found earlier by Showers (1959), using Marchi's method. No degeneration was found in the mammillary bodies, the hypothalamus, the septal area, or the amygdala after any cingulate lesion.

A schematic summarization of the thalamic projections to and from the cingulate cortex found by Domesick (1972) is presented in Figure 13. The anterior midline regions receive projections both from the anterior medial thalamic nucleus and from the dorsomedial thalamic nucleus. In 1969, Leonard reported that the cortex near the midline of the brain in front of the genu of the corpus callosum receives strong projections from the dorsomedial nucleus of the thalamus. Therefore, this cortex could be thought of as bearing a similarity to the dorsolateral prefrontal cortex of primates.

The organization of the midline cortex in the rat seems to be based on a dorsoventral distinction. The *ventral* portions of this cortical region seem to receive projections from the anterior thalamic group: the anterior medial nucleus rostrally and the anterior dorsal and anterior ventral nuclei caudally. The dorsomedial nucleus of the thala-

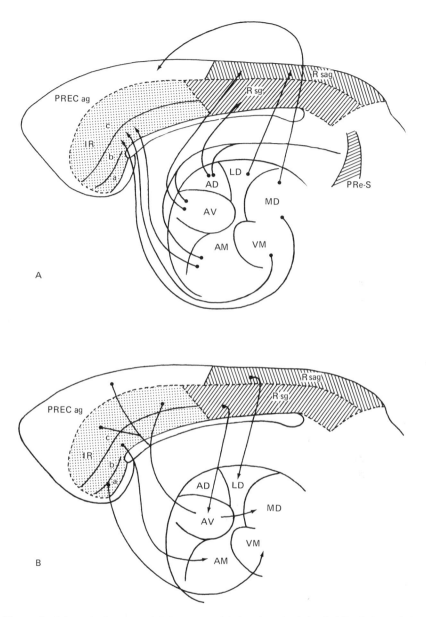

Figure 13. Schematic diagrams of thalamocortical (A) and corticothalamic (B) relations of cingulate cortex of rat. Both area infraradiatae and area retrosplenialis are considered cingulate cortex. The size of the thalamus has been greatly exaggerated relative to the cortex. Abbreviations: AD, anterodorsal nucleus of thalamus; AV, anteroventral nucleus of thalamus; AM, anteromedial nucleus of thalamus; LD, laterodorsal nucleus of thalamus; MD, dorsomedial nucleus of thalamus; VM, ventromedial nucleus of thalamus; IR, area infraradiatae; R sg, area retrosplenial granularis; PREC ag, area precentral agranularis; R sag, area retrosplenial agranularis; a, b, and c, subdivisions of area infraradiatae; PRe-S, presubiculum. Drawings based on Domesick (1972).

mus projects to the *dorsal* portions of the midline cortex (the upper shoulder of this tissue) rostrally, while the lateral dorsal nucleus projects to this shoulder region in the caudal portion. Since both the ventral and the dorsal portions of the midline cortex are considered cingulate cortex, the rat may be unusual in having its cingulate cortex receive projections from several sets of thalamic nuclei. On the other hand, multiple innervation of cingulate regions may be found in other species in future studies.

Beckstead (1979) has pursued the earlier work of Leonard (1969) with the tracing of efferents from the cortical areas receiving projections from the dorsomedial nucleus using autoradiographic methods. Cells in these areas project to the retrosplenial nucleus, the entorhinal nucleus, the lateral septal nucleus, the nucleus accumbens, and the deep layers of the olfactory tubercle, as well as to the pretectal area and the superior colliculi. Projections from these areas reach the subicular regions, which are the transitional regions to the hippocampus over the cingulum bundle. Other projections to the caudate and the thalamic regions correspond in essence to those reported by Leonard and others.

The relationship between the cingulate cortex and the cingulum bundle is not easily understood. Domesick (1970) has presented evidence that the cingulum should be considered a projection system for thalamic fibers in the rat. In primates, it is likely that the fiber system includes a greater number of fibers contributed from the prefrontal neocortex, and Adey and Meyer (1952) have suggested that there are substantial contributions made to the cingulum bundle from the frontal cortex that terminate in parahippocampal regions. The fiber system described by Domesick leaves the anterior thalamic nuclei, travels forward, and turns to pierce portions of the callosal system. It turns somewhat toward the midline of the brain to become the cingulate fasciculus. This upturning of the thalamocortical fibers occurs at levels anterior to the genu of the corpus callosum. This cingulate bundle sends off fibers along its course, especially into the medial (cingulate) cortex and into the presubicular cortex. In the rat, few, if any, fibers join the cingulum bundle from other cortical areas. As mentioned above, there is evidence that the cingulum bundle does accept fibers from other regions in some species. For example, fibers from the amygdala have been shown to join the cingulum bundle at the pregenual level in the cat and the monkey (Lammers & Lohman, 1957;

Nauta, 1961). Catecholamine-containing fibers from cells in the brain stem also join the cingulum bundle.

The failure to find degeneration in the hypothalamus, the septal area, and the amygdala after lesions of the cingulate cortex makes it unique among structures of the limbic system. All of the other structures of the limbic system have strong projections to at least one other limbic region and the hypothalamus. The main anatomical basis for the inclusion of the cingulate cortex in the limbic system seems to be its indirect association with the mammillary bodies.

The main efferent fibers from the mammillary nuclei are fibers that extend dorsally and at some distance above the mammillary bodies, dividing into a mammillothalamic tract and a mammillotegmental tract. It is uncertain whether this division is produced by a bifurcation of axons so that one branch of the axon reaches toward the anterior nucleus of the thalamus and the other toward the tegmentum, or whether the axons running in each direction have independent cells of origin. The mammillotegmental portion of the fibers reaches to the dorsal tegmental nucleus. Destruction of the mammillary body produces degeneration in both the dorsal and the ventral tegmental nuclei. It is thought that the degeneration in the ventral tegmental nu-

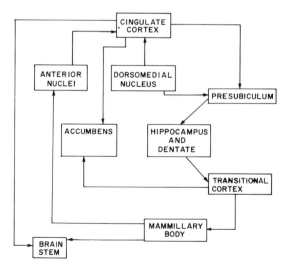

Figure 14. Schematic modern version of Papez's circuit. The "transitional cortex" shown in the figure is used to designate the subicular and entorhinal areas.

cleus is produced by terminals whose axons arrive over the mammillary peduncle. The mammillopeduncular tract is a small bundle of fibers that runs from the medial mammillary nucleus, and also from the interpeduncular nucleus, to end in the ventral tegmental area.

Based on the recent advances in our knowledge of the anatomy of areas involved in the original Papez circuit, the "wiring diagram" for it must be expanded. A schematic representation of a more adequate Papez circuit is shown in Figure 14. This version indicates the fact that the hippocampal formation influences distant regions primarily by its actions on cells located in the subiculum, that the cingulate cortex receives multiple thalamic input, and that an important basal ganglia target for the major cortical areas of the circuit, the hippocampus and the cingulate, is the nucleus accumbens. Whether this more detailed version of Papez's anatomical circuit for the emotions will add to its usefulness remains to be seen, but it does offer a new route for influencing behavior: a link with the basal ganglia, in particular the nucleus accumbens. The importance of this connection is stressed in the final chapter.

2

The Hypothalamus

Neural systems of the hypothalamus influence many types of behavior, but the most frequently studied behaviors are those closely related to physiological functions (e.g., food and water ingestion and sex behavior). This is true because many areas in the hypothalamus are involved in the regulation of the thermal, hormonal, osmotic, and nutritional balances of the body, and cells in this area are responsive to information arising in the internal and external environments. In addition, however, the hypothalamus is involved in the regulation of somatic activities and modulates activity in other forebrain regions of the brain.

However, the limbic system's influences on behavior extend far beyond those actions directed toward the maintenance of particular physiological conditions or balances. They involve many subtle aspects of learning, memory, motivation, and performance. They include effects that may be described in terms of cognitive acts, strategies, and hypotheses. Because of the intimate relationships of the septal area, the amygdala, the hippocampus, and other limbic regions with the hypothalamus, it may serve us well to begin our study with this area, where all of the limbic structures' influences converge.

Because of my view that it is important to break with traditional ways of looking at the hypothalamus only as a regulator of physiological systems, I will begin with a landmark in research on brain functions that also helped to change prominent theories of behavior: the discovery of pleasure centers in the brain.

PLEASURABLE REACTIONS

In 1953, Drs. James Olds and Peter Milner began a whole new approach to the analysis of brain activities as related to behavior with their discovery of rewarding effects produced by electrical stimulation of the brain. I have heard that at the time of their discovery, Olds and Milner were attempting to determine the behavioral effects of electrical stimulation of "arousal systems." While testing their animals in a tabletop enclosure, they noticed that the animals seemed to be attracted to the corner of the enclosure in which they had received the stimulation. The animals seemed to "like" this area. This observation led Olds and Milner to give the animals an opportunity to make responses that would produce their own brain stimulation. Simply enough, they arranged a situation in which the animals could depress a lever in an operant chamber. Pressing the lever activated control devices that sent small amounts of electrical current between the electrodes implanted deep in the animal's brains, exciting nearby tissues. The report of this experiment is now a milestone in the history of brain–behavior research (Olds & Milner, 1954).

This experiment was a turning point in the theoretical analysis of brain–behavior relationships. Until the time of the Olds and Milner experiment, the analysis of the brain's effects on behavior was dominated by behavioristic approaches. These included those developed and made popular in the world of experimental psychology by Clark Hull, Kenneth Spence, B. F. Skinner, and their associates. These theories were based on the assumption that behavior could be explained by the development of rules describing the relationship between the stimuli affecting the organism, the responses made by the individual, and the conditions under which rewards were obtained. Behavior was to be explained on the basis of measurable events: stimuli, responses, and rewards. The theories were barren of any reference to the individual's plans, experiences, or beliefs.

The discovery of brain regions that, when electrically stimulated, seemed to produce rewarding effects began an era of greater freedom in the scientific description of behavior. It did so because the behavior of the animals seemed most easily explained on the basis that the animals would perform responses of several different kinds to obtain electrical stimulation in certain brain regions. The goal of their efforts was most easily described in terms of obtaining a pleasurable experience. Thus, the experiences of the organism had to become a factor in describing or explaining behavior. *Pleasure* and *pain* became accepted as legitimate terms, once again, for scientists trying to discover the neural bases of behavior. In short, the results of Olds and Milner helped break down the strong theoretical fortress of artificial concepts developed by learning theorists. Olds and Milner's results justified explanations of experimental data in hedonistic terms.

At first, the report of Olds and Milner, as well as subsequent publications dealing with self-stimulation phenomena, was criticized as being "nonbehavioristic." Critics argued that better explanations of the behavior could be found within the stimulus–response (S–R) framework and that "feelings" of "affective experiences" need not be attributed to the animals whose brains were being stimulated. Nevertheless, as experiment mounted on experiment, it became evident that the most useful way to describe the behavioral effects of the brain stimulation was indeed in terms of the elicitation of positively rewarding, or pleasant, experiences. Reports from people whose brains had been stimulated in the reward regions have indicated that the experience obtained is, in fact, pleasant (Bishop, Elder, & Heath, 1963).

The change of orientation of scientists in the brain–behavior area should not be interpreted as an overthrow of a strict scientific methodology for a looser and less demanding one. It was an overthrow of a theoretical structure that was too narrow and imposed too many constraints on the ideas that could be investigated. It is always important to be able to define precisely what is done in an experiment and to have theories in which the variables manipulated can be defined and understood by others. The fact is that as yet, we do not have truly satisfactory theories of brain functions or of behavior, but progress toward better theories should not be inhibited by the dogmatic acceptance of inadequate ones.

THE LOCATION OF PLEASURE REGIONS

Olds and Milner first discovered rewarding or pleasant effects by stimulation of the septal area. But further investigations soon found sites in many areas of the brain that produced positively rewarding effects when electrically stimulated. These include some parts of all of the structures of the limbic system and some of the surrounding transitional cortical areas. There are many areas that do not produce reward reactions when electrically stimulated. Indeed, the majority of the forebrain is "silent" in regard to emotional or affective reactions. This discovery led to the view that there were certain collections of neurons that were essential to rewarding or pleasurable reactions. Some of the regions that produce positively rewarding effects when stimulated are now well established. These include the lateral septal area, certain portions of the amygdala, some parts of the hippocampus, and the lateral hypothalamus. In addition, self-stimulation has been reported to occur in the dorsal-frontal cortex and various brain stem regions of the rat. As a rule of thumb, it can be said that most limbic areas will support self-stimulation behavior, although there is considerable variation in the apparent intensity of the effects among areas. Also associated with self-stimulation behavior are the major catecholamine systems ranging from their sites of origin in the brain stem to their terminations in the forebrain.

The most "rewarding" regions of the brain are found along the base of the brain in the general region of the lateral hypothalamus and the medial forebrain bundle (Olds & Olds, 1963). Perhaps the strongest pleasurable effects are produced by electrical stimulation at posterior reaches of the hypothalamus, just ahead of the mammillary bodies. Boyd and Gardner (1967) have suggested that there are multiple hypothalamic pathways involved in the mediation of rewarding effects and that lesions in any one of them would produce a reduction in, but not a total abolition of, self-stimulation effects. This view is supported by the finding that lesions of the lateral hypothalamic-medial forebrain bundle region do not disturb self-stimulation for all forebrain regions (Valenstein & Campbell, 1966).

The early observation that self-stimulation could be found along the course of the medial forebrain bundle was extended by further work to associate such sites with the forebrain projections of the larger catecholamine projections. As newer techniques allowed better detection of catecholamine locations, these were also found to be correlated with self-rewarding effects. Indeed, it has been suggested that the amount of catecholamine concentrations in tissues at the tip of the electrode is correlated with the rate of self-stimulation (German & Bowden, 1974). However, the relationship between the catecholamines and behavior is by no means settled. There are disputes about experimental observations, conflicting data, and difficulties in the interpretation of what is known. For example, if norepinephrine were to play an important role in support of self-stimulation behavior then it would be expected that stimulation of the locus ceruleus should produce reward effects. Some authors report such effects (e.g., Segal & Bloom, 1976a,b), but others do not (Amaral & Routtenberg, 1975). Destruction of the dorsal or ventral tegmental bundles over which most of the noradrenergic fibers reach forebrain sites does not eliminate self-stimulation behavior.

Self-stimulation has been reported for the cell bodies of the dopaminergic systems in the brain stem (Crow, 1972; Phillips, Carter, & Fibiger, 1976), and since the projections from these cells course through, and nearby, the medial forebundle projection system, they could be implicated in the strong self-stimulation behavior seen from this region. Once again, however, there are conflicts among experimental reports about the relationship of dopaminergic systems to reward behaviors. For example, some researchers report self-stimulation behavior from forebrain targets of the dopamine projection regions, the caudate and the nucleus accumbens (Phillips, Brooke, & Fibiger, 1975; Phillips, Carter, & Fibiger, 1976), while others have reported results at variance with these observations (M. E. Olds, 1970; Routtenberg, 1971). In addition, an extreme reduction of forebrain dopamine by neurotoxin injections into ascending pathways only caused transitory reductions in self-stimulation (Clavier & Fibiger, 1977).

Despite intense efforts in many laboratories, it has not been possible to relate unequivocally either noradrenergic or dopaminergic systems to hypothalamic self-stimulation. It has been postulated that the noncatecholaminergic fibers running in the medial forebrain bundle regions are the ones essential to reward functions (Stiglick & White, 1977). Investigations based on the disruption of self-stimulation by pharmacological means present difficulties because of their nonspecific effects on performance (Atrens, Ljungberg, & Ungerstedt, 1976; Fibiger, Carter, & Phillips, 1976). A summary of the relationship between self-stimulation, reward effects, and the catecholamines is available (Wise, 1978). In it, Wise pointed out the need for more studies in which the effects of naturally occurring rewarding events and self-stimulation are compared. Certain attempts have been made in this direction (e.g., Hernandez & Hoebel, 1978), but much more needs to be done.

Another recent direction of research into the mechanisms underlying hypothalamic stimulation relates to the role played by the endogenous opiate systems. Stein and Belluzzi (1979) have proposed that the enkephalins may be the transmitters involved in the reward or pleasure systems of the brain. This opinion was based on studies in which animals responded to provide themselves with the delivery of enkephalin to the brain and the fact that the opiate antagonist naloxone reduced the rate of responding for electrical stimulation. This effect was found, however, at a high dose level of the opiate antagonist, and the electrodes were not in the hypothalamus. Others have not found naloxone effects on hypothalamic self-stimulation (Lorens & Sainati, 1978b). Naloxone apparently reduces the effects of drugs that enhance rates of lateral hypothalamic stimulation, such as ethyl alcohol or minor tranquilizers, but does not affect lateral hypothalamic self-stimulation *per se* (Lorens & Sainati, 1978a). These results would suggest that the endogenous opiates may exert a modulatory influence on self-stimulation but may not play a critical role in the basic behavior. A similar role has been suggested for endorphin fragments (Dorsa, Van Ree, & De Wied, 1979).

Self-stimulation behavior and the effects of rewards more generally seem to be closely related to hypothalamic mechanisms, but in ways that are almost as obscure as they were almost 30 years ago when they were first discovered. The modulation of these effects by drugs and by opiate mechanisms are of potential practical value but seem to speak only softly about the neural basis of pleasurable reactions.

PAIN AND PUNISHMENT

About the time that Olds and Milner were discovering that rewarding effects could be produced by electrical stimulation of the brain, Delgado, Roberts, and Miller (1954) were finding behavioral effects produced by brain stimulation that indicated that an aversive or painful state had been produced. Hungry animals were shown to avoid food associated with such stimulation, but, more important, the stimulation could serve to motivate the learning of an avoidance task. In this way, the stimulation was comparable to the effects of noxious electrical stimulation applied to the periphery of the body. It became reasonable, therefore, to regard these stimulation effects as aversive to the animal.

An interesting result stemming from brain stimulation studies is that animals will work both to turn on the electrical stimulation of the brain and to turn it off if it is left on long enough (Bower & Miller, 1958; Roberts, 1958). This sort of result has been found in most of the brain regions that have been studied. The most positively reinforcing zones, namely, in the posterior aspects of the lateral hypothalamus–medial forebrain bundle, seem to be ones in which the animal will accept prolonged periods of stimulation without acting to turn it off. But for most other areas, the animal seems to prefer limited amounts of electrical stimulation. These observations led to the notion that electrical stimulation of certain brain regions can activiate both a positively rewarding "pleasure system" and a negatively rewarding "punishment system." In those instances where an animal will act both to turn on brain stimulation and to turn it off, it might be assumed that a reward system is activated first by the electrical stimulation but that when stimulation continues, the punishment system becomes activated. When this happens, the rewarding effects become antagonized by the activation of the punishment system. Rewarding brain stimulation can mask the effects of peripheral pain in humans (Heath & Mickle, 1960) and animals (Cox & Valenstein, 1965), as well as attenuate the effects of stimulation of aversive regions (Routtenberg & Olds, 1963). Margalit and Segal (1979) found that the amount of analgesia produced by electrical brain stimulation was correlated with the rate at which the animals self-stimulated. The analgesia was reduced by naloxone. Stimulation of aversive regions can attenuate the behavioral effects produced by the stimulation of reward areas (Olds & Olds, 1962).

It might well be asked if any brain stimulation that influences behavior has some positive or negative affective quality. At least for their work with tegmental sites, Olds and Peretz (1960) have suggested that there can be three types of systems of effects produced by electrical stimulation. Two of these are related to the affective reactions of the organism: the positively and negatively rewarding systems. The third system is one that produces changes in arousal.

Certain portions of the tegmentum produce both behavioral and electrical signs of arousal when stimulated. This stimulation is without affective tone since the animals do not act to turn it on or off. Thus, there may be systems that modulate the arousal of the animal without necessarily producing pleasure or pain. It is likely that the stimulation of most regions of the brain produces some combinations of activity of the affective and the arousal systems.

THE LOCATION OF PAIN-RELATED REGIONS

The midbrain central gray and periventricular regions, the region of the medial lemniscus in the midbrain, and the ventromedial nucleus of the hypothalamus all seem to produce the strong aversive reactions (Delgado *et al.*, 1954). At least some of the aversive effects can be blocked by the administration of morphine (Kiser & German, 1978).

The central gray of the midbrain can also produce strong analgesia when electrically stimulated (Reynolds, 1969). Other effective sites are the periaqueductal and periventricular regions (Mayer & Liebeskind, 1974). The analgesic effect seems to be an active process since (1) it depends on normal levels of monoamines (Akil & Liebeskind, 1975; Akil & Mayer, 1972); and (2) lesions in the area do not produce analgesia (Liebman, Mayer, & Liebeskind, 1970).

The stimulation of central gray in the human produces effective analgesia, but it is accompanied by unpleasant sensations such as vertigo and sensations of smothering and nausea (Richardson & Akil, 1977a). Stimulation of other structures, such as the parafascicular nucleus of the thalamus, can produce pain relief with fewer untoward side effects (Richardson & Akil, 1977a,b). Stimulation in this nucleus tends to produce feelings of well-being and relaxation.

It is possible that the aversive qualities found resulting from central gray stimulation are a consequence of the more diffuse unpleasant qualities described in the human reports, which represent unpleasant side effects to the analgesic effects.

The stimulation-produced analgesia in humans (Richarson & Akil, 1977b) and animals seems to be dependent on the endogenous opiate systems, since the effects are blocked by naloxone. Microinjections of morphine into the periventricular region (Tsou & Jang, 1964), as well as into the rostral periaqueductal gray and the posterior hypothalamus, produce analgesia (Jacquet & Lajtha, 1973). Both electrical stimulation of the periaqueductal gray and the administration of narcotics seem to affect activity in a system that descends through the nucleus raphe magnus into the spinal cord and inhibits pain signals there (e.g., Liebeskind, Giesler, & Urca, 1976). Some of the diencephalic regions associated with the pain-suppressive systems are the dorsomedial and the ventromedial hypothalamic nuclei (Rhodes & Liebeskind, 1978). The entire system, or multiple systems, may act as a feedback mechanism from the forebrain, which operates to limit the occurrence of painful stimulation both by internal neural mechanisms and by behavioral reactions. Viewed in this light, stimulation of the pain-suppressive reactions induces not only analgesia as an internal reaction against pain, but also escape and aversion responses that relate to the situation in which the experience occurs and, in the case of stimulation of the ventromedial nucleus, a correlated rage reaction.

The relationship of the hypothalamus to aversive systems cannot be considered in terms of a simple formulation of affective mechanisms existing independently of one other. Hoebel and Thompson (1969) have shown, for example, that escape reactions and self-stimulation rates produced by lateral hypothalamic stimulation are influenced by the animal's weight. If an animal is made overweight by forced feeding, its escape reactions to brain stimulation increase and its self-stimulation rates decrease. It is as if making an animal overweight reduces the rewarding aspects of lateral hypothalamic stimulation and enhances the negative aspects.

These observations point out that the effects of brain stimulation must be considered in terms of the internal environment of the animal. But the external environment and the animal's past experiences also play determining roles. For example, in one experiment, cats with electrodes implanted in the diencephalon were trained to make a response that caused a door to open between two compartments. One compartment was "dangerous," since the animal received electrical footshocks in it. The other was "safe," since the animal was never punished in it. After the response that opened the door between the compartments and allowed the cats to gain access to the "safe" compartment was well established, they were given identical electrical brain stimulation in both compartments. Stimulation applied to the animal while it was in the dangerous location produced the learned response that opened the door to safety. The same stimulation applied in the safe compartment made the animal relax and go to sleep. This is the "dual effect" of brain stimulation described by Grastyán (see Grastyán, 1968).

The effects of hypothalamic stimulation also depend on constitutional factors related to the individual animal. Genetic variations appear in the rates of self-stimulation of the lateral hypothalamus in both rats (Lieblich & Olds, 1971) and mice (Cazala & Guenet, 1976). It appears that this genetic characteristic is related to the tendency of hypothalamic or septal area lesions to induce hyperemotionality (see pp. 137–141). Lieblich, Cohen, Ben-Zion, and Dymshitz (1980) found that either type of lesion induced reduced emotional reactions in low self-stimulation lines, but more typical responses were found in the high self-stimulation lines. Increased food intake after ventromedial nucleus lesions in the hypothalamus was equivalent in the two self-stimulation lines. This finding suggests a functional differentiation between hypothalamic systems related to food incorporation and emotionality. Regardless of this issue, however, genetic analysis represents a powerful method for the analysis of characteristics that "go together" after brain stimulation or brain lesions. Characteristics may hang together in ways that are unexpected as, for example, in Lipp's (1979) report of a genetic association between avoidance behavior and self-stimulation.

ELICITED BEHAVIORS

Electrical brain stimulation can produce very specific behavioral acts that occur at the time the brain is being stimulated. A location from which such behaviors can be readily elicited is the lateral hypothalamus.

Elicited behaviors are typically measured in open situations where the animals can roam freely. What happens when the brain of an animal is stimulated at a lateral hypothalamic site in this open situation, one in which many kinds of responses can be made? One of the most common elicited behaviors is simply a general increase in locomotion, sometimes accompanied by orienting movements. Frequently, however, the elicited behaviors are more specific. They could be licking from a water bottle, eating a food pellet, gnawing on a block of wood, drinking water from a dish, or a sexual or aggressive act. Often these behaviors are produced by electrical stimulation at intensities too low to obtain reward effects.[1] Elicited behaviors are not consequences of the activation of a motivational system. To be sure, eating and drinking can be reliably produced by electrical stimulation in hypothalamic areas. Nevertheless, these behavioral acts are not actions directed toward the alleviation of induced motives for food or water. They seem to be patterns of behavior that are elicited without regard to the satisfaction of particular motives.

Important behavioral sequences that frequently occur must be organized at the midbrain, the brain stem, or the spinal cord levels, since no known lesion of any nucleus or tract rostral to these regions alters these acts to any appreciable degree. The contribution of the hypothalamus, and other forebrain areas, is to modify and regulate the expression of these organized behavioral sequences. The term *command area* can be used to describe the brain stem and spinal cord systems responsible for organized acts such as eating, gnawing, licking, lapping, sexual acts, aggression, and many other types of unlearned behaviors. These command areas are fully organized neural systems that are capable of coordinating the many subcomponents of behavioral acts, taking into consideration the sensory feedback arising from each of the subcomponents. The subcomponents are woven into the fabric of a complete behavior sequence. The job of understanding behavior must include the question of the neural mechanisms of the forebrain's selectively facilitating or inhibiting the many different command areas at different times.

In this light, stimulation of the hypothalamus could be seen as selectively activating a command area governing the expression of one behavioral sequence when an elicited behavior is produced. Influences from the stimulated area could be funneled into the midbrain and the brain stem through fibers of the medial forebrain bundle. As a result, it would be expected that, from time to time, electrodes in the hypothalamus would be in the immediate vicinity of nuclei or fiber tracts that exert a special influence on one or another command

---

[1] The entire volume 2, issue number 4 (1969) of *Brain, Behavior and Evolution* is recommended to the reader. It contains theoretical reviews by Valenstein, Cox, and Valenstein; by Roberts; and by Caggiula.

area. However appealing this concept may be because of its simplicity, it is incorrect.

Behaviors elicited by hypothalamic stimulation depend on the bias of the individual animal to exhibit a particular response rather than the accidental placement of the electrode in a group of cells or fibers that facilitate a one-or-another behavior. This effect has been shown in several ways. For example, animals with electrodes at several hypothalamic sites tend to exhibit the same behavior after stimulation (Valenstein, Cox, & Kakolewski, 1970). Animals fitted with movable electrodes often exhibit the same behavior when stimulated at different points over distances as large as 1.5 mm (Wise, 1971). Finally, animals in which large lesions have been made around the electrode site exhibit the same behavior pattern following stimulation as before, even when most of the tissue originally stimulated has been destroyed (Bachus & Valenstein, 1979). The persistence of the behavior after the lesions indicates that the particular elicited behavior exhibited cannot be explained on the basis of the activation of interwoven local circuits at the electrode tip.

The individual differences found in elicited behaviors are related to the genetic makeup of the animals. Although these differences have not been intensively studied, Bachus and Valenstein reported that only 10–30% of Sprague-Dawley rats exhibit elicited drinking behavior when stimulated in the hypothalamus, while this behavior is found in 80–90% of Long Evans rats. Genetic factors, therefore, contribute to the tendency of animals to respond to electrical stimulation in a particular way, at least initially.

Changes in Elicited Behaviors

If an electrode is placed in a hypothalamic region that, when stimulated, reliably produces a particular behavior, it might be thought that electrical stimulation of this region would continue to produce this response forevermore. However, this is not the case. For example, if the elicited response is licking water from a drinking tube, the question can be asked, "What would happen if the electrical stimulation were applied when a drinking tube was no longer in the animal's environment?" A theory based on the idea that a predisposition to exhibit a licking motor response would predict that a licking response would be made to any object available. A motivational theory that regards the elicited behavior as indicating the induction of thirst would predict that the animal would engage in some other form of behavior directed toward the incorporation of fluids. In fact, however, the removal of the drinking tube eliminates the licking response during periods of electrical stimulation but fails to elicit other forms of water-oriented behavior, such as lapping water from a dish. Therefore, the behavior produced by the electrical stimulation of the brain is dependent on the available objects in the environment and cannot be explained by the induction of particular physiological motives.

If an animal has been stimulated in an environment containing many types of objects and has demonstrated a particular elicited behavior, then the removal of the object supporting this behavior causes a disruption of the elicited behavior. The behavior is tied to a specific environmental support object. Even though no other behavior immediately becomes prominent when the environmental support object is removed, the animal can develop a new behavior correlated with the electrical stimulation and directed toward a different support object. This new elicited behavior is often quite different from the one made formerly. The change in elicited behaviors can be produced by stimulating the animal over a prolonged period of time while it is in the presence of other objects. For many animals, at least, a new behavior will emerge that cannot be predicted from the original elicited behavior. For example, an animal originally drinking from a drinking tube when electrically stimulated might start gnawing wood or eating food just as readily as lapping from a water dish after a prolonged bout of stimulation without the drinking tube available. If the original environmental support object is replaced in the animal's environment, the animal does not give up the new behavior sequence it has developed in place of the initial elicited behavior. The electrical stimulation of the brain without the preferred support object has changed the animal. It has a new and relatively permanent behavior associated with the brain stimulation.

The hypothesis that the behavior elicited by hypothalamic stimulation is a result of a "prepotent" or dominant behavioral tendency based on the characteristics of a particular animal is attractive, yet it presents certain difficulties. According to this theory, if each of two pairs of electrodes were placed in a behavior-facilitating system, the same "dominant behavior" should be elicited through both pairs of electrodes. Valenstein, Cox, and Kakolewski (1969) found that electrical stimulation of the lateral hypothalamus through different pairs of electrodes does *not* always elicit the same response. For example, a specific elicited behavior is often produced at one electrode site, while general exploratory activities are elicited at the other (Cox & Valenstein, 1969). In some cases, it is possible to change the behavior elicited from one site so that it is similar to that produced at the other location. Gallistel (1969) found that when a posterior hypothalamic electrode elicited sexual behavior and a lateral hypothalamic electrode elicited eating, later retesting indicated that both behaviors could be elicited from each placement.

It is not possible to establish a stimulus-bound behavior simply by pairing electrical stimulation of the brain with the spontaneous occurrence of a behavioral response or by stimulating the animal while it is under the influence of a particular biological motive. Valenstein and Cox (1970) found that stimulating the hypothalamus while the animal was eating did not establish elicited feeding. Repeated pairings of a behavior and the electrical stimulation are of help only when the electrical stimulation *was* able to elicit the response in the first place.

It should also be noted that some investigators have found more specificity in the response to localized lateral hypothalamic stimulation than reported by Valenstein and his co-workers. However, many of these studies have used different species. Examples of greater specificity come from the work of Roberts, Steinberg, and Means (1967) with the opossum, of Flynn, Vanegas, Foote, and Edwards (1970) with the cat, and of Martin (1976) with the guinea pig.

Well-organized, aggressive acts are frequently observed after hypothalamic stimulation. The most extensive work with such behaviors has been done on cats and was first reported in the pioneering studies of hypothalamic stimulation by Hess (1949). The rage responses exhibited during stimulation were very similar to those found in natural conditions of rage and attack. The induced attacks were real, and sometimes the observer would be the object attacked. Other observations, however, indicated that hypothalamic stimulation could lead to some peripheral signs of rage, but the cats failed to exhibit attacks. Rage and well-directed attack behaviors are most likely to be found after the stimulation of lateral hypothalamic areas in the cat. More medial sites may produce partial or sham rage. In extending these early results, Flynn (1967) found two forms of aggressive behaviors after hypothalamic stimulation: *affective attack* and *quiet, biting attack*.

In the first form, signs of sympathetic arousal, hissing, and snarling are observed. In the second, the animal is quieter and resembles an animal stalking its prey. The quiet, biting attack systems of the forebrain seem to follow the medial forebrain bundle back to the ventral tegmental region, but a large number of anatomical sites can produce this type of behavior when stimulated: the posterior thalamus, the lateral preoptic area, the midbrain reticular formation, portions of the periaqueductal gray, the pontine tegmentum, parts of the cerebellum, and the ventral tegmental area (e.g., Flynn, 1976). At least some of these sites are interconnected, as evidenced by the fact that stimulation at one location can influence the excitability of another (Bandler & Fatouris, 1978). However, the interaction of only a few regions was investigated in this study.

Electrical stimulation of the hypothalamus does more than elicit specific behaviors. It also changes an animal's reactions to sensory stimulation. For example, Flynn (1967) noted changes in a cat's responsiveness to stimulation applied around its face when the hypothalamus was stimulated. He regarded the stimulation as both potentiating the sensory reactions and increasing the effectiveness of the stimulation in initiating responses related to eating and aggression. The potentiation of responses can be quite specific. Certain points in the hypothalamus of a cat elicit attacks on the experimenter but not on a rat. Stimulation at other hypothalamic points leads to attacks on a rat but not on the experimenter. Nevertheless, these different responses could be caused by effects produced in the animal that are not as specific as might at first appear. The extent to which the animal is afraid might help determine whether attack would be directed toward a large (experimenter) or a small (rat) stimulus. In addition, it is difficult to determine the relative contribution of response and sensory mechanisms to an observed behavioral act. Does the exaggerated tendency to respond to a stimulus applied to the cat's muzzle indicate a facilitation of the sensory input, the effectiveness of the input in directing behavior, or the response mechanisms involved? These questions are difficult to unravel experimentally.

Self-Stimulation, Arousal, and Elicited Behaviors

Since animals will press levers or perform other acts to obtain electrical stimulation of the hypothalamus, they can be said to be "motivated" by the brain stimulation. Since stimulation can be used as a reward for learning or performance in many types of situations, it must also have reinforcing properties. Therefore, electrical stimulation of the hypothalamus has both reinforcing and motivating qualities. The question arises whether these components can be separated anatomically or physiologically. The distinction between the motivational and the rewarding properties of brain stimulation has been emphasized by several authors (e.g., Deutsch & Howarth, 1963; Gallistel, 1964).

Huston (1971) has reported studies in which he measured the amounts of electrical stimulation needed to affect three types of "motivation-sensitive" behaviors: (1) the production of stimulus-bound eating, drinking, or copulating; (2) the facilitation of operant response rate on a fixed-ratio schedule; and (3) the "release" of a previously extinguished response. Then, he compared the current levels required to obtain these behaviors with the current required to support self-stimulation at the same electrode sites. The thresholds for all three types of motivation-sensitive behaviors were well below the threshold for self-stimulation. This finding could be interpreted to mean that self-stimulation effects depend on the activation of a high-threshold reward system that is independent of the lower-threshold motivation-sensitive systems.

Rolls (1971) has pointed out that two fairly clear patterns of behavior are associated with self-stimulation in different brain regions. The behavioral syndrome produced by medial-forebrain-bundle–lateral-hypothalamus stimulation includes hyperactivity, a high rate of responding in an operant situation, a lack of habituation to the stimulation, and sometimes the production of elicited behaviors. This pattern is similar to that described by Huston for his motivation-sensitive effects. Self-stimulation induced in other brain regions, including some limbic locations, is associated with reduced activity, low rates of operant response, rapid habituation of response rate, and sometimes poststimulus "rebound behaviors" (see Milgram, 1969). These results suggest the possibility of two (or more) reward systems in the brain.

When rats are to be trained to run through a straight runway to obtain electrical brain stimulation, they must be "primed" by stimulation given in the start box before every trial (Gallistel, 1969), but priming of a behavior rewarded by electrical brain stimulation does not require the use of the electrical stimulation of the *brain*. Peripheral electrical stimulation of the animal's feet will also work (MacDougall & Bevan, 1968). This finding suggests that stimulation of the medial forebrain bundle could produce rewarding effects by facilitation of one neural system and could produce increased behavioral activation by facilitation of a different system. In fact, Rolls and Kelly (1972) suggested that the hypothalamic stimulation could antidromically excite cells in the brain stem whose collaterals reach other cells in the same area. The brain stem cells affected in this secondary fashion could be responsible for the activation and arousal produced by the hypothalamic stimulation. On the other hand, Keene and Casey (1970) have shown that electrical stimulation of the lateral hypothalamus produces orthodromic excitatory effects on neurons in the brain-stem reticular formation that are also influenced by noxious peripheral stimulation.

From these studies, it is clear that stimulation of the lateral hypothalamus produces at least three quite distinctive effects: (1) specific behavioral acts; (2) the activation of behavior, reflected in several ways, including increases in the rates of responding and the release of previously extinguished behaviors; and (3) rewarding effects. A dissociation between general arousal and rewarding effects is emphasized by the fact that self-stimulation can be obtained by stimulation in regions that, when stimulated, produce few, if any, signs of behavioral or electrographic arousal. Changes in performance occurring as a consequence of limbic or hypothalamic stimulation or lesions could be due to effects produced on either the arousal or the reward systems but must always be considered in the context of the animal's internal and external environment.

RELATIONS OF THE HYPOTHALAMUS WITH THE AUTONOMIC NERVOUS SYSTEM

For many years, the anterior hypothalamic regions have been associated with parasympathetic activities in the autonomic nervous system and the posterior regions associated with sympathetic activities. This generalization comes from observations by many investigators of the effects produced by the stimulation of hypothalamic sites. Like many generalizations, however, it is inaccurate in several ways. The simple dichotomous breakdown into anterior and posterior regions is misleading, since these regions are well organized into different nuclear groups. The parasympathetic and sympathetic zones are by no means as discretely localized as was thought earlier. Furthermore, autonomic responses elicited from the hypothalamus are often discrete reactions, such as urinary bladder contraction, rather than a part of a total bodily response of one division of the autonomic nervous system.

The hypothalamic modulation of autonomic activities may be mediated by the synaptic intervention of brain stem areas, such as the midbrain reticular formation but some direct pathways from the hypothalamus (dorsomedial nuclei, paraventricular nuclei) to preganglion nuclei of the sympathetic and parasympathetic branches of the autonomic nervous system have been demonstrated (Saper, Loewy, Swanson, & Cowan, 1976). Hess (1949) pointed out that stimulation of the hypothalamus always elicits both autonomic and somatic changes. Therefore, he proposed the terms *trophotropic* and *ergotropic* to describe the effects of stimulation of the anterior and posterior hypothalamus, respectively. *Trophotropic* effects would include parasympathetic activities and in addition the correlated activities of the somatic musculature associated with the conservation of bodily energies and with activities of the internal organs related to digestion and elimination. The term *ergotropic* is used to include reactions of both smooth and striate muscles directed toward the mobilization and expenditure of the body's resources.

The terms *trophotropic* and *ergotropic* emphasize that the effects produced by hypothalamic stimulation extend beyond the autonomic nervous system and even beyond the somatic nervous system. Trophotropic reactions include changes in the electrical activity found in the neocortex that indicate decreased arousal. Ergotropic reactions include the desynchronization of the electrical activity of the cortex. Speculations about the role of the ergotropic and trophotropic systems in behavior have been advanced before by Gellhorn (e.g., 1970).

The ergotropic reactions mediated by the hypothalamus may play an important role in activating and maintaining behavioral sequences. Such a role would be comparable to the "motivational effects" produced by hypothalamic stimulation described above. I have suggested that an ergotropic balance activity may be essential to the initiation and the continuation of behavioral episodes and that the hippocampus provides one means of adjusting this balance (Isaacson, 1972b). (See also pp. 175–176.)

The ergotropic and trophotropic systems are thought to cooperate to maintain a balance between them appropriate to the environmental circumstances. Normally, the greater the activity in one, the less activity there will be in the other, since the two stand in a mutually inhibitory relationship. However, this balance can be upset so that great amounts of activity can occur in both systems at the same time. This simultaneous activation of the two systems is found during convulsions.

While the terms *ergotropic* and *trophotropic* suggest unitary anatomical or functional systems, this need not be the case. Each "system" is probably a collection of specific neural subsystems that share the potential of increasing or decreasing the components of behavioral arousal. Each of these subsystems could act to provide degrees of somatic and autonomic activation appropriate to its own actions.

THE SUPRACHIASMATIC NUCLEUS

On the basis of the observations that lesions of the suprachiasmatic nuclei abolish the usual rhythms of locomotor activity, eating, drinking, adrenal corticosterone activity, and pineal N-acetyltransferase activity in rats (e.g., Stephan & Zucker, 1972; Moore & Eichler, 1972; for a review, see Rusak & Zucker, 1979), these regions have been considered a central pacemaker or biological clock for the animal (Pittendrigh, 1974).

Lesions of the suprachiasmatic nuclei not only abolish behaviors entrained to synchronizing environmental stimuli (*Zeitgebers,* usually but not necessarily light–dark periods), they also abolish the free-running circadian rhythms of physiological and behavioral activities (Zucker, Rusak, & King, 1976). Damage to this area also disturbs sleep rhythms (Coindet, Chouvet, & Mouret, 1975). In addition, the lesions eliminate the normally increased heart rate found in periods of darkness during the day–night cycles (Saleh & Winget, 1977) and induce a condition of permanent estrus without ovulation in female rats (e.g., Brown-Grant & Raisman, 1977). The effects of the lesions cannot be explained simply on the basis of an overall depression of behavior or function, since the effect of the lesions is to redistribute behaviors over time but not to reduce the total amount of activity. Furthermore, while other lesions, such as those of the lateral hypothalamus, can influence circadian behaviors, none produces as profound an effect as those following suprachiasmatic lesions.

Even though free-running circadian rhythms are abolished by suprachiasmatic lesions, some rhythms persist if they are entrained to rhythmic occurrences of environmental events. For example, restricted feeding schedules induced a 12-hour phase shift in body temperature and corticosteroids that remained after lesions of the suprachiasmatic nucleus (Krieger, Hauser, & Krey, 1977). Stephan, Swann, and Sisk (1978) extended these observations by showing that activity increased before food was made available and that this activity rhythm could survive, at least for a short time, after the animals were taken off the food deprivation schedule. However, these entrainment-to-deprivation effects were not found when the animals were water-deprived (R. Y. Moore, 1980). This finding may reflect differences in the effects of food and water deprivation, but the effects could also be due to the shorter period of time that Moore's animals were subjected to the deprivation schedule. In general, several types of behaviors or physiological reactions can be entrained to environmental cues other than the light–dark cycle. Restricted food and/or water availability are powerful cues for entrainment. Some exceptions are found. The pineal gland enzyme, serotonin-N-acetyltransferase, does not appear to be entrainable to environmental conditions after suprachiasmatic lesions.

The behavioral changes that occur after syprachiasmatic lesions are not reproduced by the blinding of the animals. While visual input to these nuclei is essential for the entrainment of behaviors to visually mediated environmental cues, the nuclei themselves are essential for the generation of rhythmic events—at least those of a circadian nature and possibly others as well. The mechanisms by which the suprachiasmatic nuclei influence cyclic behaviors are unknown as yet. The most likely hypothesis is that their caudally directed fibers related to the periventricular and median eminence regions are important because of the association of these regions to neuroendocrine function. A related question pertains to the nature of endogenous oscillators in neural tissue. This question, however, is so complex at both the neurological and the theoretical levels that resolutions will not soon be found.

LESIONS OF THE LATERAL HYPOTHALAMUS

Lesions of the lateral hypothalamus produce aphagia and adipsia (Teitelbaum & Epstein, 1962). Animals with such lesions will die unless they are tube-fed after the operation. If this is done, however, the animals can, over time, begin to eat food and ultimately to drink water. Usually, the animals begin to eat food spontaneously before they begin to drink water spontaneously. Teitelbaum and Epstein described four stages in the recovery of animals with lesions of the lateral hypothalamus. These recovery stages can be described as follows: In Stage 1, the animals will eat some wet and palatable food. In Stage 2, the animals will spontaneously regulate their food intake and body weight on the wet and palatable foods. (In Stage 1, the animals will not eat enough to provide themselves with the necessary metabolic requirements.) In Stage 3, the animals will eat dry food, provided that they have an appropriate water balance. The animals have to be hydrated artificially by stomach tubes in order to eat dry foods and maintain themselves in a reasonable nutritional state. In Stage 4, the animals will drink water spontaneously and will survive on a dry food diet. Teitelbaum, Cheng, and Rozin (1969) have suggested that the recovery process that occurs after lateral hypothalamic lesions represents a behavioral recapitulation of the mechanisms responsible for the development of regulated food intake after birth.

Recovery is never really complete. For example, even in Stage 4, the animals drink water only after eating. The animals seem to be wetting their mouths in order to eat the dry food. In addition, these animals are always finicky about their food. They reject food that has been adulterated with an unpleasant substance more readily than normal animals do. Animals that have recovered from the lateral hypothalamic damage do not reach the same body weights as normal animals despite normal levels of food intake.

It should be noted that lesions of the lateral hypothalamus produce a variety of changes in the animals, many of which may be directly or indirectly related to aphagia and adipsia. These include disruption of saliva secretion (Epstein, 1971) and changes in thyroid activity (Szentagothai, Flerko, Mess, & Halaz, 1968), oxygen consumption (Stevenson & Montemurro, 1963), and body temperature (Harrell, de Castro, & Balagura, 1975). Gastric lesions have also been found. The extent of the gastric pathology is correlated with the length of time of aphagia found after the hypothalamic damage. Furthermore, the food restriction regimes provided the animals before the brain lesions determine the degree of gastric anomalies and the length of aphagia (Grijalva, Lindholm, & Schallert, 1976). Gradual reductions in food intake produce fewer gastric disturbances and a shorter period of aphagia. The beneficial effect of prelesion starvation occurs only under a gradual restriction of diet and may be mediated by reduced gastric effects. Some of these effects may be mediated through the vagus nerve, but transection of the vagus does not mimic lateral hypothalamic weight loss (Opshal & Powley, 1977).

Powley and Keesey (1970) have pointed out that the aphagic and adipsic condition following lateral hypothalamic lesions can be greatly reduced if the subjects are food-deprived before the lesions are made. In some cases, prelesion weight reduction can even prevent the usual aphagia and adipsia. Some animals actually overeat after the lesion. Powley and Keesey suggested that the effect of the lateral hypothalamic lesion is to reset bodily mechanisms for a new ideal "target weight" (probably reflected in the amount of fat in the adipose tissues), which is less than that of normal animals. The effect of a ventromedial hypothalamic lesion could be to establish a new target weight that is higher than that of normal animals. Therefore, the aphagia or hyperphagia that follows hypothalamic destruction could be explained as attempts of the animals to reach their new target weights. Animals made overweight before ventromedial lesions show only slight overeating afterward (Hoebel & Teitelbaum, 1966).

When animals are fed intragastrically after the lateral hypothalamic lesions are made, they are usually maintained at something approximating their preoperative weight levels. According to the Powley and Keesey position, keeping the body weights elevated by artificial means just postpones the inevitable. It is worth noting that the theorized "recovery" does not occur after the hypothalamic lesions. After the lesions, the animals merely start to eat, or do not eat, to attain their "ideal" weights. Furthermore, if lesions of the lateral hypothalamus result in the setting of a lower target weight and lesions of the ventromedial hypothalamus result in the setting of a higher target weight, then it might be possible for lesions in each to offset each other, at least to some extent.

The feeding systems of the brain have been associated with neural systems that use adrenergic transmitters (see Grossman, 1960; Slangen & Miller, 1969; Leibowitz, 1970). It is perhaps not very surprising, therefore, that the injection of norepinephrine into the ventricles can restore the drinking of milk in aphagic and adipsic animals with lateral hypothalamic damage (Berger, Wise, & Stein, 1971). The place in which direct adrenergic stimulation is most effective in inducing eating in the hypothalamus seems to be the paraventricular nucleus (Leibowitz, 1978). It is possible that feeding elicited from other sites by adrenergic agonists, such as the perifornical region and the dorsomedial and ventromedial nuclei, arises from spread of the drug to the paraventricular region. The effects of the intraventricular injection of norepinephrine are also probably mediated by this region.

New interpretations of the effects of lateral hypothalamic damage have been offered by Stricker (1976) and by Wolgin, Cytawa, and Teitelbaum (1976). Stricker reported that the usual deficits in water intake found in thirsty animals "recovered" from lateral hypothalamic damage were not found if the period of water availability was lengthened. Stricker argued that the problem for the lesioned animals was an inability to respond to the challenge or stress of the thirst induction procedures. He also noted that the most effective lateral hypothalamic lesions were not confined to that region but extended into far lateral areas, areas containing the ascending dopamine fibers from the substantia nigra (see Ungerstedt, 1971). Indeed, many of the symptoms of the lateral hypothalamic syndrome can be produced by a selective destruction of nigrostriatal fibers. Even unilateral nigrostriatal lesions produce major changes in food and water intake (Baez, Ahlskog, & Randall, 1977). It is possible that recovery from lateral hypothalamic damage involves increased efficiency in the use of the remaining fibers in this system (e.g., Zigmond & Stricker, 1973). Stricker, Cooper, Marshall, and Zigmond (1979) have found that reducing dopaminergic activities by administration of the dopaminergic blocking agent spiroperidol or by synthesis reduction by α-methyltyrosine reverses recovery. However, lesions of the zona compacta of the substantia nigra do not alter ingestive behaviors (Hodge & Butcher, 1980).

Ellison (1968) has devised a technique that produces a lesion

circumscribing the hypothalamus. The technique isolates the hypothalamus and prevents its communicating with the rest of the brain.
The technique has been used in both cats and rats (Ellison & Flynn,
1968; Ellison, Sorenson, & Jacobs, 1970). If the lesion extends to include the far lateral reaches of the hypothalamus, the animals become
permanently aphagic and starve to death. Recovery does not occur
even when the animals have been maintained by forced feeding for
over 100 days. Oddly enough, the animals are not finicky about their
food. They swallow food if it is placed in their mouths. Thus, they
do not actively reject food as do animals with the lateral hypothalamic
syndrome. The animals seem to have lost the appetitive drive to seek
food, but they do not find the taste of food aversive. The aversion to
the taste of food may arise from a hyperactivity of the medial hypothalamic systems still available to animals with lateral hypothalamic
lesions.

If the lesions do not extend quite so far laterally, the animals will
accept, but not seek, food almost immediately after the lesion. Nib-
bling of food returns in a few days and spontaneous eating in a little
over a week. Eating sufficient to maintain weight returns in about
two weeks. This smaller lesion leaves some parts of the lateral hypothalamus intact and in communication with the rest of the brain.
This smaller circumscription of the hypothalamus apparently removes
the aversive components of the syndrome from being exhibited, presumably because of the isolation of the medial hypothalamus. This
isolation, in combination with some intact lateral tissue, allows the
animal to enter into "recovery" Stage 4 soon after the lesion.

Wolgin et al. (1976) and Wolgin and Teitelbaum (1978) proposed
that two factors contribute to the lateral hypothalamic syndrome:
multimodal sensory neglect and a decrease in normal activation. Both
characteristics, of course, may be related to the nigrostriatal tract
destruction thought by Stricker to be essential to the loss in abilities
to withstand stressful challenge. The sensory neglect characteristic is
considered separately in a subsequent section. The loss of behavioral
activation should be discussed in some detail.

Immediately after lateral hypothalamic lesions, the animals seem
to be asleep or in a stupor. Only very strong stimulation, like a tail
pinch, arouses them. After time passes, the animals become less
sleepy but tend to remain in one position without moving for pro-

longed periods (akinesia). At this time, they also show cataleptic behaviors. They can be aroused by intense stimulation, such as being placed in a tub of cold water, where they swim and try to escape. When placed in warm water, they just sink to the bottom. Rats with posterior hypothalamic lesions have the same loss of activation and, when placed in a warm water tank, sink to the bottom, where they engage in grooming behaviors (Robinson & Whishaw, 1974). In Stage 2 of recovery, the animals eat when aroused but remain aphagic if not aroused. Pharmacological activation with amphetamine can induce eating and spontaneous movements, as can noxious stimulation.

The question of the relative importance of damage to fiber tracts or to cellular groups of the hypothalamus in regard to the lateral hypothalamic syndrome is not entirely solved. However, it is clear that any substantial interference with the afferent or efferent connections of the caudate results in aphagia and adipsia along with other sensory and motor disabilities (Grossman & Grossman, 1971; Alheid, McDermott, Kelly, Halaris, & Grossman, 1977; Walsh, Halaris, Grossman, & Grossman, 1977). In general, it appears from studies of fiber tract sections that the constellation of behavioral changes occurring after lateral hypothalamic damage may involve a number of independent behaviors, pathways, and transmitter systems (McDermott, Alheid, Kelly, Halaris, & Grossman, 1977). Indeed, there may be several types of syndromes produced in diverse ways to produce the common results of aphagia and adipsia (e.g., Zeigler, 1976). However, certain of the sensory and motor components of the usual lateral hypothalamic syndrome, as well as overall changes in activation, are almost certainly associated with decreased dopaminergic activity in the nigrostriatal system.

Escape and Avoidance Behaviors

M. E. Olds and Frey (1971) reported that lesions in either the medial or the lateral areas eliminate escape responses elicited by electrical stimulation of the aversive systems of the midbrain. These results are somewhat surprising if one considers the lateral hypothalamus a part of a positive reinforcing system that normally acts in opposition to a pain or punishment system. A disruption of the positive reward system might be expected to produce exaggerated escape behaviors, and, in fact, there have been reports of increased reactions to painful stimuli after lateral hypothalamic lesions, as is mentioned below.

A lesion-produced disruption of the aversive system of the medial hypothalamus could reduce the effectiveness of pain in regulating behavior, but how can the effects of lateral hypothalamic lesions be explained? If the medial-forebrain-bundle–lateral-hypothalamus system is considered a region that mediates the activation of dominant behavioral sequences then the results make sense. The lesions would have eliminated or diminished the neural mechanisms that are responsible for the initiation and maintenance of the behavior. Indeed, Olds and Frey (1971) suggested this possibility: "The basis for the deficits produced by lateral hypothalamic lesions lies in the damage inflicted in the positively reinforcing system or in the excitatory forces initiating and maintaining behaviors" (p. 17).

Even unilateral lesions of the lateral hypothalamic area impair the retention of an active avoidance response (Asdourian, Dark, Chiodo, & Papich, 1977). The poor performance arises from an inability to execute the escape movements after shock or conditioned stimulus (CS) onset. Orientation toward the CS seems to be normal. Similar effects were found after 6-OH-dopamine lesions of the lateral hypothalamus, and the effect seemed to represent a failure to initiate the appropriate response (Smith, Levin, & Ervin, 1975).

Lesions in the medial forebrain bundle can produce an enhanced reflexive reaction to painful stimulation. This reaction has been shown to be a consequence of the lesion's producing a reduction in the serotonin content of the forebrain, presumably by the interruption of fibers originating from the raphe nuclei and ascending through this fiber bundle. Treatment of the animals with the immediate precursor of serotonin (DL-5-hydroxytryptophan) restores normal reactivity to pain (Yunger & Harvey, 1973). These results point out that it is difficult to ascribe the behavioral effects of hypothalamic lesions or stimulation directly to anatomical regions without taking the status of related fiber systems into account. Furthermore, the results of Yunger and Harvey make the first possible explanation offered by Olds and Frey most unlikely and leave the second as the viable alternative. In addition, this second proposal explains why stimulation of the lateral hypothalamus enhances escape responding rather than diminishing it (Olds & Olds, 1962). The hypothalamic stimulation is eliciting and energizing the dominant response of the situation. This energizing or activating effect could involve the nigrostriatal system, whose role in this aspect of behavior has been emphasized by Stricker and his associates.

Other behavioral changes found after lateral hypothalamic damage include reduced locomotion in open fields but not in the home cage (Young, Ervin, & Smith, 1976). An enhanced tendency to evidence immobility or initial testing in the open field was also found. Schedule-induced and schedule-dependent behaviors are also reduced (Wayner, Loullis, & Barone, 1977). Unilateral lesions produce an effect on T-maze choice behaviors if the animals are required to turn to the same side as the brain lesion (Dark, Chiodo, Papich, Yori, & Asdourian, 1977).

Sensory Neglect

Rats with unilateral damage to the lateral hypothalamus fail to orient their heads toward visual, tactile, and olfactory stimuli that impinge on the opposite side of the body. Stimuli arriving ipsilateral to the lesion elicit assentially normal reactions (Marshall, Turner, & Teitelbaum, 1971; Turner, 1973). Motoric abilities involving the limbs contralateral to the lesion are also affected. After bilateral damage, rats and cats show bilateral impairments in limb movements and orientation (Teitelbaum & Wolgin, 1975), but, of course, these animals are also aphagic, adipsic, and akinetic, as described above in connection with the lateral hypothalamic syndrome. The failure to orient toward or pay attention to stimuli arising from stimulation contralateral to the lesion has been termed *sensory neglect*. This term seems to have been first used to describe the striking neglect of contralateral stimulation by human patients with parietal, cingulate, or frontal lobe damage (see Heilman & Watson, 1976, 1977). This inattention can be as dramatic as patients' "not seeing" half of their dinner plates or believing that their own arm or leg belongs to another person (Heilman, personal communication, 1976). The patient can even try to throw the unrecognized arm or leg out of bed, complaining to the nurse that another patient had gotten into his or her bed.

Recovery from the sensory neglect that follows lateral hypothalamic damage proceeds in a rostral-caudal direction in animals. Sensitivity on the face and snout recover first, followed later by areas of the midsection and the flank. Sensory neglect has been found for many types of stimuli. Food was less frequently approached and eaten when presented on the side contralateral to the lesion than when presented on the ipsilateral side. The elicitation of mouse killing was nonexistent when the mouse was on the contralateral side, even in established mouse killers. The animals did not use information arriving from the side opposite that of the lesion to accept food or to initiate attack behaviors. Marshall *et al.* (1971) interpreted their results in terms of the ability of the rat to integrate the sensory information with effective behavior patterns of biological significance to the animal. Turner (1973) also found a transient contralateral neglect to arise from unilateral lesions of the amygdala and argued that there is presumptive evidence that these effects are mediated by amygdalohypothalamic fibers coursing through the ventrofugal fiber system.

Other subcortical lesions can produce neglectlike syndromes. These include the nigrostriatal fibers, the substantia nigra, the midbrain reticular formation, the globus pallidus, and the subthalamic area. Destruction of these regions also induces aphagia and adipsia. Destruction of the superior colliculus, on the other hand, produces a sensory neglect without these other behavioral changes (Marshall, 1978).

It now appears that the neglect that follows the destruction of the lateral hypothalamus is due to the disruption of fibers that run to or from basal ganglia regions and dopamine cell groups in the tegmentum and that pass through the far lateral hypothalamus and portions of the adjacent internal capsule. After destruction of cell bodies in the lateral hypothalamus with kainic acid, disturbances of eating and drinking were produced, but not neglect (Grossman, Dacey, Halaris, Collier, & Routtenberg, 1978). In addition, Feeney and Wier (1979), studying cats, found that lesions to the lateral hypothalamus that failed to include the far lateral–internal capsule areas produced only a mild and transient sensory neglect.

VENTROMEDIAL HYPOTHALAMIC LESIONS

The most prominent effect reported to follow lesions of the ventromedial nucleus of the hypothalamus is a permanent hyperphagia and obesity (e.g., Heatherington & Ranson, 1942). Similar results have been observed in cats, dogs, monkeys, and even birds (Anand & Dua, 1956; Rozkowska & Fonberg, 1971; Snapir, Yaakobi, Robinzon, Ravona, & Perek, 1976). Reports have been made of obesity (and other symptoms) in the human where there is suspected damage of medial hypothalamic regions (e.g., Killeffer & Stern, 1970; Reeves & Plum, 1969). While the general effects of ventromedial lesions were first described in terms of a reduction in the effectiveness of a satiety mechanism (Epstein, 1960; Teitelbaum & Campbell, 1958), there are a number of surprising behavioral and physiological changes found in animals following such lesions. Not all of them fit in with any simple explanation of the lesion effects. One such change is that while animals with such lesions overeat and gain weight, they are finicky about the taste of their food (Teitelbaum, 1955). They will turn away from food adulterated with quinine or other distasteful substance at levels that will not deter normal animals. For many reasons, the notion of the ventromedial nucleus as a satiety center must be rejected (e.g., Rabin, 1972).

There are two phases of the hyperphagia that follows ventromedial lesions. The first is a brief dynamic phase in which food intake doubles, followed by a prolonged static phase in which the greatly increased body weight is maintained by nearly normal food intake. The food intake occurring just after the lesions are produced is voracious and ravenous and may begin even before the anesthesia has completely worn off. This period of greatly increased eating is correlated with increased activity and emotionality, which also last two to three days. The exact plateau of weight gain found in the static phase depends on a variety of situational and experimental variables (see Powley, 1977, for a review of these variables). The animal in the static phase is obese almost entirely because of increased fat deposits, and there is a corresponding reduction in lean body weight (Bernardis & Skelton, 1966/1967). The increased disposition to fat increases relative to lean weight occurs even if normal amounts of food intake are allowed (Rabin, 1972).

The lesion-induced obesity seems to be a consequence of hyperinsulinemia coupled with increased gastric secretions, gluconeogenesis, serum triglycerides, and cholesterol. There is a reduced rate of oxygen consumption. Sectioning the vagus nerve, which eliminates the hyperinsulinemia, also eliminates the enhanced fat deposits after ventromedial nucleus lesions (Powley & Opsahl, 1974).

Powley (1977) has suggested that the ventromedial nucleus acts to modulate reflexes related to food incorporation that originate in the forebrain either through the activation of specialized receptors or through intrinsic activities of the brain. When the ventromedial area is damaged, these reflexes become exaggerated. The reflexes he proposed to be increased include salivation, insulin secretion from the pancreas, and a shift in internal metabolism toward fat storage. In essence, the attractive sights, smells, and tastes of that lead to food incorporation elicit overpreparation for food intake, and, indeed, this overreaction actually causes the animals to eat more in order to counterbalance the exaggerated secretions of the exocrine and endocrine glands. In essence, Powley proposed that the ventromedial-lesioned animal overeats because it oversecretes.

Furthermore, the finickiness of these animals is explained by a lesion-induced overresponsiveness to negative attributes. Bitter tastes, as well as other aversive stimuli, can induce ejection or rejection responses to food-related materials. Since these responses are enhanced by the hypothalamic damage, finickiness is increased beyond normal limits.

Although there have been reports that animals with ventromedial lesions will not "work" to obtain the additional food requirements (e.g., Miller, Bailey, & Stevenson, 1950; Teitelbaum, 1957), more recent evidence suggests that they do behave as if they were hungrier than nonlesioned control animals. Kent and Peters (1973) tested their subjects postoperatively on a variable-interval schedule of reinforcement in an operant task under various food-deprivation levels. The lesions did not enhance responding when the animals were tested at 80% of their preoperative weights. As food deprivation was lessened, however, the control animals reduced their response rates, while the rates of lesioned animals remained high. Under low to moderate food deprivation, the lesioned animals started to run a straight alley for food rewards more quickly than did control animals, and their rate of food ingestion in their home cages was higher under all conditions of deprivation. Kent and Peters suggested that other authors may have inadvertently confused the heightened emotionality of the animals, which was exaggerated by the training conditions, with a diminished interest in working to obtain food. Powley (1977) would explain these results on the basis of the degree to which the food ingestion reflexes had been conditioned to the cues of the situation and the degree to which food was associated with the responses. The greater the conditioning and the more food was associated with responding, the more the lesioned animal would show enhanced reflexive activation and, as a consequence, the more abnormal would be the behavior. As emphasized by Powley, the lesioned animal's behavior is strongly regulated by taste factors, so much so that if the taste of food is removed by intragastric feeding, the animals will fail to depress the lever in an operant task to feed themselves (McGinty, Epstein, & Teitelbaum, 1965).

Most of the studies that have shown the reluctance of animals with ventromedial lesions to respond effectively for food in situations in which they must "work for it" have used what are called *lean schedules* of reinforcement in operant chambers. Lean schedules mean that animals must make many responses to obtain a small amount of food. It now seems clear that some of the behavior impairment can be attributed both to the aversive quality of lean schedules and to the obesity of the lesioned animals. Two different types of manipulations tend to offset the usual poor performance on lean schedules. Pretaining on the lean schedule before surgery helps animals overcome the aversive nature of the schedule, as does the careful matching of body weights among lesioned and control animals (see King, 1980).

It is also the case that certain of the behavioral deficits found after ventromedial lesions are hard to account for on the basis of taste or other food-related changes. For example, ventromedial-lesioned rats show a deficit in thirst-motivated as well as hunger-motivated tasks when tested in operant situations on intermittent schedules of reinforcement (King & Gaston, 1976a). The animals are also impaired in active avoidance responding in lever-press tasks (King & Gaston, 1976b; King, Alheid, & Grossman, 1977).

However, lesions of the ventromedial nucleus produce a facilitation, not an impairment, in the acquisition of a conditioned avoidance response (Grossman, 1966, 1972). Lesions of the ventromedial nuclei of the hypothalamus have also been reported to produce an impairment in passive avoidance behaviors (Kaada, Rasmussen, & Kveim, 1962; McNew & Thompson, 1966; Sclafani & Grossman, 1971). Gold and Proulx (1972) found that these lesions also produced an impaired ability to avoid a saccharin solution that was associated with sickness produced by injections of apomorphine. Lesions that interrupt descending influences from the medial areas of the hypothalamus have also been shown to enhance components of the copulatory response in male rats, reducing the postejaculatory interval and allowing ejaculations to occur after only a few intromissions (Heimer & Larsson, 1964, 1966–1967).

The data mentioned above indicate that the ventromedial lesions may produce behavioral and physiological changes specific to food incorporation and metabolism and also ones affecting behavior in a more general fashion. In this regard, Rowland, Marshall, Antelman, and Edwards (1979) have reported that the hyperphagia that follows ventromedial lesions can be eliminated by destruction of the ascending dopaminergic pathways, although this procedure did not affect the hyperreactivity or the hyperemotionality also found after the lesions.

If hyperphagia is the most prominent behavioral characteristic found after destruction of the ventromedial nuclei, savageness and aggression must rank a close second. Both effects can occur together. Indeed, one of my own most striking memories is of huge, fat, and extremely hostile cats with ventromedial hypothalamic lesions, which I observed many years ago at the University of Iowa. When they observed laboratory visitors through the bars—thankfully, strong bars—of their cages, they appeared to have a singular interest in attack. They gave every sign of dedication to the goal of destroying the visitor. Their great size made the threat something not to be taken lightly. Reports of such fierce attack behavior after ventromedial hypothalamic lesions have been reported in rat, cat, and monkey (Eclancher & Karli, 1971). However, rage and attack are not always found after lesions of the ventromedial nucleus, and sometimes only a relatively minor increase of aggression is found. There is a possibility that hyperphagia and aggression are correlated consequences of lesions in the ventromedial nucleus, but different mechanisms may be involved.

A dissociation of the mechanisms responsible for active avoidance learning and intraspecies aggression was reported by Grossman and Grossman (1970). Transverse cuts through the anterior hypothalamus reduced aggressive acts but did not affect avoidance performance. Aggressive behaviors were not affected by the posterior sections that did influence avoidance behaviors despite the massive amount of fiber destruction involved. The measurement of changes in aggressive behaviors is undoubtedly a complex matter, and the evaluation of the anatomical systems involved will be no less difficult. In the cat, Chi and Flynn (1971) have described separate anatomical pathways descending into the midbrain related to quiet biting attacks and to the more full-scale aggressive reactions.

THE NEUROCHEMISTRY OF EATING

In studies where the limbic system has been stimulated chemically, adrenergic stimulation has elicited feeding responses and cholinergic stimulation has elicited drinking (Grossman, 1960, 1969; Fisher, 1969). One subsequent direction of research has been the attempt to refine the understanding of the regulation of feeding behaviors. Some investigators have postulated that there is an antagonism between the α- and β-adrenergic systems in the hypothalamus (Leibowitz, 1970, 1976). The α-adrenergic system is thought to be involved with the initiation of eating, while the β-adrenergic system is thought to be involved in the suppression of eating; this involvement with the termination of feeding leads to a possible association with the medial hypothalamic satiety mechanisms. Evidence for such a view comes from the fact that the intrahypothalamic injection of α-adrenergic agonists produces eating, while β-adrenergic agonists injected into the same area inhibit eating, even in food-deprived animals. The injection of an α-adrenergic antagonist blocks eating, while the injection of a β-antagonist seems to reduce "satiety." Leibowitz believes that α-adrenergic terminals inhibit medial satiety neurons, thus releasing feeding centers in the brain stem from the normal suppression after eating. The β-adrenergic terminals are thought to be inhibitory on lateral hypothalamic feeding neurons.

The paraventricular nucleus of the hypothalamus seems to be the most effective location for the stimulation of ingestive behaviors in the rat (Davis & Keesey, 1971; Leibowitz, 1978). Norepinephrine injected into this region induces the largest amount of feeding and also preprandial drinking. Other, less sensitive, sites may exist in perifornical, ventromedial, and dorsomedial hypothalamic regions. Food deprivation increases both the strength of the norepinephrine-induced response and the size of the area around the paraventricular nucleus from which feeding effects can be elicited. The paraventricular nucleus may be the focus of a feeding-oriented system that radiates from it, crossing traditional nuclear boundaries. The norepinephrine-related feeding system is apparently modulated by circulating adrenal steroids (Leibowitz, Chang, & Oppenheimer, 1976) and the norepinephrine feeding response is abolished by sectioning the vagus nerve (Leibowitz, unpublished observations, cited in Leibowitz, 1978). This procedure affects the pancreatic secretion of insulin as mentioned previously.

The suppression of food consumption seems to involve the lateral perifornical area in the rostral and middle hypothalamus. Both dopaminergic and β-adrenergic receptors seem to mediate this suppression (Leibowitz & Rossakis, 1978a,b). These systems seem to be involved in the neural mediation of amphetamine-induced anorexia.

A similar, but not identical, system is thought to hold for the lateral hypothalamic neurons. This area is thought to contain β-adrenergic-sensitive cells and to project their influences to cells in the brain stem by an unknown transmitter system. The adrenergic brainstem cells affected by the lateral hypothalamic neurons then send axons to the ventromedial hypothalamic area and release their α-adrenergic substances there. Thus, the effect of the ventromedial nucleus on the lateral hypothalamic cells is direct, while the effect of the lateral hypothalamus on the medial is indirect and includes a relay in the brain stem. Despite this difference in the two systems, lateral and medial, they are postulated to stand in a mutually inhibitory relation to each other.

Margules (1970a,b) has presented a different theory of feeding, which is also related to α-adrenergic and β-adrenergic activities. In his theory, the β-adrenergic system is thought to mediate the inhibition of eating on the basis of taste factors. The α-adrenergic system is also thought to be an inhibitory system. It inhibits eating on the basis of physiological satiety, and it regulates eating on the basis of caloric requirements rather than on the taste of the food. Heightened activity in either system can inhibit eating behavior.

Margules's experimental approach differed from that of Leibowitz in several ways—in particular, the nature of the materials used for measuring food intake and the times of testing. Rats were generally taken from their home cages during the night portion of the day–night cycle and tested for the incorporation of sweetened canned milk. In contrast, Leibowitz usually measured the daytime incorporation of standard laboratory rat chow. The importance of diurnal factors in the effect of brain stimulation was emphasized when it was found that norepinephrine injected in the same amounts at the same brain location inhibited milk intake at night but enhanced it during the day (Margules, Lewis, Dragovich, & Margules, 1972). As a consequence, it seems clear that norepinephrine systems must interact with the light–dark behavioral regulators or with circadian oscillator systems to produce different effects under different testing conditions. Interactions of drug effects with times of the day are not uncommon (see Reinberg & Hallberg, 1971). Results supporting the interaction of norepinephrine-related behavioral changes have also been reported by Stern and Zwick (1973). Norepinephrine-depleted animals overeat during the night but not during the day (Ahlskog & Hoebel, 1973; Ahlskog, Randall, & Hoebel, 1975). When the effects of serotonin depletion produced by administration of parachlorophenylalinine are examined, it appears that the effects are observed during daytime hours. Therefore, while the relation of adrenergic mechanisms related to food incorporation is far from explained, it is now clear that the influence of day–night cycles, and perhaps the amount of ambient light provided during testing, may be critical in determining the effects of neurochemical manipulations.

Specific catecholamine pathways that run to or through the hypothalamus have been involved with the regulation of food intake. These include the ventral noradrenergic bundle (Ahlskog, 1974; Ahlskog & Hoebel, 1973) and the nigrostriatal tract (Ungerstedt, 1971). It appears that interruption of the ventral noradrenergic bundle can induce increased feeding, but it differs from the hyperphagia found after ventromedial hypothalamic destruction (Ahlskog, 1976; Ahlskog, et al., 1975). There is also no doubt that damage to the nigrostriatal tract does induce drastically reduced food and water intake. After neurochemical lesions of this pathway, recovery occurs that follows the pattern of recovery after traditional lateral hypothalamic lesions. Both types of lesions seem to induce an inability to deal with severe stressors, as well as sensory neglect. The question remains whether there is any specific food-related dysfunction remaining after lateral hypothalamic or nigrostriatal tract lesions beyond the behavioral changes related to the alterations in the sensory or stress-reaction areas.

The pharmacology of food-intake modulation has been reviewed by Hoebel (1977), who concentrated primarily on the study of drugs derived from the basic catecholamine configuration. From the study of structure–activity relationships, it is possible to derive relationships between molecular alterations and behavior. These offer promise of new therapeutic interventions and also a new understanding of the receptor systems being affected.

Despite the current interest in the monoamine transmitter systems in the regulation of food intake, there are several other possible neurochemical modulators. For example, there are suggestions that the brain or certain portions of it may be sensitive to cholecystokinin. This gastrointestinal tract hormone could function as an inhibitor of feeding. Cholecystokinin-like peptides have been found localized in cortical neurons, and the brains of genetically obese mice contain much less of these peptides than the brains of nonobese littermates (Straus & Yalow, 1979). In all likelihood, other peripheral hormones or enzymes from stomach, gut, or liver will be found to have the capacity to alter neural activities related to food and water incorporation.

THE NEUROCHEMISTRY OF BEHAVIORAL SUPPRESSION

The application of some forms of norepinephrine to limbic structures can release behaviors that have been suppressed by punishment. Margules (1968) demonstrated this phenomenon with injections into the amygdala in rats. The damage caused by the introduction of the cannulae into the amygdala produced passive avoidance deficits, but these deficits were enhanced by the application of norepinephrine through the cannulae. Margules interpreted these results as meaning that the amygdala is under the inhibitory control of adrenergic fibers that originate in the brain stem and that pass through the medial forebrain bundle system. The function of the norepinephrine is to inhibit ongoing activities of the amygdala and thus indirectly to release behaviors being suppressed by the amygdala. L. Stein (1969) has suggested that all of the noradrenergic fibers going to limbic areas are inhibitory. According to his view, the unlearned tendencies to approach stimuli in the environment are suppressed by the limbic system. When the limbic system is inhibited through activation of the medial forebrain bundle, this inhibition is accomplished through the noradrenergic components of the system.

This theory, and others like it, regard the limbic system as being all of a piece—as exerting inhibitory or facilitatory influences on another system in a homogenous way. This is probably too broad a generalization. Furthermore, limbic system damage, at least in some regions, has the effect of potentiating the animals' reactivity to low doses of amphetamine. It is not clear that this reaction could be adequately explained only as a reduction of facilitation supplied to the periventricular system as proposed in Stein's model.

In the 1972 version of their theory, Stein, Wise, and Berger considered the possible significance of the fact that the ascending noradrenergic system has two major branches. The dorsal branch reaches the neocortex and the hippocampus. The ventral branch projects mainly to the hypothalamus and the ventral forebrain regions (Fuxe, Hökfelt, & Ungerstedt, 1970). Both of these adrenergic pathways are thought to be involved in the mediation of rewarding effects. The ventral pathway is thought to be concerned with the motor acts of the individual, activating and supporting them to completion. The dorsal pathway is thought to be associated with facilitating *thought* (italics mine). The reader cannot help but be struck with the realization of how openly respected neuroscientists, like Stein and his colleagues, talk about "thought," using it as an accepted psychological term in experimental and biological contexts. This is an excellent example of how far the biobehavioral sciences have turned away from a hidebound stimulus–response behaviorism and toward terms found in common language and in theories with a cognitive or humanistic basis.

Carlton (1969) has emphasized the role of the cholinergic system in the suppression of responses. One example of response suppression is the decline in the magnitude of responses over repeated trials referred to as *habituation*. Carlton argued that the cholinergic system is responsible for habituation. Habituation can be related to the difference between rewards and reinforcements. For example, if the effects of rewards are resistant to habituation while those of reinforcements are not, then reinforcements could be transmuted into rewards by decreasing the effective cholinergic supplies.

The role of response suppression in the learning of new responses is of major importance. For example, in the original learning of a problem, an anticholinergic drug should enhance acquisition. The response to be learned would be less likely to be suppressed by moment-to-moment changes of the animal relative to the environment. This effect should be most prominent at the beginning of training. But once a response has been acquired, there should be a disruption of performance, since animals given anticholinergic drugs should not be able to achieve as high a stable level of performance as animals not given the drug.

A muscarinic cholinergic blocking agent placed in ventromedial hypothalamic regions increases the number of responses made to activate a milk dispenser, an acquired food-related response, but it does not tend to increased milk intake (Margules & Stein, 1967). Margules and Stein thought that the blocking agent interrupted cholinergic systems normally related to response suppression.

Changes in the willingness to perform acquired responses leading to food incorporation, or even acquired responses in general, may be the basis of studies in which there is an apparent drug tolerance developing. For example, if animals are given repeated daily administration of amphetamine, the resulting anorexia appears to diminish over the testing days. The gradual lessening of the anorexic effects could be due to induced changes in cholinergic systems or catecholamine systems, *or* to the fact that the animals perform more food-approach and eating responses during the times that food is available. That this interpretation has merit is indicated by the observation that amphetamine given daily *after* eating rather than before does not produce amphetamine tolerance in later tests (Carlton & Wolgin, 1971). Therefore, it is important to understand the behavioral changes occurring during drug-related studies and to take into consideration manipulations that make responding more or less likely to occur. A case in point would be the contribution of obesity in animals with ventromedial area lesions. The obesity is required for the observation of changes in performance in active and passive shock-avoidance behaviors, whether running or lever-press responding is required. Lean animals with virtually identical hypothalamic damage do not show such changes. Furthermore, the effects cannot be attributed to a general loss of motor abilities due to the fatness (King *et al.*, 1977). Some factor associated with the fat deposits must interact with central nervous mechanisms to affect performance in a general fashion. The degree of alteration found after the lesion is dependent on the testing circumstances (King & Grossman, 1978).

THE MAMMILLARY BODIES, THE MAMMILLOTHALAMIC TRACT, AND THE CINGULATE CORTEX

The mammillary bodies are a special collection of nuclei at the posterior boundary of the hypothalamus. Most of the studies directed toward understanding their contribution to behavior have investigated the effects of sectioning one of the pathways arising from them, the mammillothalamic tract. Since this tract is the initial component of a system reaching the anterior thalamic nuclei and progressing, after synaptic "relay," to the cingulate cortex, these structures will be considered together. However, it should be noted that the behavioral studies that involve sections of the mammillothalamic tract disrupt only one pathway from the mammillary nuclei. The other major efferent pathway, the mammillotegmental tract, leading to the tegmentum, is usually unaffected by the lesion.

Lesions of the Mammillothalamic Tract

Caution must be observed in the interpretation of the effects of lesions made in the mammillary bodies because of the likelihood of interrupting other fiber systems passing through the area, including the ventral noradrenergic bundle and the medial forebrain bundle. Lesions of these systems can cause substantial depletion of monoamine supplies to large areas of the forebrain. In addition, the mammillary bodies are difficult to approach surgically without doing damage to other neural areas above them. The mammillothalamic tract is small and compact, and many other fiber systems lie close to it.

In his dissertation a the University of Illinois, Krieckhaus (1962, 1964) studied the effect of mammillothalamic tract (MTT) lesions in cats, extending observations made earlier by two of his mentors, Thomas and Fry. He found, as they had before, that either complete or partial destruction of the MTT (produced by ultrasound) adversely affected the retention of a two-way active-avoidance task. A much less striking deficit was found after MTT lesion in a one-way active-avoidance task. At that time, Krieckhaus interpreted his results in terms of an enhanced tendency of the lesioned animals to "freeze," that is, to crouch and become immobile under the stress of his testing situation.

Subsequently, Thomas, Frey, Slotnick, and Krieckhaus (1963) found that ultrasonic lesions of the MTT failed to affect the retention of a visual discrimination learned for a positive reward. They also trained lesioned animals in the two-way active-avoidance task. This was a study of the postoperative acquisition of the avoidance problem as opposed to previous studies in which the retention of the problem was examined. They found rather mixed results. Of the 11 animals studied, 7 acquired the problem within the number of trials usually required by intact animals, but 4 animals failed to learn the task at all. This study indicated that disruption in "memory," as a global concept, could not account for the behavioral changes produced by the MTT lesions, although the question of the effects of the lesions on the postoperative acquisition of the avoidance problem was not answered definitively. Ploog and MacLean (1963) found that lesioned squirrel monkeys performed normally in a two-way avoidance task even when a delay was imposed between the CS and the time at which a response had to be made.

In 1965, Krieckhaus found that the behavioral changes produced by MTT lesions in the rat mimicked those found previously in the cat. The lesions reduced the retention of the two-way active-avoidance task. He also found that the performance of the lesioned animals could be greatly improved by the administration of amphetamine before testing. It had been shown before that amphetamine improves the active avoidance performance of normal animals as well as of those with hypothalamic lesions (Cardo, 1960). The drug also enhances locomotor behavior and reduces "freezing." Therefore, Krieckhaus believed that the beneficial effect of the amphetamine was primarily to reduce the enhanced freezing response of the lesioned animals, which, in turn, produced a beneficial effect on the avoidance behavior.

Later, Krieckhaus and Chi (1966) began to question the explanation of the avoidance task deficits based on an enchancement of the freezing response. They reported data that showed that the retention deficit could be found in animals that did not have any exaggerated signs of fear or freezing. They also found that when the cats with MTT lesions were subjected to training conditions that should have increased fear, their performance actually improved. Later, Krieckhaus (1966) reported that conditioned emotional responses were not enhanced by the MTT lesions. He concluded that the increased occurrence of freezing found in previous studies had been a consequence rather than the cause of the retention deficits.

Krieckhaus and Lorenz (1968) found that cats were much differently affected by MTT lesions when trained in a lever-press task to avoid shock than when they were trained to press a lever to acquire milk. This finding suggested that the deficits were not due to an inability to perform the required response but were linked to the motivational systems required to avoid the punishing electrical shocks. Krieckhaus, Coons, Greenspon, Weiss, and Lorenz (1968) also found that the deficit produced by the MTT lesions was unrelated to the difficulty of the task. The retention deficits seemed to be related to the willingness of the animals to undertake the required response, since once the animal was induced to begin a behavioral sequence in a T-maze, it made the correct choice in a successive-brightness-discrimination problem. This reluctance to undertake a behavioral response was also found in a study by Krieckhaus and Randall (1968). These authors found that MTT animals were not impaired in learning a spatial discrimination for a water reward using a T-maze, either in terms of the number of trials required for learning or in terms of errors. The animals were, however, slower in leaving the start box at the beginning of a trial.

R. Thompson (1964) and Thompson, Langer, and Rich (1964) have reported that lesions of the MTT or the mammillary bodies *per se* resulted in an impairment of the ability to perform a spatial discrimination in a T-maze in order to avoid electrical foot shocks. The results of Krieckhaus and Randall, discussed above, point out that animals with the MTT lesions are not generally impaired in such tasks, since they can perform them when working to obtain water when thirsty. However, the behavior of animals with MTT lesions can be altered in tasks other than those based on avoidance of shock. Krieckhaus and Randall (1968) found data supporting earlier results obtained by Thompson, in that the MTT lesions improved performance on a reversal task even when the water reward was used.

Smith and Schmaltz (1965) found that small electrolytic or penicillin-induced lesions in the mammillary bodies produced marked impairment on DRL-20 operant tasks. Impairments were found with both types of lesions in mice that were different from those found after hippocampal ablation. No increase in response rates was found after the mammillary body lesions.

At the present time, it appears that lesions of the MTT lead to disturbances of certain types of behaviors learned on the basis of punishment and that the impairment cannot be described as a general loss of memory, since some tasks learned from positive rewards are unaltered by the lesions. The most significant observation is that animals with MTT lesions are slow or reluctant to begin new behavioral acts. This observation must be considered in the context of related changes in behavior caused by lesions of the limbic system that affect the animals' willingness to initiate or continue behavioral sequences.

The Cingulate Cortex: Avoidance Tasks

Most of the early observations made of animals with lesions of the cingulate cortex failed to find any behavioral consequences. Such disturbances as were found were described as "transient, apparently minimal, and difficult to appraise." (Pribram & Fulton, 1954, p. 39). The lesions made in Pribram and Fulton study were restricted to the anterior cingulate regions. Performance was measured in a delayed response task and in a visual discrimination problem, and no effects were found. A reduction in the duration of retreat and withdrawal behaviors was noted when the expected reward was omitted after a correct response, but a similar reduction in this emotional reaction was found after other types of prefrontal lobe lesions, too. Pribram and Weiskrantz (1957) found more rapid extinction of a two-way active-avoidance task after anterior cingulate lesions when the lesioned animals were tested after a one-week recovery interval. Reconditioning of the active avoidance task was also impaired. Shortly afterward, other types of behavioral deficits resulting from cingulate lesions came to be reported in the literature. For example, Brutkowski and Mempel (1961) found that dogs with anterior (but not posterior) cingulate lesions seemed unable to restrain their responding to a nonrewarded stimulus. The ability to respond correctly to the positive stimulus was retained. These authors interpreted their results in terms of a loss of the "inhibition" required by the animals to refrain from responding on negative trials (i.e., those trials on which a response did not lead to a reward).

Lubar (1964) reported that anterior cingulate lesions did not affect the learning of a one-way avoidance task and actually potentiated the learning of a passive avoidance response, at least as measured by how many trials were required to extinguish the avoidance response. Furthermore, these effects of cingulate destruction were antagonistic to the effects of septal area destruction, which diminished an animal's ability to form a passive avoidance response. Combined cingulate–septal area lesions produce an animal with essentially unchanged passive avoidance behavior. Lubar proposed a direct antagonism between the influences mediated by the cingulate cortex and the septal area.

If there is such an antagonism, it should be reflected in the learning of a two-way active-avoidance task. F. A. King (1958) was the first to report a facilitation in the acquisition of this task after septal lesions, and now there are reports of impairments in the task produced by cingulate destruction (Peretz, 1960; Thomas & Slotnick, 1962; McCleary, 1961). Lubar and Perachio (1965) found an impairment in two-way active-avoidance conditioning in cats after cingulate lesions. They noticed enhanced freezing responses in the animals with cingulate lesions and advanced the hypothesis of an enhanced fear response to account for their observations, as Krieckhaus had done to account for effects of damage to the MTT. However, once again, this hypothesis has not been confirmed in subsequent studies. Kimble and Gostnell (1968), for example, failed to find any evidence of an enhancement of fear after cingulate lesions, using two different behavioral measures, although a substantial impairment in active avoidance conditioning was found.

Lubar, Perachio, and Kavanagh (1966) suggested that the impairment found after cingulate cortex lesions was due to damage of the visual neocortical areas of the cat brain incidentally produced when these areas were undercut as the cingulate lesions were made. However, the actual observations made by Lubar et al. were that damage to the lateral or posterolateral gyri could produce deficits in two-way active-avoidance conditioning. A direct experimental test of their hypothesis was not undertaken in this study.

The explanation offered by Lubar et al. (1966) for the impairment of avoidance conditioning (i.e., damage to the visual cortex) may have merit for the cat but does not seem appropriate for studies in which the rat cingulate cortex is destroyed. In some studies using the rat, cortical control lesions were made that were more likely to interrupt the visual system than were the cingulate lesions. These control lesions were ineffective in altering two-way active-avoidance behavior (e.g., Kimble, 1968). In addition, Trafton, Fibley, and Johnson (1969) found that lesions of several different regions of the anterior cingulate areas, far removed from the visual system, were effective in impairing the active avoidance conditioning. Therefore, while the "visual cortex" of the cat may participate in the regulation of some of the behavioral mechanisms underlying avoidance behavior, the anterior cingulate regions make their own contributions.

The avoidance impairment produced by cingulate lesions is not absolute. For example, if animals are trained in an avoidance task under conditions of food deprivation, the usual deficit may be substantially reduced (Thomas & Slotnick, 1963). This effect could well be mediated by an alteration in the motivational or the arousal level of the organism, so that the heightened arousal produced by the lesions actually "offsets" the effect of the lesion.

Other Behavioral Contributions of the Cingulate Cortex

Lesions made in the cingulate cortex lead to the disruption of the orderly sequencing of behaviors. For example, Stamm (1955) has shown that the sequential organization of the behavioral acts used by rats to produce an appropriate nest and to retrieve their young pups was disturbed if the rat "mothers" had cingulate damage. Both anterior and posterior cingulate lesions were reported to disrupt the sequential behaviors of an ethologically significant nature. On the other hand, Wilsoncroft (1963) found that the greatest behavioral effect was produced by lesions of the anterior cingulate region.

The most extensive analysis of the effects of cingulate damage on maternal behaviors has been made by Slotnick (1967). In general, the lesioned animals appear to be confused. They go out to retrieve pups, to gather nesting materials, or to engage in other nest-building operations, but they fail to complete the behavioral sequence normally. The animals may drop a pup halfway back to the nest or bring the pup back to the nest and then remove it again. Recently, similar reduction in the duration of spontaneously occurring behaviors has been noted after hippocampal destruction (Reinstein, Hannigan, & Isaacson, in press). Perhaps the reduced duration of behavioral acts found by Slotnick is not restricted to maternal behaviors.

Barker and Thomas (1965, 1966) studied the acquisition of a single runway problem in which rewards were provided only on alternate trials. The animals with lesions in the anterior cingulate areas were greatly impaired in the mastery of the problem. Animals with pos-terior cingulate lesions were not. For animals with the anterior cin-gulate lesions, the degree of retrograde destruction in the antero-medial thalamic nuclei was correlated with the behavioral im-pairment. Subsequently, Barker (1967) found an impairment in the performance of the alternation of bar-press responses in an operant situation.

An appealing suggestion related to one aspect of the behavioral deficit produced by cingulate damage comes from a study by Glass, Ison, and Thomas (1969). They proposed that the lesioned animals are unable to anticipate the emotional consequences of their behaviors both for rewards and for punishments.

This interpretation is related to the forecasting of future, stressful events and could be related to the mobilization of the body's resources in preparation for them. Several years ago, I was associated with the beginnings of research aimed at testing this possibility more directly. Using a paradigm for evaluating the reduction of circulating eosino-phils as a measure of stress (Gollender, Law, & Isaacson, 1960), Gol-lender (1967) was able to show that cingulate destruction eliminated or reduced the conditioned stress response but did not change the unconditioned response. Pursuing this general idea in a different way, Liebeskind (1962) found that animals with neocortical damage could become adapted to the stress of being tumbled in a Noble-Collip drum. Destruction of the cingulate areas, however, impaired the abil-ity of the animals to profit from prior stress experiences.

In humans, surgical disruption of the cingulate system has been attempted for the relief of pain (Foltz & White, 1962). Apparently, this procedure is of value to some patients, but it is not uniformly successful. In tests of cognitive function after cingulectomy, the great-est changes observed were in nonverbal tasks that required temporal ordering or sequencing (Faillace, Allen, McQueen, & Northrup, 1971). This result would be expected on the basis of the results obtained from animals. Earlier reports that destruction of the cingulum bundle was without effects on cognition were based on verbal testing pro-cedures alone, and it may be that the destruction of the cingulum influences only certain nonverbal processes. Supporting this lack of effect of cingulum destruction on verbal behavior is the report of Fedio and Ommaya (1970) that bilateral lesions of the bundle did not affect tests of intelligence or memory even though electrical stimulation of the left (but not the right) cinguium did so before the coagulation that produced the ultimate destruction. These authors suggested that the stimulation-produced memory effects are a result of indirect stimulation of structures at a distance from the site of stimulation via interconnecting fiber systems.

Earlier, Foltz and White (1957) and Foltz (1959) in monkeys and Foltz and White (1962) in humans reported that lesions of the cingulum bundle decreased withdrawal reactions to morphine. In a study with rats, Trafton and Marques (1971) found that rats with anterior cingulate lesions failed to show behaviors that were indications of addictive behavior. The behavior of the lesioned animals was less opiate-oriented than that of rats with control lesions (some of which included the septal area) both during the period when the addiction was being formed and after total drug withdrawal. However, not all subsequent reports have shown beneficial effects of cingulum lesions on drug dependence. For example, Wikler, Norrell, and Miller (1972) found that cingulum lesions did not alter the signs of specific morphine withdrawal in the rat. These signs include "wet-dog" shaking and a decrease in temperature measured in the colon. Therefore, the effects obtained in these several studies could reflect the attenuation of the anticipation of future pleasures or punishments while leaving unaltered the fundamental physiological alterations induced by the morphine.

Lesions of the mammillothalamic tract seem to be related to the initiation of behaviors, and once the animal starts performing a task, it can learn, remember, and perform it. The deficit in initiating behaviors seems to be specific to the motives used to induce the behavior. An impaired ability to utilize spatial aspects of the environment may also be found in animals with damage to the tracts. Neither type of deficit should be regarded as uniquely associated with the mammillothalamic tract, since similar effects can be found after damage to other parts of the limbic system.

The effects of lesions of the cingulate cortex depend on the subregions affected. Anterior cingulate lesions are more related to impairments in withholding or suppressing responses than are those of the posterior region. As noted in the preceding chapter, the anterior and posterior subregions of the cingulate cortex receive different projections from the anterior nuclear group of the thalamus. An interaction with treatments that affect the arousal of the animals is also implied on the basis of the behavioral changes induced in the lesioned animals by amphetamine administration and by changes in the motivational circumstances under which the animals are tested.

Studies of the effects of cingulate lesions in the rat have involved the production of midline cortical damage. Unfortunately, as reported in the previous chapter, the midline cortex of the rat is not comparable to the midline cortex of other animals as defined on the basis of the fibers it receives from the thalamus. In addition, lesions of the midline cortex, whether in the rat or in other species, are likely to interfere with fibers of the neural systems in or near it. These include the cingulum bundle and the supracallosal fibers of the fornix. Norepinephrine-containing fibers also pass through this region in or near the cingulum bundle. These fibers ascend through the anterior dorsolateral septal area and turn up and back to pass through the midline regions and innervate the entire medial cortex (Morrison, Molliver, & Grzanna, 1979). Lesions in this area reduce the norepinephrine distribution throughout the rostrocaudal extent of the medial cortex. A similar problem results from destruction to the anterior cortical regions. Lesions in that region could reduce the norepinephrine supplies of the entire dorsolateral cortex. Therefore, it becomes difficult to evaluate separately the effects of destruction of the cingulate cortex, the cingulum bundle, or the superior fornix, either behaviorally or anatomically.

REFLECTIONS AND SUMMARY

Even with the massive intervention in ongoing hypothalamic activities produced by the electrical stimulation of this structure, the effects obtained depend on the genetics, the history, and the environment of the animal. Repeatedly, it has been found that the effects of stimulation or lesions are conditioned by such factors regardless of the type of events measured, for example, in Mendelson's (1972) demonstration that the preferred duration of rewarding brain stimulation is affected by the objects in the animal's environment. This sort of behavioral modulation should not be considered a unique event. Similar factors have been found to influence the effects of stimulation or lesions of both cortical and subcortical regions, and similar observations are reported for other regions of the limbic system in subsequent chapters.

The results presented in this chapter indicate that the hypothalamus is indeed a "head ganglion" of those systems that are directed toward maintaining a favorable internal environment both through the regulation of the internal organs and through the behavior of the entire organism. But the hypothalamus does not act as if it were a motor command center. Rather, it acts to bias and modulate other systems. In turn, activities and conditions in the periphery influence the activity of the hypothalamus.

Therefore, the appropriate view of the hypothalamus is that it is a relatively small brain region that interacts with almost all other brain regions, with the goal of maintaining suitable conditions for mental actions and for behavior. These conditions and behaviors are suitable or not depending on the status of the individual as reflected by internal conditions. A possible way for the modulation to occur is through the modification of reflex circuits by the hypothalamus.

As will be found in regard to other limbic regions, the hypothalamus tends to exert its influences on other brain areas by altering the tendency to begin behavioral acts. In a sense it influences the willingness of the animal to stop ongoing behaviors and to undertake different ones. Once again, this is a characteristic shared by other limbic regions.

3

The Amygdala

As with other regions of the limbic system, the amygdala has close ties with the hypothalamus, although it differs from other limbic structures in also having a close relationship to the basal ganglia. Thus, the amygdala has a special place among the subcortical nuclear masses in being intimately involved in both limbic and striatal activities. However, a clear division among nuclear groups in terms of being more "limbic" or more "basal ganglionic" is not possible. Rather, many nuclear groups seem to have their own special characteristics, and functional divisions appear to cross lines among nuclei. However, there are certain general changes in behavior that seem to follow the destruction of large portions of the amygdala.

GENERAL AND SPECIFIC EFFECTS PRODUCED BY AMYGDALA STIMULATION OR LESIONS

In the context of this chapter, and certain subsequent ones, I will distinguish the *general* from the *specific* effects produced by lesions or by stimulation. By these terms, I do not mean to imply more than that some of these effects, the "general" effects, can be observed in a wider range of situations than others, the "specific" effects. For example, stimulation of the amygdala might produce heart rate changes in many situations. If it did, then it would be considered a general effect. But if the heart rate effect were found only in a particular type of situation—say, when the animal was tightly restrained—it would be considered a specialized change. It will be admitted that all behavioral effects produced by lesions or by stimulation are probably neither general to all situations nor entirely specific to one situation, but it is helpful to organize the available literature on this basis.

Autonomic Effects

Electrical stimulation of the amygdala does produce effects on autonomic activity, including heart rate and respiration. Both bradycardia and tachycardia have been produced by stimulation of the amygdala (e.g., Koikegami *et al.*, 1957). The slowing of the heart rate produced by amygdala stimulation can be abolished by atropine or vagotomy, whereas the tachycardia effects are not influenced by section of the vagal nerves. The increase in heart rate response is presumed to be of sympathetic origin, whereas the bradycardial reaction is thought to be secondary to the interruption of normal reflex functions induced by the stimulation (Reis & McHugh, 1968). The location of the electrodes in the amygdala is important in determining the direction of the heart rate changes, as is the anesthetic used in the experiment (Mogenson & Calaresu, 1973). Presence of afterdischarges induced by the stimulation can influence the intensity of the reaction, but not the type of effect that occurs. For example, if the electrode is in a region of the amygdala that produces a bradycardial response, this response will be greatest if an afterdischarge is elicited. Changing the frequency of stimulation or reducing its intensity so as not to produce afterdischarges will change only the magnitude of the heart rate slowing (Reis & Oliphant, 1964). In paralyzed animals, Bonvallet and Bobo (1972) found that decreases in respiration were obtained from stimulation of the lateral parts of the central nucleus, the lateral nucleus, and the small cell division of the basal nucleus. A decrease in heart rate often accompanied a corresponding respiratory change. Respiratory increases, frequently associated with cardiac acceleration, could be produced by stimulation of the amygdala; however, there seemed to be no clear pattern of localization of these effects. Stimulation of the magnocellular portions of the amygdala produced an initial decrease in respiration followed by a "rebound" increase. The heart rate changes were closely associated with the changes in respiration.

Changes in the galvanic skin response (GSR) have also been found to result from stimulation of the amygdala and the subsequent afterdischarges (Lang, Tourinen, & Valleala, 1964). The "middle regions" of the amygdala have been found to be the most effective in producing the GSR effects. These observations on the galvanic skin response were substantiated by observations in which the GSR was decreased or abolished by lesions of the amygdala (Bagshaw, Kimble, & Pribram, 1965). Lesions of the amygdala tend to eliminate the autonomic, but not the somatic, components of the orienting reflex in monkeys. In addition to a reduction of the GSR, heart rate and respiratory reactions were not found even though the lesioned animals could still exhibit orienting reflexes. Somatic reactions and activation of the cortical EEG associated with the orienting reaction remained after the lesions (Bagshaw & Benzies, 1968). The association of the amygdala with the orienting response, or portions of it, is related to the observations that stimulation of the amygdala can produce orienting reactions (Ursin, Wester, & Ursin, 1967; Ursin, Sundberg, & Menaker, 1969).

The amygdala may be involved in the modulation of temperature experience. Chin, Pribram, Drake, and Greene (1976) found that stimulation of either the orbitofrontal cortex or the amygdala interfered with temperature discriminations in monkeys. The amygdala effects were subject to habituation and were associated with enhanced response latencies. These authors view the amygdala as influencing the intensity dimension of many of the sensory modalities.

Damage to the amygdala does not seem to interfere with normal food and water intake (Kemble & Nagel, 1973). Such effects found after amygdala lesions can probably be explained on the basis of incidental damage to the internal capsule, the globus pallidus, or the entopeduncular nucleus (Dacey & Grossman, 1977).

Orienting, Habituation, and Exploration

The orienting reflex or reaction is, of course, of great significance to all animals. The complete orienting reaction includes the suppression of ongoing behaviors, the orienting of the body and receptor toward the new stimulus, changes in the peripheral autonomic nervous system, and, perhaps less obviously, preparations for associating the new stimulus with memories from the past and expectancies of the future.

In a study using a camera to record eye fixations on visual targets, Bagshaw, Mackworth, and Pribram (1972) were able to demonstrate that when responses to particular visual stimuli were not rewarded, monkeys with destruction of the amygdala made fewer observing responses than normal monkeys. Visual orientation toward unfamiliar stimuli was greatly reduced by amygdala damage. These results suggest that the lesions produce animals that pay less attention to their visual environment and that react less to changes in the visual world around them. On the other hand, when the animals with amygdala lesions are rewarded for attending to visual stimuli, as in visual discrimination problems, they can learn them as readily as normal animals (Schwartzbaum & Pribram, 1960), despite their apparent inattentiveness. Lesions of the inferotemporal cortex, on the other hand, produce animals that have great difficulty in learning visual discriminations but that exhibit more visual orienting responses than intact animals in nonrewarded conditions. The monkeys with inferotemporal lesions also react to novel conditions in a visual display in the same fashion as do normal subjects. It may be that amygdala lesions alter the animals' willingness to respond to novel events unless there is a substantial reward for doing so. This idea is supported by previous studies in which the behavior of the animals with amygdala lesions could be explained on the basis that the lesion altered the willingness of the animal to undertake new responses (Pribram, Douglas, & Pribram, 1969). In essence, the lesioned animals can orient toward new stimuli but are reluctant to do so.

Destruction of the amygdala alters the rate of habituation of locomotor activity, while not influencing its peak levels. Furthermore, the locomotor activity of animals with amygdala damage is not overly enhanced by external stimulation, as is sometimes found after damage to the frontal lobes. Monkeys with amygdala lesions do not exhibit the incessant pacing often found in animals with frontal lobe damage. The failure of locomotor activity to habituate is confined to tests made when the amygdala-lesioned animals are placed in unfamiliar circumstances. The animals are not overactive in their home cages (Schwartzbaum, Wilson, & Morrissette, 1961). Lesions of the amygdala in the rat do not seem to reduce open-field locomotion (e.g., Corman, Meyer, & Meyer, 1967). Indeed, there are a number of reports of hyperactivity following amygdala damage in several species, including rats (Corman *et al.*, 1967; Schwartzbaum & Gay, 1966), cats (Glendenning, 1972; Schreiner & Kling, 1953), and monkeys (Schwartzbaum *et al.*, 1961). Some authors have found hyperactivity only when lesions are made before adulthood (Eclancher & Karli, 1979; Thompson, Bergland, & Towfighi, 1977). There are reports of enhanced exploration of novel objects (White & Weingarten, 1976). This enhanced object exploration is not found after lesions of the stria terminalis or the piriform cortex (Coulombe & White, 1978). Indeed, both of these lesions reduce object exploration. White and Weingarten suggested that lesions of the amygdala disinhibit responses to salient environmental stimuli. They found that the response enhanced in the lesion animal was related to the motivational context in which testing occurred.

Turner, Mishkin, and Knapp (1980) found that each of the sensory association areas sends afferents to the amygdala selectively. The input from these association areas is dovetailed into portions of certain amygdalar nuclei. These authors suggested that sensory influences on the emotional systems are mediated by the amygdala in an autonomically specific fashion for each sensory modality.

Emotional Changes

Fonberg and Delgado (1961) studied the reactions of cats both to short periods of amygdala stimulation and to chronic stimulation of the structure lasting over 24 hr. They found that the brief periods of stimulation could interrupt certain kinds of behaviors. These included eating and the responses learned to obtain food. The interruption of behaviors produced by amygdala stimulation was specific to food-oriented behaviors. Related studies have found that lesions of the amygdala can produce voracious attacks on food in some animals, including humans (Pribram & Bagshaw, 1953; see Pribram, 1971). If the stimulation applied to the amygdala by Fonberg and Delgado did not produce afterdischarges or obvious motor effects, it would not disrupt playing behaviors or alert the animal if it was resting. Chronic stimulation of the basolateral nucleus that lasted for periods of 24 hr produced decreased activity and food intake. In general, the animals seemed to be relaxed and purred a great deal. They were not impaired on previously learned avoidance behaviors unless afterdischarges or obvious motor effects were produced by the electrical stimulation.[1] However, the animals adapted to this type of stimulation and came to eat, as well as to bar-press for food, over the course of the 24-hr period.

On the basis of studies of animals with lesions in different regions of the amygdala, Fonberg (1973) believes that there are two antagonistic divisions relative to eating and emotional reactions: (1) a dorsomedial region that, when lesioned, results in a loss of emotional tone and (2) a lateral division that, when lesioned, produces an enhancement of pleasure. The net effect of a lesion in the amygdalar complex is determined by the extent to which the balance of impulses over the two systems is affected. If a lesion were to affect the two amygdala areas equally, the balance of activities would be unaltered and no change observed. However, it is possible that lesions or stimulation of the dorsomedial regions might involve portions of the internal capsule, the entopeduncular nucleus, or the globus pallidus and produce symptoms characteristic of the interruption of systems passing through the region, including portions of the ascending dopaminergic systems. The result would be signs of emotional deficits and aphagia.

Emotional changes were also observed as a function of lesions in the two systems. After lesions of the dorsal-medial region, dogs ceased to be friendly and became fearful, sad, and sometimes aggressive. After a second lesion of the lateral area, the dogs became happy, played, showed affection, and enjoyed eating again. The balance between the two amygdala systems had been restored, according to the Fonberg interpretation.

In another type of study, stimulation of the amygdala was found to suppress aggressive activities in the animals, including aggression induced by hypothalamic stimulation (Egger & Flynn, 1962). However, regional differences within the amygdala again must be considered. Whether attack and aggressive behaviors are facilitated or inhibited by stimulation of the amygdala is related to the region in which the electrode is located.

Ursin and Kaada (1960) stimulated the amygdalar complex with chronically implanted electrodes. They found a dissociation of fear

---

[1] In contrast, prolonged stimulation of the cingulate cortex produced increased activity, signs of anxiety, and hyperirritability.

(flight) and aggressive behaviors. Flight and fear responses could be obtained from the rostral regions of the amygdala, including the lateral nucleus, the periamygdaloid area, and the central nucleus. Defense or aggressive reactions could be obtained from the medial and the caudal aspects of the amygdala. These regions in the cat, as mapped out by Ursin, are shown in Figure 15. As can be seen, the flight and defensive regions do not correspond to the established nuclear division of the amygdala. F. A. King (personal communication, 1981) was able to show that the attack behavior elicited by stimulation of the amygdala differed from that elicited by stimulation of the hypothalamus. The attack behavior elicited from the hypothalamus began immediately, with the onset of stimulation, and terminated as soon as the stimulation was ended. On the other hand, the amygdala stimulation produced a gradual buildup of aggressive behaviors. These behaviors gradually subsided after the stimulation was terminated. In addition, using subthreshold levels of current, King was able to find additive effects of stimulation at the two sites. Thus, subthreshold stimulation of the amygdala would summate with subthreshold stimulation of the hypothalamus to produce a suprathreshold aggressive response. King also found that septal stimulation applied before either hypothalamus or amygdala stimulation could prevent the occurrence of the aggressive behaviors.

Stimulation of the medial hypothalamus can produce directed attack behaviors, and the electrical threshold for such effects can be lowered by environmental manipulations, such as by disturbing and provoking the animal. Lesions of the amygdala can raise this provocation-induced lowered electrical threshold for aggressive acts (Maeda & Hirata, 1978). Thus, the aggressive behaviors influenced by stimulation or by destruction of limbic areas should be thought of not merely as automatic acts but as reflecting biases placed on reactions to naturally elicited behaviors. These results, and those of King, point to the interaction of diverse limbic areas in producing such effects.

Arousal and Social Reactivity

Destruction of the amygdala often produces a sluggish animal. Weiskrantz (1956) coined the term an "amygdala hangover" to describe this behavioral syndrome. For a period of time after the lesion, the lesioned monkeys of Weiskrantz were droopy and paid little at-

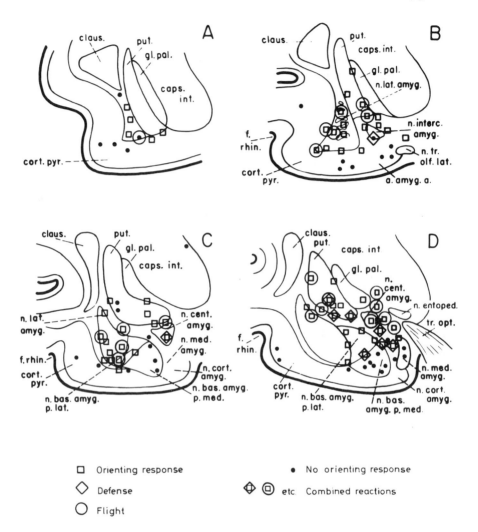

Figure 15. *Diagrammatic representations of the locations within the amygdala that, when electrically stimulated, produce orienting, defensive reactions, flight, or combinations of these responses. Abbreviations: claus., claustrum; put., putamen; gl. pal., globus pallidus; caps. int., internal capsule; cort. pyr., pyriform cortex; n. lat. amyg., lateral nucleus of amygdala; n. tr. olf. lat., nucleus of lateral olfactory tract; a. amyg. a., anterior amygdaloid area; f. rhin., rhinal fissure; n. cent. amyg., central nucleus of amygdala; n. med. amyg., medial nucleus of amygdala; n. cort. amyg., cortical nucleus of amygdala; n. bas. amyg. p. med., medial portion of basal nucleus of amygdala; n. bas. amyg. p. lat., lateral portion of basal nucleus of amygdala; n. lat. amyg., lateral nucleus of amygdala; n. cent. amyg., central nucleus of amygdala; n. entoped., entopeduncular nucleus; tr. opt., optic tract; n. caud., caudate nucleus (tail); fim., fimbria; hip., hippocampus; v. lat., lateral ventricle. Courtesy of Dr. Holger Ursin.*

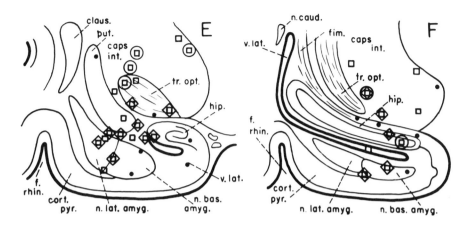

tention to what was going on around them. In the cat, Ursin (1965) found that this "hangover" results primarily from lesions made in areas of the amygdala from which flight reaction can be elicited by electrical stimulation, whereas in the dog, Fonberg (1973) found it to follow lesions in dorsomedial areas. For the most part, animals with lesions in the amygdala become very tame. This result has been shown in a wide variety of species (see Goddard, 1964b, for a listing of some 43 references on this topic). Amygdala lesions can even produce a calm demeanor in animals made rageful and hyperreactive by lesions in the septal area (King & Meyer, 1958). However, the general behavioral effects produced by lesions of the amygdala depend on the regions of the amygdalar complex damaged (e.g., Fonberg, 1973).

By and large, animals of several species with amygdala damage are low in social dominance relative to nonlesioned animals. These species include the rat (Bunnell, 1966), the dog (Fuller, Rosvold, & Pribram, 1957), and the monkey (Dicks, Myers, & Kling, 1979; Rosvold, Mirsky, & Pribram, 1954). This effect may be due to a decreased ability to respond to subtle social signals and this could also account for the fact that they often respond in what appears to be a fearless manner when in a threatening situation. When a threatening newcomer of their species is presented to them, lesioned monkeys displayed less fear than control, peer animals. The same lesioned animals were totally submissive to their control peers, who showed more submissive reactions to the stronger animals (Thompson et al., 1977).

Perhaps the amygdalectomized animals repeatedly exhibit behaviors that evoke aggression against them, evoking repeated threat–flight response sequences. It may be of interest that in this study, one of the behavioral characteristics of the lesioned animals was a rapid change from one behavior to another in the testing situation, indicating a reduced duration of behavioral acts. This type of behavioral change was found after hypothalamic damage and has been reported after hippocampal damage, too. The idea that the amygdala plays an important role in how behavioral processes become established in development is supported by the differences found between animals lesioned early in life and raised in group or isolated living conditions.

Both the Thompson *et al.* (1977) and the Eclancher and Karli (1979) studies emphasize that often the effects of amygdala lesions may not appear for a long time after surgery. In the case of studies with monkeys, behavioral effects may not appear until three years after the damage (also see Goldman, 1974). In these studies, early lesioned animals show little, if any, decrease in the behavioral effects produced by the lesions relative to adults. If there is any sparing due to the earliness of the lesions, it is specific to a few tasks on which the animal is tested and not to a general alleviation (see Nonneman & Isaacson, 1973).

Eclancher and Karli (1971) found that amygdala lesions made early in life produced hyperactivity when the animals were tested in novel environments. Coupled with observations on lesion-induced changes in mouse killing, these authors suggested that the amygdala is involved in two separate types of processes, one involving the establishment of inhibitory processes to environmental signals and the other involving the regulation of aggressive acts.

The effects of amygdala lesions can be contrasted with those produced by the septal area. Jonason and Enloe (1971) found that amygdala lesions produced a reduction in the social contacts made by the lesioned animals, while septal lesions produced an enhancement of social contacts. The authors explained this effect on the basis of an enhancement or facilitation of prepotent responses produced by septal lesions. This normal tendency toward social contacts was facilitated by the septal lesions and was reduced by amygdala lesions.

The effects of amygdala lesions cannot be explained simply as a reduction in all types of behavior. Galef (1970) studied the effects of amygdala lesions in wild Norway rats. He found these animals to be more aggressive toward humans, mice, and other rats than the domesticated laboratory animals. As would be expected, the wild rats were tamer after the lesions and exhibited fewer aggressive acts. However, the wild rats were also more timid in novel feeding situations than the domesticated laboratory animals. Thus, they did not begin eating in an unfamiliar situation as quickly as did the tamer, laboratory animals. After the amygdala lesions, however, these animals began to eat in unfamiliar circumstances more readily. As measured by the time required to begin eating in unfamiliar circumstances, they were less timid after the amygdala lesions.

In studies of free-roaming monkeys in the jungle habitat, Kling (1972) found that animals with amygdala lesions quickly became social isolates. They did not interact with others in the monkey tribe and soon wandered off, probably to die. They did not respond to the social signals given out by the other monkeys, and they did not initiate social interactions. These effects are not a unique consequence of amygdala destruction. Myers and Swett (1970) observed monkeys with anterior-temporal-lobe damage that were allowed to roam freely over an island near Puerto Rico. These lesions, which did not invade the amygdala, also made the animals into lonely, asocial creatures without affinity for their group. Their survival time in the jungle was only a few weeks, on the average. In general, the integrity of three forebrain areas seem to be essential for the maintenance of normal social interactions among nonhuman primates: the amygdala, the posterior-medial orbitofrontal cortex, and the anterior temporal lobe (Kling & Steklis, 1976).

Recordings of the electrical activities of free-roaming monkeys indicate that at least two types of electrical activities can originate from the amygdala. Slower-frequency components seem to be related to the ambiguity of the environment or the intended actions of the animal. High-frequency alterations seem to be related to the amount of arousal or activation of the animal (Kling, Steklis, & Deutsch, 1979).

Stimulation of the amygdala can produce arousal reactions of many different kinds. These arousal effects are widespread and involve many neural systems, both autonomic and somatic. In some ways, they are reminiscent of the effects of stimulation of the midbrain reticular formation (e.g., Feindel & Gloor, 1954). Kreindler and Steriade (1963) have reported that stimulation of the dorsal amygdala produced effects that were quite different from those found after stimulation of its ventral regions. High-frequency stimulation of the dorsal regions produced desynchronization of neocortical rhythms, whereas the same stimulation of ventral regions induced synchronized rhythms and sleep patterns in the neocortex. In addition, stimulation of the ventral regions could produce seizure discharges during the time of stimulation, whereas stimulation of the dorsal amygdala produced seizure discharges only after the stimulation has ended. The arousal systems of the amygdala seem to be independent of the midbrain reticular formation since the arousal effects produced by amygdala stimulation can be found after lesions of the midbrain reticular formation. The cortical arousal effects initiated by the dorsal amygdala stimulation can suppress epileptiform discharges produced by the application of penicillin to the neocortex (Kreindler & Steriade, 1964). In addition, the activation of the neocortex by amygdala stimulation can also occlude evoked potentials in the neocortex (King, Schricker, & O'Leary, 1953).

The Kindling of Seizures

The periodic electrical stimulation of a variety of subcortical regions can produce the progressive enhancement of seizure activity (Goddard, McIntyre, & Leech, 1969). This progressive development of seizure activity is called *kindling*. Stimulation well below the amount necessary to induce electrical seizures or afterdischarges will, when delivered in a distributed fashion over days, come to elicit seizure activity. Kindling has been most extensively studied in the amygdala but can also be found in frontal limbic regions, the septal region, and other subcortical regions. The forebrain commissures are not essential for kindling to occur (McIntyre, 1975), and interruption of the corpus callosum, the hippocampal commissure, and the anterior commissure actually facilitate kindling (McCaughran, Corcoran, & Wada, 1978; Wada & Sato, 1975). This effect could be due to a denervation supersensitivity induced in the to-be-kindled region or to the disruption of interhemisphere inhibition. However, the kindling of the amygdala on one side of the brain does exert a facilitative effect on the contralateral structure as measured by the time to initiate the kindling effect (McIntyre & Goddard, 1973).

Other than the development of enhanced seizure activity, the kindling of a forebrain region can produce interesting behavioral changes. Some of these changes are found in fear-motivated behaviors. Kindled epileptiform foci in the amygdala on one side of the brain of an animal with the amygdala on the other side lesioned produce a deficit in the acquisition of conditioned emotional responses (McIntyre & Molino, 1972). Bilateral kindling of the amygdala induces a deficit on a one-trial passive-avoidance test (Boast & McIntyre, 1977). These effects do not seem to be the result of a general impairment in performance, although kindled animals may evidence changes in emotionality (Pinel, Treit, & Rovner, 1977). Apparent amnesiac effects can be found when stimulation is applied during conditioned emotional-response training but only when generalized, subcortical seizure activity is produced (McIntyre, 1979). This behavioral effect is primarily found on fear-motivated tasks.

STUDIES OF LEARNING AND MEMORY

The tameness found in animals after amygdalectomy seems to reflect a decrease in emotionality, at least in response to many conditions and signals from the environment. This reduction in emotional responsiveness may be related to the changes in behavior found in the formal tasks used to study learning and memory.

Aversive Conditioning

The effects of amygdala lesions have been studied in many types of learning situations, but probably the most intensive study has been made on animals performing avoidance tasks. The learning of an avoidance task is related to the intensity of the electrical shock used as punishment or, more accurately, to how the animals experience the shock. An amygdala lesion could alter the pain sensitivity or alter reactions to pain. In the monkey, lesions of the amygdala seem to change the threshold for reactions to punishing electrical shocks (Bagshaw & Pribram, 1968). In the rat, Kemble and Beckman (1969) tested the escape reactions of animals with amygdala damage to the sequential administration of 0.5-, 0.1-, and 1.0-mA foot shocks. They found the lesioned animals to react more quickly than control animals at the low-intensity levels but more slowly at the high-intensity level. This result is very likely related to the effect of amygdala lesions on active-avoidance performance described below. In a second experiment, Kemble and Beckman found escape latencies lower than those of control animals under the 1.0-mA condition when this shock intensity was the only one given to the animals. Animals with amygdala lesions had very similar escape latencies to the first experience of electrical shock at all intensities. In other words, the animals responded with the same speed regardless of the intensity of shock employed, while the speed of the control animals' reactions changed with the shock levels used. Since impairments of avoidance learning produced by lesions are evaluated relative to the performance of control animals, the level of shock employed could be of great significance in the results obtained.

In one of the earlier studies of avoidance conditioning, Horvath (1963) found some impairment in two-way active-avoidance (shuttlebox) learning after amygdala lesions, but the effects were not large. In this study, cats with lesions of the basolateral complex were the most impaired, and indeed, there was some suggestion that damage to the corticomedial group could attenuate the effect of the basolateral damage. Horvath also found that the retention of the two-way active-avoidance response was reduced after the basolateral lesion. No lesion effect was observed on a passive-avoidance task or on one-way active-avoidance problems. The effect of the amygdala lesions on the retention of the shuttlebox task found by Horvath is somewhat surprising since Fonberg, Brutkowski, and Mempel (1962) failed to find a retention deficit on a well-established preoperative avoidance response in dogs after damage to the amygdala.

King (1958) failed to find any debilitation on the two-way active-avoidance task in terms of the number of responses made, although there was an effect on the speed with which the responses were made. The animals with the amygdala lesions were much slower in making the avoidance response, barely accomplishing it in the interval between the onset of the conditioned stimulus and the onset of the shock. This is an important point, since there is evidence to suggest that one of the major difficulties of animals with amygdala lesions is their reluctance to initiate behavioral acts.

Deficiencies on the two-way active-avoidance task as a consequence of amygdala lesions in the cat have been observed by Kling, Orbach, Schwartz, and Towne (1960). The animals showed a deficit in terms of the number of trials required to begin making avoidance responses. Once the animals had begun to make avoidance responses, learning seemed to progress naturally and at the same rate as found in the intact animals. Suggestion of a similar deficit was found in the rat after lesions of the stria terminalis by Fred Pond and me (unpublished observations, 1967). Animals with lesions involving the stria terminalis were found to require more trials to begin avoidance responding, but once avoidance responding had been initiated, learning progressed as in normal animals.

Although the large majority of published studies indicate an impaired acquisition of two-way active-avoidance behaviors after nearly complete amygdaloid lesions (e.g., Campenot, 1969; Robinson, 1963; Werka, Skår, & Ursin, 1978), some exceptions have been noted. The results of F. A. King (1958) were mentioned above. Grossman, Grossman, and Walsh (1975) found that amygdala lesions facilitated avoidance learning on one- and two-way active-avoidance problems. They attributed the deficits found on two-way active-avoidance tasks to encroachment on the nearby piriform cortex. However, the foot shock used by Grossman *et al.* was very low. As described above, amygdala-lesioned rats are more responsive to low levels of foot shocks than controls. This could account for their unusual results. Studies showing impaired active-avoidance performance after amygdala lesions have used higher foot-shock intensities. Eclancher and Karli (1980) found impaired two-way active-avoidance deficits after large amygdala damage that failed to damage the piriform cortex. These authors also reported that amygdala damage created in the 7-day-old rat failed to influence two-way active-avoidance learning in adulthood, even though other behavioral characteristics of the lesion were found. Lesions of the centromedial area affect avoidance learning in different ways, depending on postoperative rearing.

Yeudall and Walley (1977) also found deficits in active-avoidance learning after amygdala lesions but also reported that when given methylphenidate, the animals quickly began to perform as well as controls. In fact, they may have responded in a superior fashion, given the previous numbers of training trials that had been given. The lesioned animals had formed associations between the (CS) conditioned stimulus and the (US) unconditioned stimulus in the situation but had not performed on the basis of the knowledge until the drug was given. A month later, in a retention test, the drug-treated groups exhibited greater retention than the nondrug lesioned groups.

In a related study, Bush, Lovely, and Pagano (1973) found that sub-cutaneous administration of ACTH can eliminate the avoidance deficits found after amygdalectomy. Therefore, it appears that the destruction of the amygdala influences nonassociative performance variables in certain fear-motivated test situations but not learning or memory *per se*.

In general, amygdala lesions do not change behavior on passive-avoidance tasks (e.g., McNew & Thompson, 1966), although there are exceptions (see Nagel & Kemble, 1976). Nagel and Kemble found that the effect of amygdala lesions on performance on passive-avoidance problems was "task-specific"; that is, it depended on the particular method and procedures being used. Ursin (1965) found that lesions of the medial nucleus of the amygdala produced an impairment in passive-avoidance behaviors. Specific details of training are important. A deficit in one-way active-avoidance behavior was found by McNew and Thompson, as well as by Ursin, using a task in which the animals were not picked up between trials. The influence of handling between trials is important and probably adds to the emotionality of the animal in the training task. Tasks without handling between trials probably allow the animals to be evaluated at lower arousal or emotionality levels than when they are handled between trials. Handling between trials may also produce some disorientation of the animals or may distract the animals from the specific requirements of the task. In any case, task parameters are of great significance in the evaluation of avoidance deficits after amygdala lesions. Such deficits are not a necessary consequence of amygdala damage. For example, no decrement in avoidance behavior was found in a bar-press avoidance task for either a tone or a visual signal following amygdala lesions (Di Cara, 1966).

One important observation made by Ursin in his study of the one-way active-avoidance problem was that the animals failed to initiate their responses despite "fullblown" emotional reactions in response to the CS. The lesions were in the flight zone (fear zone) of the amygdala. This finding suggests more evidence for a dissociation between the expression of behavior and what has been learned.

Animals with amygdala lesions are frequently loath to begin responses under certain conditions and are often quick to give them up. Rapid extinction of two-way active-avoidance tasks and panel-pressing avoidance reactions has been observed in monkeys (Pribram

& Weiskrantz, 1957; Weiskrantz, 1956; Weiskrantz & Wilson, 1955, 1958). Moreover, animals with amygdala lesions often simply refuse to respond to two-choice maze problems. This effect has been found when training the animals in reversal procedures. The lesioned animals seem to have an enhanced tendency to stop all responding when confronted by disrupting events and nonreinforcement, although they exhibit more "vicarious trial-and-error" movements at the choice point of the maze (Kemble & Beckman, 1970).

Lesions of the amygdala also disrupt the formation of conditioned emotional responses. In this task, the emotional reaction is measured by the extent to which operant responding is suppressed during the presentation of a tone or a visual stimulus that was associated in the past with some form of noxious stimulation, usually electrical foot-shock. The degree of suppression of the response during the presentation of the tone is a measure of the degree to which an association has been made between the signal and the painful stimulation. Usually, it is thought that the animals become "afraid" of the signal and that this fear produces responses incompatible with bar pressing. These incompatible responses lower the rate of bar pressing for food or water. However, in brain-damaged animals when a conditioned emotional response cannot be established or is less than in control animals, this does not mean that the lesioned animals are less fearful of the stimulus. It could be that the brain-damaged animals are just as afraid of the stimulus as their normal counterparts but have lost the ability to suppress ongoing behaviors. A seeming dissociation between emotional responses and the expression of the emotions in behavior was noted by Ursin after amygdala damage (mentioned above). Furthermore, explanations of the conditioned emotional response based entirely on the failure of animals to consolidate or incubate a fear response are inadequate. Using a bar-press avoidance task, Campenot (1969) found that animals with amygdala lesions performed poorly on the task the first day of training but that on the second day, they showed anticipatory responses to the signals in a normal fashion. On the second day, they did learn the task, but as training continued on the second day, the animals' behavior began to deteriorate once again. The interpretation of this behavior cannot be based on the failure of the animals to consolidate the fear response on the first day of training, since it was expressed quite well in behavior on the second day. Campenot suggested that the more adequate explanation must be based on an alteration in the animals' ability to suppress previously learned behavior sequences. The interruption of conditioned emotional-response formation reported by Thompson and Schwartzbaum (1964) to follow amygdala lesions could represent a change in emotional reactivity or response inhibition or both. A debilitation in the suppression of responses not based on the conditioning of a fear response has also been reported by Schwartzbaum, Thompson, and Kellicutt (1964).

Goddard (1964a) studied the effects of continuous stimulation of the amygdala on several types of behavioral problems.[2] He found that stimulation of the amygdala impaired two-way active-avoidance behavior but failed to have any influence on the learning of a Lashley III maze for a food reward. Normal acquisition of a one-way active-avoidance response was observed, although this response extinguished more rapidly than it did in normal animals. There was also a disruption of the formation of conditioned emotional responses. To further investigate the effect of amygdala stimulation on the formation of conditioned emotional responses, in one group of subjects Goddard applied the stimulation only during the period during which the CS was presented and in another group for 5 min after the painful shock, which was paired with a tone. He found that the pairing of the tone with the amygdala stimulation did not affect the formation of the conditioned emotional response, whereas stimulation of the amygdala after the painful shock did. At that time, he proposed that stimulation of the amygdala produced a disruption in the "consolidation" or the "incubation" of the fear response.[3]

In 1969, Goddard modified his previous hypothesis on the basis of new information. In this more recent study, he stimulated the amygdala with injections of carbachol and found disruption in con-

[2] The stimulation used by Goddard was a 60-cycle/sec stimulus ranging in current level from 3 to 13 µA. The stimulation was applied the entire time the animal was in the training situation. The stimulation was adjusted so that it was below threshold for any observable motor effects.

[3] Pellegrino (1965) reported that noncontingent continuous stimulation of the amygdala interfered with the learning of a passive avoidance response. Lidsky, Levine, Kreinick, and Schwartzbaum (1970) challenged the results of Pellegrino on the basis of probable artifactual interactions between the grid shock and the brain stimulation circuit. The issue of such interactions was discussed by Schwartzbaum and Donovick (1968) and by Schwartzbaum and Gustafson (1970).

ditioned emotional responses and on a passive-avoidance task but found no effects on behavior in the one-way active-avoidance response. The disruption of the passive-avoidance behavior occurred only when the training had been distributed over several days and not when massed training was given to the animals. Goddard noted that retention was impaired only when the animals were required to suppress previously learned behaviors. The ability to withhold responses on the basis of associations with noxious events seemed to be lost. The carbachol injection into the amygdala seemed to eliminate the ability of the animals to inhibit responses based on fear motivation.

The performance of avoidance responses can be influenced by ACTH and certain of its shorter fragments (see de Wied, 1974). Administration of $ACTH_{4-10}$ prolongs extinction in pole-jump avoidance tasks, for example. Van Wimersma Greidanus, Croiset, Bakker, and Bowman (1979) found that lesions of the amygdala eliminated this neuropeptide effect. This finding suggests that the effects of amygdala lesions and stimulation could be mediated by alterations in neuropeptide release or activities, a possibility that needs much further study.

Changes in the neuropeptides may also underlie alterations in the retention of learned performances after amygdala stimulation. Posttraining electrical stimulation of this structure has been found to impair the retention of passive (Gold, Edwards, & McGaugh, 1975; Gold, Macri, & McGaugh, 1973; Kesner & Conner, 1974) and active (Handwerker, Gold, & McGaugh, 1975) avoidance tasks. Impaired retention has also been found in a shock-motivated visual discrimination task (Gold, Rose, Hankins, & Spanis, 1976). These amygdala effects could result from "widespread effects" due to alterations in neuropeptides (Gold & Van Buskirk, 1976) or to alterations in neurotransmitter systems (see Reis & Gunne, 1965). However, if this is the case, the location within the amygdala of sites that produce such effects vary as a function of time after training. Gold et al. (1976) and Gold, Hankins, and Rose (1977) found that the location within the amygdala that produces the greatest impairment in retention changes with posttraining time. It is also known that the effect of stimulation of the amygdala on ACTH release depends on the conditions under which the animal is tested: release is facilitated during low-stress states but is inhibited under high stress (Matheson, Branch, & Taylor, 1971). Regional differences within the amygdala are also to be found.

Since the animal's state of arousal and stress changes progressively after training, it would be expected that the stimulation of different areas would produce different hormonal and behavioral changes when applied at various posttraining intervals.

Response Suppression in Appetitive Tasks

The ability of animals with destruction of the amygdala to inhibit responses has been studied on many types of tasks in which the animals work to obtain positive rewards. These studies should be considered in the context of the changes related to food and water regulation that may follow amygdala lesions. Unfortunately, the data available in the literature are not consistent. There are about as many reports of decreased food intake as of increased food intake after amygdala lesions (see Goddard, 1964b). In some cases, a decrease in food intake is found immediately after the lesion and is replaced by an increase later on. In addition, lesions of the amygdala can also lead to indiscriminate incorporation of inedible objects, such as in animals with the Klüver-Bucy syndrome (Klüver & Bucy, 1939), which results from extensive damage to the temporal lobes (Rosvold, Fuller, & Pribram, 1951).

Animals with amygdala lesions do not become overly motivated to obtain food. Rather, there is some evidence that cats and monkeys are less motivated to obtain food after amygdala lesions (Masserman, Levitt, McAvoy, Kling, & Pechtel, 1958) and are relatively insensitive to conditions of food deprivation and rewards (Schwartzbaum, 1960, 1961). Kemble and Beckman (1970) found that animals with amygdala lesions seemed to be less sensitive to the amounts of the incentives provided than were control animals, but they suggested that this effect was due to a perseveration of the fast speeds of responding first acquired under initial incentive conditions.

A comparison of the ability to inhibit responses following amygdala or hippocampus lesions was undertaken by Schwartzbaum, Thompson, and Kellicutt (1964). These investigators found that animals with amygdala lesions increased the number of responses made during conditions when reinforcements were not being obtained. These results tend to indicate an inability of the animal with amygdala damage to withhold responses under conditions of nonreinforcement. This effect was not found after small lesions of the hippocampus (a reasonable control lesion), a finding that indicates that the effect did not follow all limbic lesions, although this does not mean that such changes would not occur after more radical destruction of the hippocampus.

Schwartzbaum and Poulos (1965) found that amygdala lesions impaired the acquisition of successive reversals and learning sets in monkeys. In this experiment, the monkeys were unable to withhold responses to irrelevant aspects of the stimuli and had trouble suppressing responses that had been learned in the past but that no longer led to rewards. Reactions to the new "situations" presented by the reversal and learning-set conditions lasted longer than in control animals. These results are not unlike those found after orbital frontal lesions in monkeys (Butter, Mishkin, & Rosvold, 1963). These similarities in lesion-produced effects could be expected on the basis of the strong interconnections between the amygdala and nearby temporal lobe areas and the orbital frontal regions of the monkey neocortex. A learning-set impairment has also been found by Barrett (1969). Eleftheriou, Elias, and Norman (1972) found impaired learning of successive reversals in the deermouse following lesions in the cortical or basolateral amygdala, but not after lesions of the medial nuclear group.

In a subsequent study, Elias, Dupree, and Eleftheriou (1973) found that lesions of a particular area of the amygdala do not always produce the same kinds of behavioral effects in different strains of mice. Mice of the C57B1/6J strain with damage to the lateral nucleus evidenced an impairment in learning the second reversal after damage to the medial nucleus, while mice of the BALB/cJ strain were impaired in learning the first reversal. This finding indicates that an appropriate analysis of lesion effects on behavior must include consideration of the animal strain used and the exact anatomical structures destroyed, as well as of the behavioral requirements of the task.

Henke, Allen, and Davison (1972) trained animals on two different reinforcement schedules in the same operant situation. The animals responded on two "signaled" variable-interval (VI) schedules each day. After behavior had become stable on the two concurrent schedules, one of the signaled VI schedules was changed to extinction. Normal animals showed greatly enhanced response rates in the periods during which they could obtain reinforcements on the remaining VI schedule and stopped responding in the nonrewarded periods.

The animals with amygdala lesions did not show an increased rate of response during periods of reward on the remaining VI schedule but did stop responding in the nonrewarded periods. Henke *et al.* believe that the increase in responding found in the normal animals reflects a heightened emotionality or arousal resulting from the frustration induced by the change of one of the VI schedules to extinction. The amygdala-lesioned animals respond less because their emotional reactivity is decreased by the lesion. However, the failure to increase responding on the still-active VI schedule could also be interpreted as perseveration of the previously acquired rate of responding. The emotional reactions of the animals with amygdala lesions could be as great as those of normal animals, but their behavior need not reflect these reactions. The same issue arises in connection with experiments in which an incentive is made less attractive. N. White (1971) has shown that animals with lesions of the amygdala perseverate in drinking a water solution adulterated with quinine to a greater extent than normal animals. This finding could be interpreted as an example of perseveration of behavior in the face of an unpleasant consequence of the response, although an explanation in terms of the raising of a threshold for unpleasant tastes could also explain these data. However, this threshold explanation cannot be applied satisfactorily to all types of situations in which perseverative behaviors are found after amygdala lesions.

Acquired Taste-Aversions

Animals with damage to the amygdala have been reported to have difficulty in forming acquired aversions to a taste when the animals are made ill after experiencing the taste (McGowan, Hankins, & Garcia, 1972; Kemble & Nagel, 1973; Nachman & Ashe, 1974). The effect is not absolute, however, since if sufficiently large doses of the poison (usually LiCl) are given and the animals are made extremely sick, the impairment in acquired taste-aversion can be overcome (Rolls & Rolls, 1973). Furthermore, the deficit seems to be reduced when longer postoperative recovery periods are given the animals before testing (Nachman & Ashe, 1974). Mikulka, Freeman, and Lidstrom (1977) found that amygdala lesions did not produce a conditioned taste-aversion when a two-bottle procedure was used. With this procedure, the animal could choose either of two tastes: one taste had preceded a LiCl-induced illness; the other had not. Consistent with other reports, these investigators found that when a one-bottle technique was used, the amygdala-lesioned animals did show an impairment. The authors believe that in the one-bottle test, the inability of the lesioned animals to withhold approach responses produced behaviors that looked like a failure to acquire the taste aversion but that really was not. A very stable and prolonged retention of the aversion was found in animals with amygdala lesions. This finding indicates that the problem of the animals was not one of acquiring the association but was one of executing performance based on it. Furthermore, animals with amygdala lesions apparently do not have difficulty in recognizing taste cues to sugar (Freeman, Mikulka, Phillips, Megarr, & Meisel, 1978). This finding also indicates that the taste–sickness association can be acquired by the lesioned animals even though whether it is expressed in behavior depends on the nature of the tests given the animals.

Transfer and Transposition

In a series of experiments, the ability of monkeys with lesions of the amygdala to transfer what had been learned on one task to a somewhat modified training condition was studied. Some of these studies involved the use of a "transposition paradigm." For example, monkeys have been trained to respond to the lighter of two gray panels for a food reward. After acquisition of this problem, they were tested with the previously rewarded light gray panel paired with an even lighter gray panel. The normal monkeys responded to this altered condition by pressing the lighter of the two gray panels. They behaved as if they had learned to respond to the relative brightness of the two gray panels. However, the animals with lesions of the amygdala distributed their responses equally between the two gray panels when tested with the new, lighter gray panel. This type of behavior would be expected if the lesioned monkeys perceived the changed test conditions as an entirely new circumstance, one unrelated to the former conditions of training (Schwartzbaum & Pribram, 1960). A similar observation was made by Bagshaw and Pribram (1965). They found that while normal monkeys trained to respond to the larger of two squares selected the larger of two new circles, amygdalectomized monkeys responded equally to the two new stimuli. Of special interest is the fact that animals with lesions of the amygdala generalized their responses in a normal fashion when tested for stimulus generalization.

Douglas (1966) has raised some serious questions about the conclusions drawn from the transposition experiments mentioned above. He has pointed out that the study by Bagshaw and Pribram was actually an investigation of postoperative retention, with all of the training being given before surgery. The transposition tests were made after the removal of the amygdala. Douglas also pointed out that the transposition deficit found by Schwartzbaum and Pribram occurred in only one of two experiments reported in their article. The results of the second experiment with the same animals could be interpreted as indicating an exaggerated degree of transposition. The animals in the second experiment were given half the trials with a medium gray matched against a light gray, and on the other half of the trials, they were given the medium gray with a dark gray. Responses to the medium gray were always reinforced. Normal monkeys quickly learned to respond to the medium gray, whereas the amygdalectomized animals made many more mistakes when the light gray and the medium gray were paired and few mistakes with the medium-gray–dark-gray pair. It was this pair that had been used in the original training of the discrimination. Douglas argued that an enhanced degree of transposition would have led to the larger numbers of errors during testing with the two light shades of gray. In the first Schwartzbaum and Pribram procedure, only a few (12) test trials for transposition were given. To study the problem further, Douglas tested animals with amygdala lesions, animals with hippocampus lesions, and control animals in a transposition test in which acquisition training was given postoperatively and more test trials were given. He found no evidence of a transpositional deficit in either group of lesioned subjects. For various reasons, Douglas believes that the seeming impairment in transpositional response found previously was due to the altered reactions to novel stimulus conditions found in the amygdalectomized animals. Errors produced by the enhanced novelty reactions were mistaken for the absence of transpositional abilities. In a subsequent paper, Douglas and Pribram (1969) reported that lesions of the amygdala produced an exaggerated distractibility to novel stimulus conditions on the first occasion that a distracting stimulus was presented, but that this overreaction soon habituated to the levels of the control animals. Changes in the position or the nature of the distracting stimulus produced renewed distractibility of the lesioned monkeys, which again declined rapidly.

If stimuli of the environment are to be used by the animal in guiding its behavior, they must be detected and evaluated. After lesions of the amygdala, or at least some portions of it, the animals give fewer signs of orienting toward unexpected stimuli (Bagshaw *et al.*, 1972) but can use the visual information if sufficient justification is provided. They can use these stimuli to form new behavior patterns and to pause in their reactions when the unexpected occurs (Douglas & Pribram, 1969). Under certain conditions, they overreact to novel stimuli, and this overreaction can interfere with the efficient performance of an ongoing behavioral act.

But what is a novel stimulus? By experimental definition, it is a stimulus that is unexpected, something added to the environment of the animal as it is engaged in a behavioral act. The performance of any behavioral act suggests that the animal has developed a set of hypotheses about its environment and the payoff of certain behavioral reactions in that environment. The animal has expectations about relevant and irrelevant aspects of the environment. The introduction of a new stimulus can be useful in obtaining rewards or relief from environmental oppressions, or it can be irrelevant to them. Therefore, reactions to the unexpected or the expected stimuli can be useful or not, depending on the relationship of the stimulus to the payoff to be found in the environment.

A novel stimulus is one for which the animal is unprepared. It has not been evaluated for possible relevancy. It has not been tested for its potential contributions to behavior. The animal with destruction of the amygdala is reluctant to undertake the evaluation of novel stimuli unless it has good justification for so doing. This justification is based on the creation of a sufficient motivational state and the induction of a belief that there is a course of action open to the animal that will lead to attenuation of the motivational conditions. Thus, if the animal is led to believe that differential responding to visual cues can improve its conditions, it can learn to respond differentially. If it finds that running will lead to escape from or avoidance of an electrical shock, it will run. It is as if the animal with amygdala damage is reluctant to take the "first step," to begin a new form of behavior. Once it does begin, it can and will learn readily to do what is consistent with the reward structure of the environment. The reluctance to begin new acts includes those related to observing and investigation as well as to new forms of learned reactions.

REFLECTIONS AND SUMMARY

The amygdala is not a homogenous structure; it is made up of a number of anatomical subdivisions, tied differentially and specifically to sensory association areas, which participate in the modulation of emotional reactions. These subdivisions participate not only in the modulation of autonomic reactions but in the somatic responses involved in orienting toward significant behavior events and in the use of this information to direct behavior. Learning and memory do not seem to be altered by lesions of the amygdala, although electrical stimulation studies have produced some evidence on the other side. However, these "memory effects" could well be due to more global, diffuse effects on the brain or could be secondary to the alterations in peripheral autonomic activities induced by the stimulation. In general, however, it is performance, not knowledge, that seems to be altered by interference with the activities of the amygdala.

Like the hypothalamus, the amygdala participates in governing behavior in such a way that the actual effects are dependent on genetic, historical, and environmental factors. There is no one abiding symptom that is always the consequence of the lesion or the stimulation. The effects obtained are contingent on the nature of the animal or the person and the situation, that is, the state of other brain systems.

It cannot be said that the amygdala acts only as a regulator or modulator of the hypothalamus, although it surely does this, However, it also plays its part in the modulation of other limbic structures, the basal ganglia, and the associated neocortical systems as well. Behavior and mental activities must represent the integrated activities of all of these systems, and it is hard to parcel out responsibility, blame, or credit for a particular type of action.

Like the hypothalamus, the amygdala seems to be especially influential in the initiation and continuation of behavioral acts. Indeed, after amygdalar or hypothalamic damage, individual acts become shorter in duration; yet under some conditions, organized sequences of behaviors seem to continue longer than usual. These are general consequences of limbic system dysfunction, since they are found after almost all types of damage to regions of the system.

4

The Septal Area

As in the previous chapter, I examine here some of the behavioral effects produced by stimulation and lesions of the septal area, beginning with those of a general nature and proceeding to ones of greater specificity. The purpose is to understand the nature and diversity of these changes and hopefully to place them in a more general context based on the relationship of the septal area to the hypothalamus and other limbic system structures.

GENERAL CHANGES FOLLOWING SEPTAL LESIONS

Emotionality

Rats and mice with lesions made in the septal area often exhibit increased rage reactions and hyperemotionality immediately after surgery. These characteristics are sometimes called the *septal syndrome* (Brady & Nauta, 1953, 1955). They disappear over time, usually lasting between two and three weeks. For some reason, these changes are not always found in all species. In particular, the golden hamster (Sodetz, Matalka, & Bunnell, 1967), the squirrel monkey (Buddington, King, & Roberts, 1967), and the rhesus monkey (Votaw, 1960) do not seem to exhibit a septal syndrome after lesions. Some hyperemotionality has been described in cats (R. Y. Moore, 1964) and rabbits (Green & Arduini, 1954). There have also been reports of hyperemotionality after septal lesions in humans (Ransom, 1895; Zeman & King, 1958),

although one difficulty in defining the human syndrome is the identification of homologues of the rodent septal area in people.

The fact that the hyperemotionality dissipates rapidly over time
after septal lesions in rodents stands in contrast to the long-lasting
hyperemotionality found after lesions of the ventromedial nucleus of
the hypothalamus (Singh, 1969) or after lesions of the olfactory bulb.

In light of the fact that many types of behavioral effects of septal
lesions are dependent on the genotypes of the animals being tested
(e.g., McDaniel, Donovick, Burright, & Fanelli, 1980), it would not
be surprising if emotional hyperreactivity were also dependent on
this factor. As far as can be determined, the relationship between
genotype and hyperemotionality has not been studied directly. However, an association between the tendency to produce electrical self-
stimulation and enhanced emotionality after septal lesions has been
reported. Using high and low self-stimulation lines obtained through
selective breeding, Lieblich, Cohen, Ben-Zion, and Dymshitz (1980)
found that damage to the septal area (or the ventromedial nucleus of
the hypothalamus) produced greater emotionality in the high than
in the low self-stimulation lines.

While the septal syndrome becomes diminished after surgery,
time is not the only essential factor. The more the animals are handled,
the faster the hyperemotionality abates. Gotsick and Marshall (1972)
found that with daily handling normal, emotionality could be
achieved as early as 6 days after surgery. If the animals were not
handled for 6 days postsurgically, they were hyperemotional for the
1st day of handling (the 7th postoperative day), but not afterward.
Some animals were handled 12 times on the 1st postoperative day,
and within this day, no decline in hyperemotionality was detected.
This finding suggests that the reduction on hyperemotionality is due
to a combination of handling and the simple passing of time. It is of
special interest that when the animals had returned to "normal levels"
of emotionality, they were actually easier to pick up and remove from
their cages than normal animals. Other factors that influence the
duration of hyperemotionality include preoperative experience (Nielson, McIver, & Boswell, 1965), the time of day at which testing occurs
(Seggie, 1970), and the capture procedures employed (Max, Cohen,
& Lieblich, 1974).

The age of the animals at the time of lesion also affects the hyperemotional reactions of the animals. Lesions made shortly after

weaning in Wistar rats produced only a transient period of hyper-emotionality, whereas lesions made at 55–65 days of age produced more persistent effects (Phillips & Lieblich, 1972). Castration of the animals early in life prevented the enhanced emotionality from occurring after the septal lesions. However, for castration to be effective, it had to be accomplished before the 30th day of life. Castration in adulthood produced no effect on the rage syndrome. Furthermore, testosterone replacement after juvenile castration failed to reinstate the rage syndrome (Lieblich, Gross, & Cohen, 1977).

While septal-lesioned animals do indeed bite, there is some reason to believe that the aggressive responses are part of exaggerated defensive reactions (see Blanchard & Blanchard, 1977; Grossman, 1978). This interpretation is based largely on the fact that the lesioned animals try to avoid unfamiliar stimulation and conflict, if possible. Lesioned animals engage in increases of the boxing, freezing, and ultrasonic vocalizations typical of defensive animals. Reflexive fighting as exhibited by septal-lesioned animals is an expression of defensive acts (Blanchard, Blanchard, Lee, & Nakamura, 1979). This view would be supported in part by the observation that septal lesions decreased the dominance of animals that had been socially dominant before surgery, although the behavior of previously submissive animals was not affected (Gage, Olton, & Bolanowski, 1978).

Animals with septal lesions are hyperresponsive to handling, puffs of air, pokes with a stick, foot shock, skin temperature changes, shifts in ambient temperature, and sounds. (For reviews, see Fried, 1972, and Olton & Gage, 1974. See also Gage, Armstrong, & Thompson, 1980, for a novel approach to the analyses of changes in reactivity.) Probably because of these changes and their heightened tendency toward defensive behaviors, they are harder to capture than controls. In other experiments, septal lesions have been found to produce an increased sensitivity to light. Lesioned animals exhibit an exaggerated photophobic reaction (Donovick, 1968; Green & Schwartzbaum, 1968). Flashes of light presented to animals with septal lesions produce enhanced levels of locomotor activity that are relatively resistant to habituation. When tested in circumstances in which a bar press turned a light on or off depending on whether it was on when the response was made, rats with septal lesions had the light on less over a 24-hour period than controls but actually pressed the bar to produce changes more frequently than controls

(Zuromski, Donovick, & Burright, 1972). Thus, while septal lesions produce an aversion to light, lesioned animals seek changes in environmental stimulation.

A decreased habituation of the cardiac component of the orienting responses to auditory stimulation has been reported (Sanwald, Porzio, Deane, & Donovick, 1970). The lateral septal area, and not the medial area, seems to be the important area in which lesions disrupt habituation of the orienting response and locomotion in an open-field setting (Köhler, 1976). It is also of interest that while the lesioned animals exhibit exaggerated motoric reactions to light flashes, they exhibit progressively reduced visual evoked potentials, and on this basis, the animals would be described as having greater habituation (Schwartzbaum, DiLorenzio, Mello, & Kreinick, 1972; Schwartzbaum, Kreinick, & Levine, 1972). This finding indicates that the effects of septal lesions on behavior and on electrical potentials may be quite different. Looking at either measure of "reactivity" alone would be misleading, revealing only one aspect of the effects produced by the septal lesions.

Exaggerated motor responses to various types of stimulation may characterize the animal with septal area destruction, as suggested by the increased reactivity to foot shock described above, but this general overreactivity does not imply that the animals are more ready to interact with their environment. Carey (1969) showed that lesions of the posterior septal area produced animals that seemed to be *less* motivated in operant tasks, based on responses produced to obtain a water reward, despite their well-established increase in *ad libitum* water consumption (see below). This finding suggests that while septal area lesions may change the animals' reactivity to external stimulation, they may not change the animals' readiness to engage in actions aimed at relieving or alleviating the stimulating conditions.

The issue of what portions of the septal area are responsible for rage, hyperemotionality, and hyperreactivity is not resolved. Some studies have reported that placidity and submissiveness result from restricted damage to the medial or dorsolateral septal areas (Clody & Carlton, 1969; Poplawsky & Johnson, 1973; Thomas & Van Atta, 1972), and others have indicated that areas ventral to the septal area must be damaged for irritability to be expressed (Turner, 1970; Thomas & Van Atta, 1972). There is considerable evidence on the opposite side, indicating that these effects can result from damage to the medial and lateral septal areas (Gotsick & Marshall, 1972; F. A. King, 1958;

R. W. Reynolds, 1965). The failure of some authors to find rage-like effects after septal lesions may be due to bilateral asymmetries of the lesions or to special conditions of presurgical handling or experience.

Schnurr (1972) found that small lesions of the anterior or middle septal area caused hyperactivity, but that lesions in the posterior regions did not. This finding was supported by Albert and Richmond (1975), who also found that hyperactivity occurs when damage ventral to the septal area is produced. Lesions restricted to the septal area proper produce only modest increases in reactivity. Damage to regions ventral to the posterior septal area considerably enhance the activity, and damage to the area between the anterior commissure and the vertical arms to the diagonal band of Broca is associated with the rage or defensive aspects (Albert & Chew, 1980). Since it is now thought that the medial septal nucleus and the nucleus of the diagonal band can be considered a functional entity, it is possible that the amount of hyperactivity could be a function of the amount of this joint nuclear region destroyed. However, a special contribution of nucleus accumbens in conjunction with the damage to the septal region cannot be discounted.

Destruction of either the major input pathway from the hippocampal formation, the fornix, or the major efferent pathways before the septal lesion can ameliorate or eliminate the septal syndrome (Olton & Gage, 1974). The fornix lesions can be made days or minutes before the septal area damage, but simultaneous lesions are not effective. The area in which the hippocampal damage produces this effect is the dorsal portion. Lesions of ventral hippocampus or adjacent entorhinal tissue do not produce this effect (Gage & Olton, 1975).

Water Consumption

An increase in the amount of water consumed by animals with septal lesions has been frequently observed (e.g., Harvey & Hunt, 1965; Donovick & Burright, 1968). It may be related to changes in the taste of various substances produced by the lesions. Beatty and Schwartzbaum (1967, 1968) found that septal lesions enhanced the animals' licking of a sucrose solution at various concentrations, and in addition, these authors showed that the increased sucrose intake could not be explained on the basis of either increased hunger or increased thirst. They suggested, as did Donovick, Burright, and Lustbader (1969), that the lesions alter the animals' reactivity to tastes by enhancing approach reactions to pleasant tastes and increasing aversive responses to unpleasant tastes. Such an observation was made by Carey (1971). In his study, animals with septal lesions took in less quinine-adulterated water, while drinking more water with saccharin in it. Carey's results could not be explained on the basis of a change in taste threshold; rather, the animals had changed reactions to the tastes. Kemble, Levine, Gregoire, Koepp, and Thomas (1972) found that these accentuated taste aversions and preferences habituated rapidly and that the differences between the lesioned animals and controls disappeared with continued exposure to the test solutions.

The increase in water consumption found after septal lesions could be interpreted as an attempt to make normal laboratory food taste better through adulteration with water. Thus, the increased water consumption would be secondary to changes in reactions to good and bad tastes. Nevertheless, some degree of hyperdipsia occurs when no food is available, as found by Harvey and Hunt. As a consequence, other supplementary explanations must be sought that go beyond those based on changes in taste alone.

Lubar et al. (1968, 1969) related the increase in water consumption found after septal lesions to a deficiency in the secretion of antidiuretic hormone (ADH). This finding suggests that the increase in water intake is secondary to an excessive excretion of water. Antidiuretic hormone is responsible for the recirculation of water through the kidneys and affects the water volume lost through urination. A deficiency in ADH results in the secretion of a more dilute urine and a greater loss of water. However, Blass and Hanson (1970) have argued that the increase in water intake found in septal-lesioned animals results from a primary effect on systems that control water intake. They showed that the amounts of water drunk by animals with septal damage were not directly related to the amount of water lost through urination, as would be expected on the basis of a deficiency in ADH secretion. In addition, they found that the drinking patterns of animals with septal lesions did not correspond to those of animals with reduced amounts of saliva (i.e., dry throats), which should occur if water volume had been depleted. Further, they found no differences in blood levels of sodium and potassium between the septal-lesioned animals and controls. This finding means that the increase in drinking could not be due to a hyponatremia (sodium deficiency). However, if animals with septal lesions do maintain serum sodium concentrations at nearly normal levels, they may not do so by the usual metabolic means. Bengelloun, Baddouri, and El Hilali (1978) reported that sodium concentrations in the internal medullary and papillary portions of the kidney and in the urine of lesioned animals were lower than those of controls. The septal-damaged animals overdrank after subcutaneous injections of polyethylene glycol. This compound reduces the total amount of an animal's plasma volume. While some data are consistent with the idea that rats with septal lesions are extrasensitive to the dipsogenic effects of angiotensin, there is no firm evidence that this sensitivity is responsible for spontaneous, unprovoked drinking under normal circumstances (Stricker, 1978). It should also be emphasized that some investigators have not found exaggerated responsiveness by lesioned animals to treatments that reduce the fluid volumes of the animals. For example, Black and Mogenson (1973) and Tondat and Almli (1975) failed to find differences in response between hyperdipsic animals and animals that drink normally after hypovolemia was induced.

Changes in both food and water consumption after septal lesions are determined in part by the strain and the prelesion experiences of the animals being tested (Donovick, Burright, Fuller, & Branson, 1975). Thus, any sweeping generalization about the mechanisms of water regulation must be considered with caution.

Social Behavior

Animals of different species do not respond in the same way to septal lesions. Rats with septal lesions tend to be hyperemotional and gregarious in open-field situations, but this reaction has not been observed in golden hamsters (Johnson, Poplawsky, & Bieliauskas, 1972). Poplawsky and Johnson (1972) have shown that the increase in sociability, as measured in increased contact time among animals and greater submissiveness, arises from medial but not lateral septal lesions. A complicating factor in interpreting these results has been introduced by MacDougall, Pennebaker, and Stevenson (1973). These authors reported that while septal area lesions enhance the social contacts made by one subspecies of the deer mouse (*gracillis*), the lesions actually reduce the social contacts made by a subspecies that is less social *(bairdi)*. This finding suggests that the effects produced by the lesions cannot be considered independently of the genetic endowments and characteristic behavior patterns of the animals. Indeed, the lesion effects may be best interpreted as potentiating the predominant behavioral tendencies of the animals, including those that are provided by their genetic endowments—and possibly also those that have been acquired.

Animals with septal lesions usually tend to interact well with other members of their species and to make a decreased number of aggressive responses to stimuli that normally induce such responses. Slotnick and McMullen (1972) found that mice with septal lesions were poor fighters. They were always defeated by normal animals. Their response to aggression exhibited by other animals was to run away, even when they had had experience in winning fighting bouts before the lesions were made. However, the septal lesion produces not an inability to fight but a reluctance to do so. For example, enhanced fighting, induced by electrical shocks, was found in rats with septal damage when they were tested 85 days postoperatively (Wetzel, Conner, & Levine, 1967). No increase in emotionality ratings was found in these animals at that time. As with the septal syndrome, the intensity of shock-induced fighting becomes less and less after surgery. The decline in the intensity of shock-induced fighting in septal-lesioned animals depends on the housing of the animals, among other things. If the animals are caged with other animals during the postoperative period, the enhanced tendency toward shock-induced fighting disappears within 17 days. On the other hand, if the animals are housed by themselves, they show this exaggerated reaction up to 45 days postoperatively (Ahmad & Harvey, 1968).

Eichelman (1971) also found that septal lesions enhance shock-induced aggressive behaviors and in addition reported a decrease in such behaviors after destruction of the amygdala. Jonason and Enloe (1971) found that animals with septal lesions spend more time in nonaggressive social contact than do controls, including animals with amygdala lesions. This effect of increased social contact seems to result from damage to the medial septal nucleus (Poplawsky & Johnson, 1973).

The stimuli responsible for intraspecies aggressive acts are quite different from those leading to shock-induced fighting. Perhaps the discrepancy found between the two measures is related to changes in the threshold of the stimulation required to elicit aggression. In studying the effects of septal lesions in hamsters, Sodetz and Bunnell (1970) found increases in the aggressiveness of their submissive subjects. The animals were still submissive after the lesions but engaged in fighting behaviors more frequently than they had before. Apparently, the lesions had not made the animals incapable of exhibiting aggression but had made most animals less likely to do so under certain conditions.

The conditions that seem most likely to elicit aggressive behaviors in animals with septal damage are those in which physical contact occurs between animals. This is especially the case when dorsal stimulation occurs as the animal is approached from the rear (Blanchard & Blanchard, 1977). This type of stimulation is very effective in producing exaggerated responses in the lesioned animals regardless of the origin of the stimulation. Of course, different methods of handling and the physical environment during testing influence the extent to which the animal is aroused and the likelihood of physical contact between animals. These factors, along with the genotype of the subjects, influence the degree of hyperactivity exhibited and the amount of stimulation-based defensive aggression. It is likely that discrepancies among reports of aggression in animals with septal lesions are due to genetic and procedural variations among experimental conditions.

Albert and Wong (1978) found increased intraspecific aggressive acts after transient chemical lesions of the septal area. Such changes were seldom seen in animals with electrolytic damage in the same area. This increase is very likely due to the fact that the temporary chemical lesions do not initiate secondary reactions in other areas that occur after permanent lesions. Secondary reactions typically occur after central nervous system damage and may be responsible for many of the behavioral consequences of central nervous system lesions (see Isaacson, 1980b).

The effect on the social dominance of animals after septal lesions probably depends on the nature of the animals before surgery. Septal lesions induce a decrease in dominance only in animals that were dominant before surgery (Gage et al., 1978). In general, the predominant effect of septal lesions has been to reduce dominance in rats and mice (Miczek & Grossman, 1972; Slotnick & McMullen, 1972), and failures to obtain such results may reflect differences in the subjects before surgery, including differences in genetic and environmental factors (e.g., Gonsiorek, Donovick, Burright, & Fuller, 1974).

Activity

There are several reports indicating that septal lesions in rats and mice reduce open-field locomotion (Brady & Nauta, 1955; Corman *et al.*, 1967; Nielson *et al.*, 1965). The decrease in locomotor activity does not seem to be a consequence of the hyperemotionality produced by the lesion (Schwartzbaum & Gay, 1966). The animals seem to exhibit less "freezing" (gross immobility) during testing than normal animals (Blanchard & Fial, 1968; Duncan, 1971; Trafton & Marques, 1971). On the other hand, animals with septal lesions have shown reduced habituation of the locomotor behavior that was associated with *higher* levels of locomotion when the animals were not exposed to the testing situation before surgery (Donovick & Wakeman, 1969; Gomer & Goldstein, 1974; Kemble & Nagel, 1975). It is likely that whether septal animals show increased or decreased open field locomotion after surgery depends on their prior experiences with being handled (Bengelloun, Finklestein, Burright, & Donovick, 1977), their conditions of rearing (Donovick, Burright, & Swidler, 1973), their diets (Donovick, Burright, & Bensten, 1975), and the conditions during testing.

Possibly related to the changes in locomotor activity after septal lesions is a persistent reduction in rearing and an increase in floor sniffing found in rats (Kemble & Nagel, 1975) and gerbils (Laughlin, Donovick, & Burright, 1975). The reduction in rearing found after septal lesions has also been found after hippocampal damage (Reinstein, Hannigan, & Isaacson, in press). The reduction in rearing after septal lesions in rats could be partially offset by an odor (isoamylacetate) placed high along the walls of the testing apparatus. Odors added to the floors influenced the control animals but not the animals with septal lesions.

In a recent study, the presence of home-cage litter shavings introduced under the floor of an open field was found to produce increases in activity in the second half of a 10-min test session in septal-lesioned animals, but this increase did not occur when clean shavings were used. Control animals in both litter-shaving conditions showed decreases in the second 5 min of the observation period (Wigal *et al.*, 1981). Olfactory stimulation appears to make important contributions to the activation of animals. The degree to which this activation depends on specific odor qualities, possibly a pheremone-like quality associated with the home cage, is unknown. However, activation of rearing was found by Kemble and Nagel using a substance that did not have pheremone-like qualities. Perhaps olfactory stimulation has general effects on the lesioned animals.

Sagvolden (1979) determined that motivational conditions play an important role in determining the activity of animals with septal lesions. In general, after surgery, the animals had lower response rates in an operant chamber in obtaining water when thirsty, but this effect was eliminated or reversed at longer deprivation conditions (48 hrs water deprivation). Locomotion away from the area of the lever in the test cage was reduced under all deprivation conditions, as was bar pressing to turn on a cue light by pressing a second bar in the test chamber. In earlier reports, Sagvolden (1975a,b) found that septal-lesioned animals tend to exhibit an apparent hypoactivity or hypo-responsiveness in that they escape less under low foot-shock levels and bar-press less for water under lower levels of water deprivation than do controls.

Using the rat, Köhler and Srebro (1980) investigated the effects of selective septal lesions on exploration in various types of situations. The lesions were small and affected only limited portions of the target areas. The effects were nevertheless dramatic in that the lateral-septal-lesion group were more likely to venture into new areas and to explore unfamiliar objects. The medial-septal-lesion group appeared frightened by novel circumstances, ventured out from their home cages less, and evidenced few signs of exploratory behaviors. Rearing and locomotion did not seem to be affected by either of the lesions in the usual open-field situation.

CHANGES IN PERFORMANCE ON LEARNING TASKS AFTER SEPTAL LESIONS: AVOIDANCE BEHAVIORS

Damage to the septal area produces many types of changes in the behavior of animals as they are trained in specific problems designed to test learning and memory. These changes are best considered in terms of the types of tasks with which the animals are confronted and the circumstances used to motivate the animals. First to be considered is the performance on tasks in which the animals attempt to avoid noxious stimulation. It is on these tasks that the behavioral effects of septal lesions have been most extensively studied.

Research on the effects of septal lesions on avoidance tasks gained significance and impetus from the work of McCleary. His hypothesis was that such lesions would impair mechanisms responsible for the suppression of behavioral acts (McCleary, 1961, 1966), although related work had begun several years earlier (e.g., F. A. King, 1958). McCleary undertook to extend the ideas of Kaada (1951), who found a facilitation or an inhibition of autonomic activities after the stimulation of many limbic system regions. McCleary had the idea that these same areas might facilitate or inhibit somatic responses and even well-defined behavior directed toward specific environmental goals.

Accordingly, he made selective lesions in various limbic system areas, among them the tissue underneath the genu of the corpus callosum, including the septal area. It was in this region that Kaada had found inhibitory effects on autonomic activities resulting from electrical stimulation. McCleary found that animals with lesions in this region were inferior to other animals in their ability to suppress behavior in certain tasks, including those in which the animals had to stop responding to avoid punishment. On the other hand, the lesioned animals were not impaired in the learning of an active-avoidance task.

Lesions in the cingulate cortex produced just the opposite effect. This finding was of interest since the cingulate area was one in which electrical stimulation facilitated autonomic activities. Thus, the combination of the results obtained by McCleary and by Kaada produced a remarkable correlation between the effects of lesions and electrical stimulation on limbic structures. Behaviorally, some lesions impaired passive, but not active, avoidance learning, while other lesions did just the opposite. The lesioned areas that caused an impairment in the passive-avoidance task were those that, when stimulated, inhibited autonomic activities. Some of these were in the septal area.

While the McCleary approach—that regions exist that globally facilitate or inhibit behavioral reactions—is tempting because of its simplicity, more recent work has shown it to be an overly simple summarization of the data. Like most wide-ranging speculations about the brain, it just won't do.

Impairments in the acquisition of passive-avoidance tasks after septal lesions have been found by many authors (e.g., Kaada *et al.*, 1962; McCleary, 1961; Lubar, 1964). There is an indication that the effect may be due to interference with lateral-septal-area systems (Hamilton, Kelsey, & Grossman, 1970). However, it must be remembered that the effect of septal lesions on the learning of both passive- and active-avoidance problems is determined by the genetic makeup of the mice being tested (McDaniel *et al.*, 1980). In addition, there remain questions about the generality of the passive-avoidance deficits observed. It is possible that such deficits are restricted to the avoidance of foot shock. Animals with septal area lesions were not found impaired when quinine (Gittelson, Donovick, & Burright, 1969), ice water (Frank & Beatty, 1974), or nausea-producing x-irradiation (McGowan, Garcia, Ervin, & Schwartz, 1969) was used as the to-be-avoided stimulation. When drinking water is adulterated with bitter substances, animals with septal lesions show a suppression often exceeding that of controls (Beatty & Schwartzbaum, 1967; Donovick, Burright, and Zuromski, 1970). The apparent discrepancies in the literature (e.g., Brown, Harrell, & Remley, 1971) are probably related to the conditions of testing the animals. The results obtained in the majority of experiments probably represent an exaggerated responsiveness to both absolute and relative taste cues (e.g., Flaherty & Hamilton, 1971) and a lowered reactivity to postingestional factors (Hamilton, Capobianco, & Worsham, 1974). In addition, Flaherty, Capobianco, and Hamilton (1973) have shown that the amount of time between the exposure to a particular taste and subsequent testing with a different taste plays an important role in determining the reactions of the animals with septal damage. These authors rewarded animals with a 32% sucrose solution and then tested them after vacations of various lengths from the training procedure with a 4% sucrose solution. The 32% solution was greatly preferred to the 4% solution. If a 4-day interval was imposed between the last day of 32% reward and testing with the 4% solution, normal animals still responded poorly to the new reward, while the animals with septal lesions did not. Flaherty *et al.* believe this finding indicates that animals with septal lesions seem to forget their experiences with the favored solution more readily than normal animals and consequently fail to show the usual depressive effect when tested with the less-preferred solution after even a few days' intermission between tests.

Time has also been found to be a critical factor in determining whether a passive avoidance deficit will be observed when an approach response to water is punished by foot shock. When rats with septal lesions experienced only one foot shock per day, they achieved criterion performance as readily as controls (Bengelloun, Burright, & Donovick, 1976). It is possible that multiple shocks interfere with the processing of information unless they are spaced out to a greater extent than for controls. This requirement could represent a severe limitation of capacity (see Isaacson, 1982), possibly due to alterations in the rate of habituation as described above. The addition of cues (changes in the house lights of the apparatus) signaling conditions of shock as the animals approached water also improved the performance of young rats with septal lesions but had less effect on older rats. Still, under the light-cue conditions, the animals with septal lesions actually performed more efficiently than the control animals (Bengelloun, Burright, & Donovick, 1977).

Septal lesions produce an enhanced acquisition of two-way active-avoidance problems. This observation was first reported by F. A. King (1958). This effect has been demonstrated in several strains of rats (Deagle & Lubar, 1971), guinea pigs (Lown, Hayes, & Schaub, 1969), mice (Carlson, 1970), and squirrel monkeys (Buddington et al., 1967). In a few studies, this facilitation has not been observed. For example, LaVaque (1966) found no difference between animals with septal lesions and normal animals in the acquisition of the two-way active-avoidance problem, and Dalby (1970) also failed to find the facilitation. In the Dalby experiment, however, a high hurdle was used to differentiate the two types of compartments. Some motor actions may be difficult for animals with limbic damage, and the motor demands presented by the hurdle could interfere with the expression of what is being learned. Kemble and Strand (1977) found that septal lesions impaired the jumping or rearing responses required in either shock-avoidance or food-motivated problems that required them to be made. Shelf-jumping responses in cats are also faulty after septal area damage (Hamilton, 1972). These motoric impairments seem to be independent of possible changes in the fear of the animals.

Another motor change found after septal damage is the reduced incidence of behavioral freezing (immobility) that occurs during stressful training or testing. While it is true that septal lesions reduce such behavior, this reduction cannot, by itself, account for the enhanced active-avoidance performance of the animals with septal lesions (e.g., Schwartzbaum & Gay, 1966). Actual punishment of intertrial responses fails to eliminate the superiority of animals with septal damage (Schwartzbaum, Green, Beatty, & Thompson, 1967). Nevertheless, the reduction in immobility produced by septal lesions can facilitate the performance of animals that respond poorly because of freezing (Poplawsky, 1978). A similar result was found after hippocampal damage in guinea pigs, which typically do not learn active-avoidance responses because of shock-induced immobility (Ireland, Hayes, & Schaub, 1969). The degree to which foot shock influences behavior is undoubtedly a function of the intensity of the shock. Sagvolden (1975a) has found evidence for a curvilinear behavioral effect of foot shock in active-avoidance tasks, with optimal performance occurring in the middle intensity range.

The cues differentiating the two compartments of the shuttleboxes used in two-way active-avoidance training are of importance. F. A. King (personal communication, 1968) found that the greater the differentiation of the compartments, the *less* the facilitation shown by animals after septal damage. When the compartments are poorly differentiated, the septal-lesioned animals show enhanced performance relative to that of the normal subjects. The same thing has been shown in animals with hippocampal lesions, which also show improvement in the two-way active-avoidance problem when the sides are poorly differentiated (Isaacson, unpublished observations, 1958). The effect of the cues provided to differentiate the two compartments is to make the problem more or less difficult for the normal animals. Normal animals learn least well when the two compartments are of the same color and best when they are of different colors. Animals with septal or hippocampal lesions seem to learn the task as quickly under well-differentiated conditions and poorly-differentiated conditions. Therefore, the best conditions for demonstrating the superiority of the animals with septal or hippocampal damage are those in which the sensory differentiation of cues is least. This differentiation affects the performance of control animals more than that of animals with septal or hippocampal damage. Animals with septal lesions may focus on one or a few specific cues and place extreme reliance on them for behavior in the situation, whereas the controls may respond to a larger number of elements or to their configuration in the testing situation (Carlson & Vallante, 1974; Gomer & Goldstein, 1974; Donovick, Burright, Sikorszky, Stamato, & McLaughlin, 1978).

While the septal lesions seem to produce animals that acquire the two-way active-avoidance response more readily than normal animals, there are also reports that these lesions interfere with the acquisition of a one-way active-avoidance problem (Kenyon & Krieckhaus, 1965; Liss, 1964, cited by Deagle & Lubar, 1971; Vanderwolf, 1964). All of these studies were done with hooded animals, and Deagle and Lubar suggested that an impairment of one-way active-avoidance conditioning is not found after septal lesions in the albino rat. This hypothesis, however, has not been supported. For example, Hamilton (1972) was able to find a substantial deficit in one-way active avoidance using albino rats. Of special interest is the fact that the animals showed deficit in terms of when the first avoidance response was made. After making the initial avoidance response, the animals with septal lesions quickly acquired the problem. This type of deficit is like that found in the learning of active avoidance tasks by animals with damage to the amygdala. In addition, Hamilton was able to show that animals with septal lesions were insensitive to manipulation of the cues provided in the training environment. This imperviousness to irrelevant environmental cues in a training situation is also found after destruction of the hippocampus and is in line with the idea that animals with septal area lesions rely on a restricted number of cues in a testing situation.

The deficit in one-way active-avoidance tasks has been attributed to several types of behavioral changes. For example, McCleary (1966) speculated that it was due to the handling that occurred between individual trials in this situation. However, elimination of this handling did not result in improved performance (Thomas & McCleary, 1974); yet this particular test situation may have made performance difficult for the lesioned animals for other reasons. Other studies have found that the elimination of handling can improve the performance of animals with septal lesions in one-way active-avoidance tasks (Bengelloun, 1979; Worsham & Hamilton, 1973).

Another type of explanation of the effects of septal lesions on one- and two-way active-avoidance behaviors is related to a reduced ability of the lesioned animals to use the spatial cues of the situation. When two compartments of an active-avoidance testing situation are physically similar, the animals may not be aware of the new, safe location. Thus, their responses would seem less likely to result in their being aware of the favorable outcome of getting away from the potentially dangerous place. In a one-way situation, it would seem as if they could not get away from the dangerous place. However, Dalby (1970) and Thomas and Thomas (1974) found either no impairment or improved performances after septal lesions when the animals were required to move spatially through a rectangular maze to avoid shock. This finding suggests that the ability of animals with septal lesions to use spatial cues as a basis of avoidance learning is adequate.

By and large, animals with septal lesions trained in avoidance tasks seem similar to animals with hippocampal destruction. Both types of animals show an enhanced rate of acquisition in the two-way avoidance task and an impairment in the acquisition of the one-way avoidance task. It should be emphasized that the changes in learning these tasks found in animals after septal-area or hippocampal destruction are always relative to the performance of normal animals.

The facilitation of performance in avoidance tasks is not restricted to the two-way problem. Duncan and Duncan (1971) found improved acquisition of operant avoidance tasks, using both signaled and unsignaled foot-shocks, in animals with septal lesions. Similar results have been reported by Morgan and Mitchell (1969) and Kelsey and Grossman (1971). The latter authors found that while the septal-lesioned animals acquired the response rapidly, they performed inefficiently in that they made many more responses than necessary to avoid all of the shocks. Sodetz (1970) found that rats with septal lesions acquired an operant avoidance task more readily than controls and that this facilitation of performance could not be accounted for on the basis of the greater number of responses made by the lesioned animals. Schwartzbaum, Green, Beatty, and Thompson (1967) showed the enhanced performance of septal-lesioned animals in the two-way active-avoidance problem to be independent of shock level (but see Sagvolden, 1975), the strength of the conditioned stimulus, the ambient level of illumination, and the gross hyperactivity of the animals. This contribution was especially important because it showed that the improvement in active-avoidance conditioning shown by such animals was not secondary to heightened locomotor activity levels in these animals. This result was supported by the results of the study of Buddington *et al.* (1967) with the squirrel monkey.

Destruction of the neocortex can produce an impairment in the two-way active-avoidance problem. However, if a septal lesion is made in animals that also have neocortical destruction, a facilitation in performance is obtained (Meyer, Johnson, & Vaughn, 1970). A similar result has been found in studies of the effect of hippocampal lesions (Olton & Isaacson, 1969). It is tempting to think that the limbic lesion somehow overrides the changes induced by the neocortical lesion. However, it is also possible that the neocortical and the limbic lesions affect quite different aspects of behavior and that neocortical damage is less influential in affecting avoidance behaviors than septal-area or hippocampal damage. This difference in interpretation could be most important. If the septal damage acted to "cure" the animal suffering from neocortical destruction, this cure would indicate a convergence of the effects of the two types of brain damage on the same output systems. If the two lesions act independently on behavior, then they probably act on different output systems. One approach to the matter would be to try to establish the specific changes in behavioral tactics or strategies produced by neocortical lesions and then to determine if these remain despite the other behavioral changes produced by subcortical lesions.

PERFORMANCE IN APPETITIVE TASKS

Impairments following septal lesions have been found by several groups of researchers when training animals to perform on schedules in which responding at a low rate is reinforced. On such schedules, animals must wait a predetermined number of seconds between responses (Burkett & Bunnell, 1966; Ellen, Wilson, & Powell, 1964; MacDougall, Van Hoesen, & Mitchell, 1969). This impairment takes the form of an inappropriately high rate of responding and a decrease in the number of reinforcements obtained under DRL schedules. If the DRL paradigm is modified to make it into a discrete trial procedure, the abilities of the lesioned animals are not improved (Van Hoesen, MacDougall, Wilson, & Mitchell, 1971). However, if the end of the delay period is originally signaled by a cue light during training and the light is then slowly faded out with further training, the lesioned animals can perform a DRL-20 task as well as controls (Ellen, Dorsett, & Richardson, 1977). Slonaker and Hothersall (1972) found that performance could also be improved with the availability in the operant chamber of wooden blocks that could be gnawed in the delay periods. Another effective remedial procedure is the gradual imposition of the DRL schedule (Caplan & Stamm, 1967). The deficits usually found on this delay schedule cannot be attributed to a general increase in activity or to an enhanced tendency to manipulate objects in the environment (Ellen, Gillenwater, & Richardson, 1977). Ellen *et al.*, however, suggested that the performance of animals with septal lesions can be predicted on the assumption that they exhibit fewer "other behaviors" in the operant chamber than do intact animals. The deficit would be one of a reduced ability to initiate responses. This line of reasoning would predict higher rates of reinforcements on "ratio" schedules, no effect on "interval" schedules, and impaired performance on delay (DRL) schedules. These predictions seem confirmed in the case of ratio and DRL schedules, but lesion effects are found, contrary to expectations, on ratio schedules as well. These effects may occur, however, only under extreme conditions of deprivation (see below). The usual impairment on delay schedules cannot be attributed to a failure of response inhibition, since Kelsey and Grossman (1971) used a shuttlebox DRL-30 task in which septal-lesioned animals made more errors of "anticipation" than of "perseveration." In this task, the animals were trained to shuttle between two compartments, alternating presses on pairs of levers placed in each of the two compartments. To make a correct response, the animals had to wait 30 sec between the time a reinforcement had been produced and the time the next response was made. An anticipatory error was made by moving into the other compartment and responding on a lever in it before 30 sec had elapsed. Kelsey and Grossman's findings suggest that the DRL impairment is not due to a simple failure to inhibit responses as would be expected on the basis of the theory of Ellen *et al.*

The connections of the septal area with the hippocampus seem important to the DRL effect found by Kelsey and Grossman. For example, the behavioral effects could be duplicated by transections of the fornix interconnecting the two structures, but not the medial forebrain bundle (Ross, Grossman, & Grossman, 1975). The section of such ventrally directed fibers did, however, reduce the weight loss and hyperdipsia found after large septal lesions.

Animals with septal lesions show altered patterns of responding on fixed-interval and fixed-ratio schedules (Ellen & Powell, 1962a,b; Lorens & Kondo, 1969; Schwartzbaum & Gay, 1966). Higher-than-normal rates of responses were found on these schedules. The behavior change is especially prominent in the higher ratios of responses to rewards (Hothersall et al., 1970). Johnson and Thatcher (1972) found that animals with septal destruction showed higher response rates on fixed-ratio schedules only when they were under stringent food deprivation. The dependency of the excessively high response rate in fixed-ratio schedules on the nature of the motivational circumstances was also supported by Harvey and Hunt (1965). These authors found that a reduction in the deprivation of the lesioned animals allowed them to exhibit more adequate performance levels on schedules where reinforcements were given intermittently.

The ability of an animal to reverse a learned habit can be considered an indicator of the ability to suppress previously acquired responses. An impaired reversal of position habits has been found in several studies (Donovick, 1968; Hamilton, 1970; Zucker & McCleary, 1964; Schwartzbaum & Donovick, 1968). Gittelson and Donovick (1968) also found a deficit in the reversal of a discrimination learned on kinesthetic cues. Furthermore, lesioned animals tested on the reversal of a brightness discrimination made more errors than controls (Chin, Donovick, & Burright, 1976), although the deficit was most apparent during the first reversal, diminishing with training with repeated reversals (Sikorszky, Donovick, Burright, & Chin, 1977). In a subsequent study (Donovick et al., 1978), animals with septal lesions were trained on problems based on brightness, spatial, or spatiotemporal discriminations. In some testing paradigms, these factors were purposefully confounded. Animals with septal lesions learned a brightness discrimination as rapidly as controls and learned a brightness *and* spatial alternation (combined) more rapidly than controls. Both animals with septal lesions and controls were disrupted by reversals in the reward significance of the cues, but the septal-lesioned animals were more affected by the brightness cue reversal than the spatial cue reversal. This finding suggests that the lesioned animals paid somewhat less attention to the spatial cue during acquisition.

Since both septal-lesioned rats and controls showed the same qualitative dependence on cues but exhibited quantitative differences to certain conditions, Donovick *et al.* believe that the greatest behavioral problem of the lesioned rats is that they focus rapidly on one aspect of the environment and are less likely to base their behavior on other cues. Kratz and Mitchell (1977) have proposed a similar idea. They suggested that the behavior of animals with septal lesions is controlled by the most salient cue available and that subtle cues are useless. Under certain—but not all—conditions, information derived from the response itself may achieve the "most salient" status.

These results indicate that animals with septal lesions need not exhibit impaired performance on reversal tests but, depending on the testing conditions, may show normal or even enhanced abilities. Dabrowska and Pluta (1978) found that when animals with septal lesions were tested on a spatial reversal under dark conditions, no deficit was found. They believe that this procedure eliminated disruptive visual cues with behavioral potencies. Cherry (1975) found enhanced performance of a simple spatial reversal problem, as well as enhanced acquisition, using a procedure in which the animals could respond at their own pace. Cherry believes that the differences in results based on an animal-based time to respond and results reporting impaired performance on spatial reversal problems (Srebro, 1973; Zucker & McCleary, 1964) lie in the fact that these experimenters used procedures in which the animals were paced by the experimenter.

A number of studies using different behavioral paradigms have shown that animals with septal lesions are slower to extinguish responses than control animals on appetitive tasks (Butters & Rosvold, 1968; Cherry, 1975; Pubols, 1966; Schwartzbaum, Kellicutt, Spieth, & Thompson, 1964; Winocur & Mills, 1970) and on the two-way active-avoidance task (LaVaque, 1966). Perhaps the most interesting report is that the degree of resistance to extinction in animals with septal lesions depends on both the motivational circumstances of the animal and its past training history (Fallon & Donovick, 1970). Furthermore, there is evidence that animals with septal lesions can, under certain circumstances, extinguish their responses as fast as, or faster than, normal animals. For example, Brown and Remley (1971) found responses made to escape from foot shock to be extinguished at the same rate by animals with septal lesions and by normal animals. In addition, Fallon and Donovick (1970) found faster extinction relative to control animals when the animals with septal lesions were tested under changed motivational circumstances.

Although animals with septal lesions have been found to exhibit prolonged, inappropriate responding on a variety of operant schedules, there is evidence that bar-press responding can be adequately suppressed (Aaron & Thorne, 1975; Atnip & Hothersall, 1975). The differences in the results obtained in various experimental studies are very likely due to differences in experimental procedures and measurement methods. Henke (1974), for example, found that prolonged training on a partial reinforcement schedule eliminated prolonged responding during extinction. Dickinson's (1972) failure to find enhanced responding after the omission of reinforcement was probably due to the use of a 6-sec time-out period after the omission.

In general, animals with septal lesions respond much more than controls on intermittent reinforcement schedules (e.g., Aaron & Thorne, 1975) and have difficulty in suppressing responses during periods in which no responses should be made, partly because of an enhancement of response rates when reinforcements are unexpectedly omitted (e.g., Poplawsky & Cohen, 1977), although the nature of prior experiences must always be regarded as a factor establishing what is anticipated.

Carlson, Carter, and Vallante (1972) found that septal-lesioned mice easily acquired differential running speeds on alternate trials in a straight runway when rewards were given only on every other trial. The lesioned animals also showed differential running speeds when rewards were given not on alternate trials but on signaled trials presented on a random basis. However, a difference was observed in the performance of lesioned and nonlesioned mice: the septal-lesioned animals learned best when a signal was given before nonrewarded trials, whereas the normal animals learned best when the signal preceded rewarded trials. Enhanced two-bar lever-press alternation (Carlson & Cole, 1970) and enhanced go–no-go alternation in an operant task (Carlson & Norman, 1971) have also been reported.

Studies of the effects of brain lesions on reasoning in rats have usually involved neocortical destruction. Only a few investigations have been made of the effects of limbic system damage on "reasoning." The experimental study of reasoning was first initiated by Maier (1932a,b) and involves three tables with three elevated pathways between them. Hungry animals are required to run from one of the tables to another, on which food has been placed. The animals learn which of the other two tables has food by previously being placed on the goal table and being allowed to see and smell the presence of food. Different combinations of food and start tables are used each day. Animals with septal lesions perform at about chance levels in this situation (50%), while controls give between 80% and 90% correct responses (Stahl & Ellen, 1973). Similar results were found by Rabe and Haddad (1969) after hippocampal lesions. Investigation of the influence of preoperative experiences on the effects of septal area lesions by Stahl and Ellen revealed that preoperative training greatly enhanced the tendency to leave the start table and to investigate the other tables, but it did not increase the percentage of correct choices. Stahl and Ellen (1979) have also found that septal damage created at 1 or 7 days after birth produces the same degree of impairment in the three-table problem when the animals were 90 days old as lesions made in adulthood. No difference in function due to the earliness of the lesion was found.

Based on observed similarities between the effects of septal lesions (Gray, 1970) and those produced by the systemic administration of minor tranquilizers, Gray has proposed that these agents produce their effects on the septohippocampal axis (Gray, Feldon, Rawlins, Owen, & McNaughton, 1978). Recent investigations of this hypothesis have used the partial reinforcement effect, which is a greater resistance to extinction when animals are trained on a partial schedule of reinforcement than after continuous reinforcement. In studies designed to determine whether damage to the medial or the lateral septal area contributes most to this effect, evidence has been reported associating lesions of the medial septal region with effects on both normal extinction and that after partial reinforcement (Feldon & Gray, 1979a,b). However, because of differences in acquisition rates and inconsistencies within the data, these results should be interpreted cautiously.

Grossman and his associates have undertaken to selectively transect fiber bundles connecting the medial septal region with others (see Grossman, 1978, for a review).

Some of the cuts made by Grossman and his associates were across the ventral regions interrupting the septal fibers going into the medial forebrain bundle, while another cut sectioned the septohippocampal fibers in the fornix. On a two-way active-avoidance task, both the septal lesions and the fornix section produced hyperactivity, but the medial forebrain bundle section did not; however, both sections facilitated the acquisition of the avoidance response (Ross, Grossman, & Grossman, 1975). Neither transection produced an impairment on the one-way active-avoidance task or on a passive-avoidance task. These results indicate that the neural substrates for the changes in one- and two-way avoidance tasks may be independent.

Ross, Grossman, and Grossman (1975) found that the fornix transection produced the same enhanced acquisition of the Sidman free-operant avoidance task as large septal lesions.

The effects of transecting the septal fibers passing through the stria medullaris or the stria terminalis were studied by Ross and Grossman (1977). Neither lesion altered one- or two-way avoidance behavior. The conflicting results reported by Van Hoesen, MacDougall, and Mitchell (1969) may have been due to the fact that their lesions (which did influence avoidance behavior) impinged on damage to the habenulopeduncular tract. Stria terminalis lesions also lead to a deficit in passive-avoidance behavior (Ross & Grossman, 1977) but are not found after sections of the fornix, the medial forebrain bundle, or the stria medullaris.

Fornix lesions, but not medial forebrain bundle lesions, interfere with performance on DRL schedules. In a two-lever situation, both animals with fornix lesions and animals with septal area lesions over-respond in an "anticipatory fashion" rather than perseverating on a lever that led to a reward just before. Stria medullaris or stria terminalis lesions fail to produce this effect.

ELECTRICAL STIMULATION OF THE SEPTAL AREA

Electrical stimulation of the septal area was found by Olds and Milner (1954) to produce what appear to be rewarding effects in rats, and similar results have been found in other species. The septal area contains many regions from which rewarding effects can be obtained when electrically stimulated. A question arises, however, about the mechanisms whereby these rewarding effects are achieved and how the septal area interacts with other brain regions that are also related to rewarding events. To study these questions, Miller and Mogenson (1971b) implanted electrodes in both the septal area and the lateral hypothalamus. Animals were trained to depress a bar to obtain electrical stimulation of the lateral hypothalamus at both low and high current levels. As might be expected, the animals responded at higher rates for the high-intensity stimulation. The animals were then tested with electrical pulses delivered to the septal area just before each pulse was applied to the hypothalamus. This procedure produced an increase in the self-stimulation rate when the hypothalamus was being stimulated with low-intensity currents, but a decrease in response rate when the hypothalamus was being stimulated by high-intensity stimulation. A similar result was found by the same authors in a study of the effects of septal stimulation on hypothalamic unit activity. Stimulation of the septal area augmented neuronal discharges when activity was low but decreased them when activity was high (Miller & Mogenson, 1971a). These investigators interpreted their data in accordance with a model in which the septal area and the hypothalamus exert mutual modulating influences on each other. The authors suggested that the different fiber systems that course between the two areas may have different functional roles. The dorsal fornix system arising from cells in the dorsal and midline septal area is thought to exert facilitative influences on the hypothalamus and the stria terminalis system, which contains fibers arising from cells in the ventral septal region thought to be inhibitory on the hypothalamus. These authors also noted that Kant (1969) proposed that two fiber systems in the medial forebrain bundle modulate the septal area antagonistically. Thus, the effects of stimulation of a large region of the septal area could activate two systems that exert antagonistic influences on the hypothalamus and other brain regions.

Some brain stimulation seems to produce pleasurable or rewarding effects, whereas stimulation applied to other brain regions produces effects that can be described as painful or aversive. What are the interactions between these two opposite effects produced by brain stimulation? In a preliminary report in 1963, Routtenberg and Olds found that stimulation of the septal area at an intensity below that required for maintaining self-stimulation attenuated escape reactions elicited by electrical stimulation of the tegmentum. This finding suggested a direct antagonism between the rewarding and the punishing effects produced by brain stimulation, at least where these two brain regions are concerned and under conditions in which the escape responses are produced by brain stimulation as opposed to peripheral shock. Subsequent investigations have extended this line of work by studying the effects of rewarding and punishing states elicited by central stimulation on aversive reactions produced by either brain or peripheral stimulation. Gardner and Malmo (1969) located sites in the ventromedial region of the septal area that produced aversive reactions when electrically stimulated. The dorsal and lateral regions of the septal area produced the pleasurable or rewarding effects on stimulation. Using these positive and negative rewarding zones of the septal area, Gardner and Malmo then studied the effect of stimulation of these zones on the time required for animals to escape from aversive stimulation induced in one of two ways: by electrical shocks applied to the skin of the neck or by stimulation of the dorsal tegmentum. These authors found that septal stimulation in the positively reinforcing zone of the septal area slowed down latencies for escape from the tegmental stimulation, whereas septal stimulation of the negatively reinforcing zones of the septal area facilitated the escape latencies. On the other hand, stimulation in either septal region shortened escape latencies when peripheral shock was applied to the skin of the neck.

The difference between pain produced by peripheral noxious stimulation and by central noxious stimulation is, of course, of considerable interest. For example, painlike responses produced by stimulation of dorsal tegmental sites do not seem to habituate, that is, decrease with repeated periods of stimulation. This type of stimulation tends to produce an "arrest reaction," or immobility. The animals seem to habituate to the painful electrical shocks delivered to the neck, and these shocks do not produce arrest or immobility. In addition, it must be remembered that electrical stimulation applied to the skin of the neck may produce quite different effects from those produced by foot shock. Breglio, Anderson, and Merrill (1970) have found a decrease in responsiveness to electrical foot shock as a result of septal stimulation.

The possibility that rewarding effects induced by septal area stimulation mediate changes in behavior found in tasks based on aversive air puffs and the experience of thirst arises from work by Klemm and Dreyfus (1975). It should also be noted that septal area stimulation is rewarding whether it produces rhythmic, slow activity or desynchronization in the hippocampus (Ball & Gray, 1971). It would appear that the possibility exists that many effects that appear to represent an inhibition of behavior after septal stimulation could be due directly to the rewarding effects that this stimulation produces.

Electrical stimulation of the septal region given before the onset of the conditioned stimulus has been shown to facilitate both one-way and two-way active-avoidance conditioning (Carder, 1971). Electrical stimulation of the septal area has also been shown to disrupt performance in spatial reversal problems (Donovick & Schwartzbaum, 1966), but not the two-bar alternation problem. In this task, animals were trained to run between two compartments. Each compartment had two levers in it. The animals had to press the bars in an alternating sequence in each compartment. In addition, as described above, the animals had to wait 30 sec between bar presses to obtain a reward. Electrical stimulation of the septal region did not affect performance on this task, whereas performance was impaired by lesions of the septal area (Schwartzbaum & Donovick, 1968).

AUTONOMIC EFFECTS PRODUCED BY SEPTAL STIMULATION

Electrical stimulation of the septal area produces several types of effects, and to this point, we have been primarily concerned with those related to behavior in learning situations or circumstances in which an animal depresses a bar or lever to produce stimulation of its own brain. These behavioral effects may be related to changes in the activity of the internal organs mediated by the autonomic nervous system. The effects of septal area stimulation on the autonomic nervous system were studied extensively by Kaada (1951). He found that septal area stimulation generally produced inhibitory effects on the autonomic nervous system in the anesthetized animal. These observations led to the general inhibitory theory of septal area function postulated by McCleary (1961), mentioned before.

One direction of more recent work has been that of Holdstock and his collaborators. In one study, Holdstock (1967) found that electrical stimulation of the septal area produced a cardiac deceleration without any effect on the galvanic skin response. This effect was reduced by the systemic administration of methyl atropine or atropine sulfate, and consequently, it was thought to be mediated by cholinergic fibers of the vagus nerve (Chalmers & Holdstock, 1969). On the other hand, Sideroff, Schneiderman, and Powell (1971) believe that the bradycardia resulting from septal area stimulation is a result of a compensatory rebound from a brief period of sympathetic activation. These authors detected increases in blood pressure resulting from septal area stimulation and viewed the delayed, more prominent, cardiac deceleration as being a parasympathetic rebound. These authors also found a difference in the effects produced by stimulation in the lateral and the medial septal areas. Stimulation of the lateral septal area produced a decrease in heart rate, whereas stimulation of the medial septal area produced a brief increase followed by a long-lasting decrease. Previously, Malmo (1965) had reported a cardiac acceleration from stimulation in the medial septal region.

Holdstock (1970) found a normal acquisition of differential heart-rate responses to different stimuli following septal lesions. He also found a clear dissociation of the increases in motoric activity from the increases in the activity of the autonomic nervous system, and he felt that a good general description of his results would be that the animals had lost normal sympathetic reactivity under certain conditions.

Stimulation of the septal area can influence drinking elicited by hypothalamic stimulation. Sibole, Miller, and Mogenson (1971) found that concurrent stimulation of the medial-septal-area region and the hypothalamus facilitates drinking, whereas electrode locations in, or near, the bed nucleus of the stria terminalis produce a reduction in drinking. These results are related to presumed differences between the fibers of the fornix and those of the stria terminalis mentioned above. Chronic stimulation of the septal area decreases spontaneous drinking, even the drinking of animals that have been deprived of water for 24 hr. Of special interest is the fact that the septal stimulation does not reduce the incidence of drinking but shortens the duration of the drinking bouts (Wishart & Mogenson, 1970b).

NEUROCHEMICAL CONSIDERATIONS

Proper understanding of the relationship of the septal area to behavior depends on an understanding of the role of the septal area in the various neurotransmitter systems of the brain. Lesions in the septal area have been found to produce decreased levels of acetyl-choline in the cortex and in the hippocampus, but not in the brain stem (Pepeu, Mulas, Ruffi, & Sotgiu, 1971). Sorensen and Harvey

(1971) found that the decrease in acetylcholine in the cortex occurred only in rats that were also made hyperdipsic by the lesions. Stimulation of the septal area has been shown to increase the acetylcholine output of the neocortex (Szerb, 1967), and Pepeu, Bartolini, and Deffenu (1970) found that the acetylcholine output does not increase in the neocortex of animals with septal lesions following the administration of amphetamine, as it does in intact animals. Kelsey and Grossman (1975) have reported that lesions of the medial septal area eliminate the effects of cholinergic drugs on DRL performances but not their effects on free operant responding.

When injected into the septal area, the cholinergic blocking agent atropine produces animals that are deficient in passive-avoidance behavior but that are unimpaired on position reversal and on the learning of a one-way active-avoidance response. This finding indicates that the cholinergic blockade of the septal area produced by the atropine reproduces some, but not all, of the effects produced by lesions (Hamilton, McCleary, & Grossman, 1968). It does not affect activity or photophobia (Kelsey & Grossman, 1969). Cholinergic blockade in the medial and ventral aspects of the septal area produces enhancement of the acquisition of the two-way active-avoidance task. This result mimics the effects produced by septal lesions. Since hippocampal lesions also produce a facilitation of two-way active-avoidance learning, this may indicate that the septal-hippocampal system that mediates these activities is cholinergic in nature. In fact, Warburton and Russell (1969) have suggested that there is a cholinergic path of reticular formation origin that courses through the medial septal area and reaches the hippocampus. Whether or not this pathway is excitatory or inhibitory relative to behavior is uncertain, since while cholinergic stimulation often affects performance in avoidance tasks this need not be a sign of a general inhibitory effect. Holloway (1972), for example, found that carbachol injections into the medial septal area reduced the number of avoidance responses made by cats and at the same time shortened the latency of the avoidance responses that were made. Greene (1968) has reported that carbachol injections into the medial septal area increased open-field locomotor activity. These observations suggest that there are effects generally considered excitatory in nature that result from cholinergic stimulation of the septal area. Most likely, the effects of chemical stimulation of the septal area can best be considered in terms of specific changes induced and not in terms of more global behavioral changes such as alterations in excitability.

Septal lesions influence a variety of neurochemical systems in the brain, and therefore, it is not surprising that such lesions influence the reaction of animals to adrenergic stimulation. There is evidence that different behavioral consequences of septal area lesions are selectively affected by amphetamine. Novick and Pihl (1969) found that the drug produced an enhancement of locomotor activity in animals with septal lesions. A dose of 3 mg/kg produced incessant exploration and pacing to a greater extent in lesioned animals than in control animals. The 9 mg/kg dose used by Novick and Pihl produced the stereotyped head-moving responses associated with large doses of amphetamine (probably owing to increased activity in the dopaminergic systems) equally in both septal-lesioned and sham-operated animals. Amphetamine did not alter the improved two-way active-avoidance performance or the impaired passive-avoidance behavior of the animals with septal lesions. At high levels of amphetamine, the drug did impair control animals in the passive-avoidance task, but it was at this drug level (9 mg/kg) that the animals had greatly reduced locomotor activity in the open-field situation. In normal animals, high levels of amphetamine decrease locomotor activity but increase reactivity to unexpected stimuli (e.g., noise, air puffs, or being captured) to a level near that of the septal-lesioned animals without the drug.

Lesions of the septal area that induce hyperreactivity have also been reported to produce decreases in whole brain norepinephrine and dopamine levels 2 days after surgery (Bernard, Berchek, & Yutzey, 1975), although other investigators have not found this result (e.g., Montgomery & Christian, 1973) at 6 days after the lesions. Donovick, Burright, Fanelli, and Engellenner (1981) failed to find decreased catecholamine levels in any of three strains of mice about 2 weeks after surgery. These investigators found enhanced norepinephrine turnover in one strain (HET), decreased turnover in another (C57), and no change in the third (RF). However, it is likely that catecholamine levels are not constant over time after a lesion and that regional differences occur. The conditions occurring before the brain samples are taken may also play a significant role in the results. For example, Brick, Burright, and Donovick (1979) found that animals with septal lesions had smaller reductions in brain norepinephrine (NE) after 3 hr of restraint stress than controls. However, the septal lesioned animals struggled more in the restraint period than controls. This behavioral difference could have led to a different degree of catecholamine utilization. In such studies it is important to distinguish direct neural causes of biochemical changes from those that may be secondary to behavioral alterations.

Bernard *et al.* (1975) found that only one of the regions they examined (i.e., the hypothalamus) had significant reduction in catecholamine levels 2 days after septal lesions. No change in serotonin levels was observed in this region. However, these authors found no change in catecholamine dynamics. Gage and Olton (1976) found that the disappearance of the hyperreactivity produced by septal lesions could be accelerated by the systemic administration of L-dopa, which enhances catecholamine availability. Septal irritability (Dominguez & Longo, 1969) and shock-induced aggression (Jones, Barchas, & Eichelman, 1976) are both rapidly reduced by the administration of *p*-chlorophenylalanine (PCPA). However, since the drug effect is so rapid in onset and the serotonin effects are so slow in occurring, the PCPA-induced effects do not imply a serotonin mediation of irritability or hyperreactivity. In fact, they suggest a catecholamine basis, since catecholamine is affected earlier after PCPA administration than is indolamine. Other catecholamine agonists share the ability of L-dopa to reduce septal-lesion–induced hyperreactivity and irritability (Marotta, Logan, Potegal, Glusman, & Gardner, 1977). Further evidence supporting a catecholamine basis for septal area hyperreactivity comes from a study in which α-adrenergic antagonists were placed directly in regions near the anterior septal area. They induced effects resembling those found after septal area damage (Albert & Richmond, 1977). Dopaminergic, cholinergic, or α-adrenergic drugs failed to do so. However, the effective sites of injection were very likely outside the septal area itself and near the edge of the nucleus accumbens. Morphine injected into the ventral hippocampus or the amygdala can attenuate the hyperresponsiveness to external stimulation produced by the septal lesions (Valdes, Cameron, Evans, & Gage, 1980). The way in which morphine influenced behavior was different in the two regions, however. Morphine injected into the posterior hypothalamus was only partly effective in altering these behavioral effects.

REFLECTIONS AND SUMMARY

The rage reaction that appears after septal area damage in the rodents and to a limited degree in certain other species has probably misled us into thinking the area to be closely associated with exaggerated emotional behaviors. However, the rage reaction is transient and leaves behind a somewhat decreased responsiveness under low or moderate motivation levels. The effect of septal area damage on social interactions depends on both the genetic inheritances of the tested animals and the specific septal areas lesioned. By and large, the dominance of animals with septal lesions is reduced, possibly due to a reluctance to exhibit aggressive acts.

Damage to the septal area often produces more rapid acquisition of a two-way active-avoidance problem and an impaired ability to acquire a passive-avoidance task. These results are generally similar to those frequently found after hippocampal damage and opposite to what occurs after large amygdala lesions. However, it must be noted that all of these effects must be tempered by the realization that what actually is found in an experiment depends on the genetics, history, and postoperative experiences of the subjects. The actual conditions of testing also help determine the effects of septal area damage.

From a variety of studies, it appears that the septal area plays a role in the use of environmental stimulation. Low-saliency stimuli are poorly used by animals with septal lesions whereas their behavior seems to be dominated by stimuli of high saliency. In normal animals the septal area helps the individual pay attention to the less significant stimuli in the environment.

The septal area is an important modulator of autonomic reactions and coordinated bodily reactions. One interesting aspect of the studies on septal area interventions has been the achievement of a dissociation of different autonomic reactions produced by stimulation in different regions of the septal area. This dissociation indicates that the septal area is heterogeneous in regard to its influence on the internal organs as well as on behavior. In this regard, it should be considered not a functional unit but a collection of coordinated nuclear groups, each with certain specificities in the regions and systems being modulated.

5

The Hippocampus

In this chapter, some of the behavioral contributions made by another of the limbic system structures, the hippocampus, are described. The approach of the two preceding chapters is followed once again. The general changes produced by hippocampal destruction or stimulation are discussed first.

GENERAL CHANGES PRODUCED BY HIPPOCAMPAL DAMAGE

Just as found after septal area damage, the consequences of hippocampal damage or stimulation depend on the genetic inheritance of the animals, on their pre- and postoperative experiences, and on the precise nature of the testing or observation conditions. Examples of the effects of these variables are given throughout the chapter. Nevertheless, it is possible to provide a general idea of the usual consequences found after hippocampal damage, given the common routines of most laboratories and the strains of animals most often used. After bilateral hippocampal damage, animals are active, seemingly eager to begin new behavioral sequences, although they often fail to persist in a particular goal-oriented activity as long as intact animals. In some ways, the changes are similar to those found after damage to the septal area, except that the transitory rage reaction is absent. The increased tendency to be active and the corresponding reduced tendency to become immobile are found in many situations.

For example, when confronted by a cat from which there is no escape, rats with hippocampal lesions tend to be more active and to exhibit fewer freezing responses than do control animals. When they can escape from the cat, rats with hippocampal damage do so more rapidly than normal animals (Blanchard & Blanchard, 1972). In normal animals, fear can lead to attempts at active escape or immobility (freezing), but the animals with hippocampal lesions are more likely to respond actively than to freeze.

The reduction in the number of freezing responses exhibited by animals with hippocampal lesions could be related to a decrease in the intensity of fear elicited by the threatening stimulus. Kim, Kim, Kim, Kim, Chang, Kim, and Lee (1971) found a reduction in aggressive acts following hippocampal lesions. These authors also reported the animals to be less fearful in general. This finding may be related to the observation that hippocampal lesions also tend to produce a reduction in shock-induced aggression, which is independent of changes in the threshold of the animals to the electrical foot shock (Eichelman, 1971). But if fear is reduced after hippocampal lesions and if this reduction is related to the reduction of the immobility response, the relationship may be complicated, since (1) a reduction in fear could cause a reduction in freezing; (2) a reduction in freezing could produce lessened fear; (3) a reduction in freezing could cause fewer behavioral signs of fear, but the animals could have internal fear responses of an intensity equal to those found in normal animals; or (4) both the decrease in the immobility response and the reduction in fear could be caused by alterations in independent neural mechanisms. Certainly, alterations in fear responses cannot account for the changes found in active-avoidance paradigms in which the animals with hippocampal lesions learn some problems (e.g., two-way active avoidance) more readily than intact animals.

Even though behavioral freezing is reduced by hippocampal damage in fear-related situations, including the reduced responding used as the index of conditioned emotional responses (e.g., Thomas, Hostetter, & Barker, 1968), not all forms of immobility are affected in the same way. Hippocampal lesions *increase* the occurrence and the duration of tonic immobility (contact defensive immobility) induced by the inversion of rabbits (Woodruff, Hatton, & Meyer, 1975). Therefore, the effect of hippocampal destruction cannot be interpreted on the basis of an increased tendency to be active.

Animals with hippocampal lesions tend to have normal circadian rhythms. However, during the daytime, when sleep is the predominant occupation of nocturnal animals, rats with hippocampal lesions tend to sleep less than control animals (Jarrard, 1968; Kim, Choi, Kim, Chang, Park, & Kang, 1970). Even though the animals sleep less during the day, the occurrence of sleep episodes and of slow-wave sleep actually increases within the daylight period. Fast-wave sleep (REM sleep) is reduced, probably because of the reduction of the length of sleep episodes. Lesions restricted to the neocortex also produce a reduction in the occurrence of REM sleep. The results of Kim, Choi, Kim, Kim, Huh, and Moon (1971) show that animals with hippocampal lesions show an increase in the frequency with which many behavior patterns, including sleep, are undertaken, but that the durations of the activities are so reduced that the total time spent in them is less than, or equal to, that of normal animals. Kim *et al.* (1970) found such effects in visitations to the food well and grooming during the evening hours. Glickman, Higgins, and Isaacson (1970) found that gerbils with hippocampal lesions tend to engage in many activities more frequently than their normal counterparts, even though the total time spent in the activities is unchanged or even reduced. Similar observations were made by Vanderwolf, Kolb, and Cooley (1978).

The greatest increase in activity of many kinds is found in the dark portion of light–dark cycles, when rats with hippocampal lesions seem greatly energized in their home cages (Jarrard, 1968). Whether this effect is due to changes in circadian rhythmicity or to conditions of illumination is not absolutely clear. The lighting conditions during testing play an important role in determining activity, as is documented below.

In an attempt to determine the behavioral effects of selective damage to various hippocampal efferents, Jarrard (1976) has found that enhanced home-cage activity increases as much after damage to the fimbria as after complete hippocampal removal. He attributed this effect to the fact that such lesions appear to interrupt the hippocampal projections to the septal area and to the nucleus of the diagonal band. If this interpretation is correct, it could be that the cholinergic input to the hippocampus from the medial septal area and the nucleus of the diagonal band becomes uncoupled from normal feedback from the hippocampus. The cholinergic systems are likely to play an important role in regulating the hippocampus, since several behavioral changes similar to those found after hippocampal damage occur after systemic administration of the cholinergic antagonist scopolamine (e.g., Douglas & Isaacson, 1966; Suits & Isaacson, 1968). However, Davis and Kent (1979) have presented evidence that interruption of the fibers of hippocampal formation origin (subiculum) that reach the anterior thalamic nucleus may also play a part in the hyperactivity found after section of the fornix system. It is possible that the increase in the activity of hippocampally lesioned animals can be induced in several ways and thus is "overdetermined." A related approach (Reinstein *et al.*, in press) indicating a role for the basal ganglia system in lesion-induced hyperactivity is presented in the next section.

Reductions in the amount of rearing displayed by animals with septal lesions has been reported (Kemble & Nagel, 1975; Laughlin, Donovick, & Burright, 1975). However, Kemble, Studelska, and Nagel (1976) were unable to find chanages in rearing after small lesions of the dorsal hippocampus. Reinstein (1981) found that rats with large hippocampal lesions rear less in open fields but rear more frequently than controls 1 or 2 weeks after surgery in a smaller, high-walled, circular test situation. Even though the animals reared more frequently at these postoperative times, their durations of rearing bouts were less, and the total duration of time spent rearing was not different from that of controls. Animals with hippocampal lesions tested 4 weeks after surgery were not different from controls in their rearing behaviors in the circular test apparatus, although they still reared less frequently in an open field. Therefore, the effect of hippocampal damage on rearing depends on both the time after surgery and the specific circumstances of testing.

It is difficult to overemphasize the importance of the time after surgery at which behavioral observations are made. Brain damage, whether it be of the hippocampus, the cortex, or the brain stem, is best seen as initiating a number of secondary changes in the remaining tissue. These secondary changes, either singly or collectively, may be responsible for the changes observed in behavior rather than the direct loss of the tissue (see Isaacson, 1976). Unfortunately, too little attention has been directed to the study of behavioral change after experimental brain damage, and the studies of clinical brain damage are often terminated after the patients leave the hospital although they have still not returned to a normal mental or behavioral condition.

Some information is available, however. Kimble and his co-workers have reported the time course of changes in spontaneous alternation, locomotor activity, and maze learning in animals repeatedly tested for extended postoperative periods following hippocampal destruction (Kimble, 1976; Kimble & Dannen, 1977). In these experiments, activity increases returned toward normal after 16 days after surgery, and there was a tendency for spontaneous alternation to increase toward normal levels. However, in subsequent studies, the effect on spontaneous alternation seems to be permanent, remaining at chance levels even 8 months after surgery (Kimble, Anderson, Bremiller, & Dannen, 1979; Kimble, Bremiller, Stickrod, & Smotherman, 1980). It is of interest that in these last two experiments, no behavioral influence of catecholaminergic axons sprouting from fibers originating from the superior cervical ganglion could be detected.

Other studies of the time course of changes after hippocampal lesions without repeated testing have been reported using spontaneously occurring behaviors (Reinstein *et al.*, in press). While the general trend of this work is similar to the results of Kimble's group, some differences do exist and are probably related to the conditions of testing and postoperative experiences.

Locomotor Activity

It is now well established that animals with hippocampal lesions exhibit enhanced locomotor activity in certain types of situations. A number of studies, reviewed by Douglas (1967) and Kimble (1968), have reported this hyperactivity in open-field situations. In general, hyperactivity is most frequently found in large, open areas and is seldom found in running wheels (Douglas & Isaacson, 1964) or in home cages (Kim *et al.*, 1970). However, this is not a universal finding. Whether or not increased locomotion is found depends on the size of the testing arena, the point in the circadian period at which testing occurs, and the lighting conditions, as well as the genetic and experiential histories of the subjects.

Isaacson and McClearn (1978) studied the effect of hippocampal lesions on the activity of mice inbred to be high or low in locomotor activity by DeFries and Hegmann (1970). Lesions of either the hippocampus or the posterior neocortex produced increased activity in the low-activity strain but a *decrease* in the activity of the high-activity strain (see Figure 16). The reduced locomotor activity found in the high-activity strain was surprising, and in an attempt to further understand these results, the level of ambient illumination was reduced from the moderate levels normally used for testing. Under the low level of ambient illumination, mice of both strains with hippocampal destruction were more active than animals with neocortical lesions or the sham-operated control animals.

In these strains of mice, neocortical destruction induced behavioral changes that were similar in direction to those found when the hippocampus was also damaged. This result is usually not found in other species (see also Jarrard & Bunnell, 1968). However, the damage in these mice with cortical "control" lesions may have included more of the entorhinal and retrosplenial cortex than in other species. Enhanced locomotor activity has been reported after damage to the entorhinal cortex. This hyperactivity develops over the first week after surgery and remains at 5 times that of control animals for several weeks at least (Entingh, 1971; Stewart, Loesche, & Horton, 1977; Lasher & Stewart, 1981). Locomotor activity increases also develop within the first week after hippocampal destruction (Lanier & Isaacson, 1975) and probably reach their asymptote by 14 days postoper-

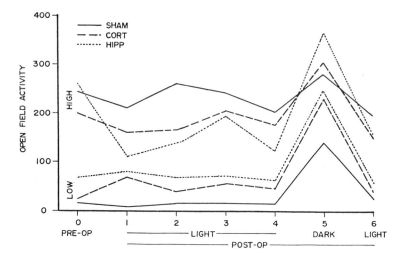

Figure 16. Open-field activity of high- and low-activity lines of selectively bred mice after sham operations (SHAM), neocortical (CORT), or hippocampal (HIPP) lesions. All testing sessions, except Session 5, were conducted in bright illumination. From "The Influence of Hippocampal Damage on Locomotor Behavior of Mice Selectively Bred for High or Low Activity in the Open Field" by R. L. Isaacson and G. E. McClearn, Brain Research, *1978, 150, 559–567. Copyright 1978 by Elsevier-North Holland. Reprinted by permission.*

atively (Reinstein *et al.*, in press). Lesions of the dorsal hippocampus induced by the neurotoxin kainic acid also induce hyperactivity in the open field (Muñoz & Grossman, 1980), although lesions made by other means restricted to the dorsal hippocampus often fail to produce this effect (e.g., Lanier & Isaacson, 1975). It would appear that disruption of activities at either the cortical or the septal end of the septohippocampal axis can induce hyperactivity when animals are tested in open environments.

The increased locomotor activity found after hippocampal lesions can be reduced by the administration of a specific type of dopamine receptor agonist (3,4-dihydroxy-phenyl-amino)-2-imidazoline (DPI) to the nucleus accumbens, a part of the basal ganglia system of the forebrain (Reinstein, 1981; Reinstein *et al.*, in press). The hippocampal formation has strong anatomical connections to this area, and the dopaminergic projections to the nucleus accumbens have been associated with behavioral changes strikingly similar to those found after hippocampal destruction. Destruction of the dopamine-containing cells that project to the frontal cortex and to the nucleus accumbens produces changes that include hyperactivity, especially during the dark portion of the day–night cycle; spillage of food while eating; and difficulties in passive-avoidance learning (Galey, Simon, & Le Moal, 1977). This cell destruction also facilitates active-avoidance learning (Thierry, Tassin, Blanc, & Glowinski, 1976). All of these changes have been found after hippocampal lesions, as well.

The increase in locomotor activity and the reductions of dopamine in the cortical and accumbens regions are highly correlated (Tassin, Stinus, Simon, Blanc, Thierry, Le Moal, Cardo, & Glowinski, 1978). Furthermore, certain of the behavioral consequences of hippocampal damage can be offset or reduced by the systemic administration of low doses of the dopamine antagonist haloperidol. This result suggests a "dopamine connection" in regard to hyperactivity after hippocampal damage. Therefore, it is not extremely surprising that the activation of dopaminergic mechanisms of the nucleus accumbens by the direct administration of DPI could influence activity levels after hippocampal destruction. It was of interest in the study of Reinstein *et al.* (in press) that the net effect of the hippocampal damage was equivalent to a reduction of the dopaminergic input to the accumbens and that enhancement of a type of dopaminergic activity could reduce this effect.

While most emphasis has been placed on the relation between

alterations of dopamine activity in the basal ganglia and activity, the frontal neocortex should not be forgotten. Frontal neocortical lesions can themselves induce hyperactivity, and the strongest correlation between dopamine content and activity was found for this tissue (Tassin *et al.*, 1978). Bär, Gispen, and Isaacson (1981) reported long-lasting biochemical responsiveness in the dorsal frontal cortex after hippocampal lesions. These changes may play a role in fostering similar alterations in the caudate nucleus after hippocampal damage—alterations that must be indirect since hippocampal–caudate interconnections have not been found.

Exploration

Despite the increases in locomotion found after hippocampal destruction, the lesioned animal may fail to make effective use of the information gained from its locomotor excursions. Kimble and Greene (1968) discovered that animals with bilateral hippocampal damage fail to use information derived from pretraining exploration of a Lashley III maze in subsequent acquisition training. While being trained to navigate the maze, animals with hippocampal destruction that had investigated the maze more actively than normal animals were no better off than animals that had not done so. The problem may be the assumption that increased locomotor activity implies a greater amount of "exploration." The term *exploration* implies an investigative attitude, an orientation toward environmental stimuli, and the processing of information derived from the activity. The problem also has to do with the ways in which exploration and its effects on the animal are measured. Suess and Berlyne (1978) found that animals with hippocampal damage were affected as much as control animals by preexposure to a complex visual stimulus as measured by the initial measurement after the preexposure but failed to show reductions across repeated testing sessions. These authors believed that this effect could be due to a failure of the experience gained in the preexposure period to be equally reflected in all forms of behavior. The dissociation of information obtained by people and animals after brain damage from their use of it has been discussed by Isaacson and Spear (in press).

Another form of exploration is the tendency for rodents to poke their heads into small holes, presumably to sample the environment on the "other side." It doesn't seem to matter if the holes are in the walls or in the floor; the response is roughly equivalent. The effects of hippocampal destruction on the tendency for rats to poke their heads through holes in the floor has recently been made by Reinstein *et al.* (in press), using a device similar to that used by File and Wardill (1975) to separate exploration and locomotion. When examined either 2 or 4 weeks after surgery, animals with hippocampal lesions investigated the holes more frequently than control animals, although their average duration of the hole-poke response was reduced by about 30%. The total time spent making the exploratory responses by animals with hippocampal lesions was not different from that of the control animals. This result is at odds with the notion put forth by O'Keefe and Nadel (1978) that animals with hippocampal damage spend less time in the exploration of an open arena. It should also be noted that contrary to the description of rats in an open field provided by O'Keefe and Nadel (p. 255), the rats with nearly complete hippocampal destruction studied by Reinstein *et al.* (in press) did not merely run around the walls in a stereotyped fashion but went into the center of the apparatus more frequently than controls and, while there, investigated the centrally located holes. Since the exploratory hole-poking response was uncorrelated with locomotion, the two responses are different aspects of behavior. Neither behavior showed a decrement over time (i.e., habituation) in the test situation.

Therefore, it appears that while animals with large hippocampal lesions explore their environments at least as frequently as controls, the question remains of how much useful information is derived from this behavior. It is possible that this information is less because of the reduced time given to each response by the lesioned animals. Therefore, it will be useful to consider the reaction to their sensory environment of animals with hippocampal damage.

Distractibility and the Use of Cues

Animals with hippocampal destruction seem to be less distractible while performing goal-oriented behavioral acts. Early studies on behavioral distractibility after hippocampal lesions indicated that these animals were less disturbed by the introduction of irrelevant stimuli into the middle of a runway while working for food rewards when hungry (Wickelgren & Isaacson, 1963; Raphelson, Isaacson, & Douglas, 1965; Gustafson, 1975). A distinction must be made between distractibility and reactivity. *Distractibility* means the extent to which a goal-oriented set of actions is disrupted by an unexpected stimulus, whereas *reactivity* means the magnitude of the animal's reactions to the unexpected. Animals with hippocampal lesions are sometimes more reactive than intact animals to unexpected stimulation. For example, gerbils with hippocampal destruction respond more intensely than normal animals to intense levels of auditory or visual stimulation in stabilimeter cages (Ireland & Isaacson, 1968). The startle responses elicited by auditory stimulation are also increased by hippocampal destruction in the rat (Coover & Levine, 1972).

Recent research has stressed the importance of the ongoing behavioral sequence in determining the degree to which animals with hippocampal lesions are distracted by novel or unexpected stimuli (Kaplan, 1968; Crowne & Riddell, 1969), but normal orientation to novel auditory or visual stimulation is found if the stimulus is presented when the lesioned animals are inactive (Hendrickson, Kimble, & Kimble, 1969).

When animals with hippocampal lesions are trained in behavioral discrimination tasks, poor performances can be due to the use of low-intensity or low-saliency cues. For example, Plunkett (1978) found that the addition of a conspicuous light to the goal area of a maze greatly improved the performance of lesioned animals relative to controls. Plunkett and Faulds (1979) reported that hippocampal damage impaired performance only on discrimination tasks in which the cues were not distinctive. Along this same line, Bauer (1974) found that performance on a discrimination task by animals with hippocampal lesions depended on whether the positive stimulus or the negative stimulus was more salient. Impaired performances occurred when the negative stimulus was more salient.

While the distinctiveness of the cues is important for adequate performance by the lesioned animals, they also process environmental information differently. When compound stimuli (light–tone) are used during training, animals with hippocampal lesions seem to form associations to both components (Freeman, 1978). When tested in a compound stimulus paradigm in which one component normally "blocks" the response to another (e.g., Kamin, 1968, 1969), lesioned rabbits and rats respond to both components (Solomon, 1977; Rickert, Bennett, Lane, & French, 1978). Rickert, Lorden, Dawson, Smyly, and Callahan (1979) have reported that animals with hippocampal damage respond equivalently to stimuli that are consistently or intermittently associated with reward in situations in which the stimulus always associated with reward usually "overshadows" and eliminates responding to the less consistent cue in intact animals. It would appear, therefore, that even when detected, stimuli are used differently by animals with hippocampal damage. This finding was confirmed in an interesting fashion by Buzsáki, Grastyán, Mód, and Winiczai (1980). Thirsty rats were trained to press a lever that turned on a tone originating from a speaker near a water delivery device. The lever was at one end of a straight alley; the tone and the water device were at the other. When, after some days of training, the speaker was moved to the middle of the alley, normal animals executed the response more slowly, indicating a "conflict" induced by the change. This conflict was not observed in animals with fornix lesions. Buzsáki et al. believe that the lesioned animals use the tone only as a trigger to release the approach response to the water dispenser, whereas the control animals learn to make approach responses both to the sound and to the dispenser. When the speaker is moved, a conflict in responding is thought to develop in the intact animals.

There are several reports of decreased habituation by rats with damage to the hippocampus (e.g., Douglas & Isaacson, 1964; Roberts, Dember, & Brodwick, 1962; H. Teitelbaum & Milner, 1963). A similar deficit was found by Douglas and Pribram (1969) in monkeys. These animals show no signs of habituation to the repeated presentation of a distracting stimulus as measured by the speed with which the response is made. On the other hand, habituation *is* found if the number of actual responses to the distracting stimulus is counted. These results point out an important difference between the response and the speed measures of distractibility and habituation.

Spontaneous Alternation

The tendency for animals to alternate visits to the two goal boxes of a T-maze on consecutive trials when a reward is not provided for responses to either goal box has been called *spontaneous alternation*. In a sense, it reflects an unlearned tendency of animals not to repeat visits to the same goal box regions on two consecutive opportunities. Douglas (1966) demonstrated that spontaneous alternation in normal animals arises from a tendency of the animal to visit alternately the *spatial locations* of the two goal boxes in two-choice T-mazes. Sherrick, Brunner, Roth, and Dember (1979) have extended Douglas's work to show that rats' tendency is to avoid repeating a direction of movement through space. On the second trial, they do not prefer a direction of movement *opposite* to that of the initial response; rather they seek to avoid repeating the direction of the first response. Animals with bilateral hippocampal destruction do not exhibit this spontaneous alternation behavior, as a rule (Roberts *et al.*, 1962; Douglas & Isaacson, 1964; Muñoz & Grossman, 1980). This finding is important because it suggests that the deficit produced by the hippocampal lesion involves the spatial organization of the animal's environment, an issue extensively pursued by O'Keefe and Nadel (1978). Ellen and De-Loache (1968) have presented additional evidence that an inability to use spatial cues is found in animals with dorsal hippocampal lesions, and this inability could result in the impaired spontaneous alternation performance. However, it must be pointed out that small electrolytic lesions of restricted regions of the hippocampus are rarely effective in altering spontaneous alternation on a long-term basis. Usually, large, almost complete, bilateral lesions are required.

Douglas (1975) believes that the close correlation found between the time of onset of behavioral alternation during development and the time of maturation of the cells of the dentate gyrus implies a causal relationship. Frederickson and Frederickson (1979) have found a sudden emergence of spontaneous alternation in the kitten at the time that the anatomical organization of the hippocampus is well progressed. This finding supports the idea that many forms of behavior emerge only when the hippocampus becomes capable of nearly adult types of function (see Altman, Brunner, & Bayer, 1973).

The work of Douglas and his associates also makes it likely that the cholinergic systems of the brain are strongly associated with spontaneous alternation. Spontaneous alternation is abolished by scopolamine (Douglas & Isaacson, 1966; Meyers & Domino, 1964). Treatment with physostigmine can induce spontaneous alternation in rabbits (Baisden, Isaacson, Woodruff, & Van Hartesveldt, 1972). A further association between cholinergic mechanisms related to the hippocampus comes from the report of Dudar, Whishaw, and Szerb (1979). They found that sensory stimulation increased the release of acetylcholine from the hippocampus and that this effect was abolished by lesions of the septal area. The sensory-induced release was abolished by a cholinergic receptor-blocking agent. A similar release of acetyl-choline by motor activity was not.

Subanesthetic doses of pentobarbital also act to reduce or elim-inate spontaneous alternation, although through mechanisms that differ from those affected by scopolamine (Douglas & Truncer, 1976). Douglas and Truncer have made a strong case for the proposal that the action of both drugs is on the hippocampal formation.

Dalland (1970) reported that animals with limbic system lesions tended to perseverate their responses in a T-maze instead of alter-nating them. This result is related to the theory of Lash (1964), who found an increase in response perseveration when the motor aspects of the response were made more discriminable. While a deficit in response inhibition cannot explain all of the behavioral debilities pro-duced by hippocampal destruction, animals with hippocampal lesions may, in fact, tend to perseverate responses in some situations, per-haps because the animals are not able to utilize information about the spatial location of the goal boxes as normal animals do and fall back on other sources of information. They must respond on the basis of less preferred cues, for example, the stimuli in the arms of the T-maze or the stimulation produced by the responses themselves. In a sub-sequent study using a procedure that isolated the effects of spatial location, cues associated with each goal arm, and the tendency to perseverate turning right or left in the maze, Dalland (1976) reported that small dorsal lesions of the hippocampus produced a persevera-tion of responses in the T-maze. In several ways, her procedures differed from those used by most investigators. They included the use of highly differentiated goal arms (black–white), group housing of the animals, the placing of the animals on a "holding board" after the first trial, small lesions, and the beginning of testing only a week after surgery. Any of these factors may be related to the response perseveration that Dalland found and that is usually not observed in other studies. Of particular interest is the fact that animals were tested in their colony room and consequently were exposed to familiar odors. Wigal, Goodlett, Eisenberg, Spear, Hannigan, Donovick, Burright, and Isaacson (1981) have found that testing septal-lesioned animals in the presence of familiar odors produces very different behavior in spontaneous alternation from testing with novel odors present.

There are several reports that animals with hippocampal lesions can exhibit spontaneous alternation behavior under changed testing circumstances. For example, Kirkby, Stein, Kimble, and Kimble (1967) confined animals for 50 min in the T-maze arm chosen on the first trial. Animals with hippocampal damage chose the other goal arm as frequently as controls on the second test. A similar result was observed by R. Stevens (1973). However, these results cannot be regarded as reflecting spontaneous alternation as normally studied with short delays. The confinement for a period of minutes could induce an aversion to the arm in all animals, or perhaps selectively in those with limbic system damage; and the choice of the other goal arm on the second test trial may only indicate an aversion to the place of confinement. The hippocampal lesions in both the Kirkby *et al.* and the Stevens experiments were also far from complete and spared a great deal of both dorsal and ventral hippocampal tissue.

Dalland (1976) also reported the enhancement of alternation in her animals with small hippocampal lesions when the animals were forced to turn right or left in the T-maze. Both hippocampally lesioned and control subjects made the response previously not forced on their next opportunity. This effect is very likely due to an aversion to the forced turn on trial 1 rather than to a true spontaneous alternation.

The question of whether spontaneous alternation can occur after large bilateral hippocampal lesions was addressed by Isseroff (1979). Previously, Isseroff and Isseroff (1978) had found an apparent return of spontaneous alternation after small dorsal hippocampal lesions when the animals were given extended postoperative testing. Isseroff extended this work by studying the return of alternation behavior in animals with larger lesions with extended postoperative testing beginning at 30 or 56 days after surgery. Both postoperative-recovery-period groups were initially impaired, but with repeated testing, there was a recovery of alternation behavior. This recovery after repeated testing, however, vanished when a 10-sec delay was imposed in the start box during testing. This start-box delay was imposed immediately after a 20-sec confinement in the arm selected on the previous trial. The failures in spontaneous alternation found initially after testing started and after the introduction of the 10-sec delay were due not to response perseveration but to chance levels of arm selection.

Several factors distinguish the Isseroff studies from others. These include the testing of the animals while they were water-deprived, the provision of water rewards in the goal arms, and the construction of the T-maze itself. In addition, the lesions were made by radio frequency electrolysis, and thus, the associated neocortical damage usually produced was reduced. However, no control animals were prepared that had puncture wounds in the neocortex that would correspond to the damage produced in lowering electrodes into the hippocampus. Nevertheless, these studies suggest that with brief intertrial intervals and extended multiple-test conditions, a return of some forms of alternation behavior may be possible, although its relation to spontaneous alternation as more commonly measured is uncertain.

In one study, the bilateral destruction of the entorhinal cortex produced a loss of alternation behavior in a T-maze in which the first trial was always forced to one goal arm (Scheff & Cotman, 1977). Recovery of alternation did occur if only unilateral lesions were made and was prominent a week after the lesion was made. The interpretation of this type of result is complicated by the fact that general stress experiences can reduce spontaneous alternation (e.g., Dokla, Kasprow, Sideleau, & Boitano, 1980), as can apparent hyperemotionality (e.g., Sherrick et al., 1979).

Since animals with hippocampal destruction are impaired in the nonrewarded spontaneous alternation tests given in a T-maze, it is natural to ask whether they can be trained to exhibit other response alternation by the use of rewards. Jackson and Strong (1969) showed that animals could learn long sequences of response alternation in a two-bar operant situation. In this task, the animals had to press first the right bar and then the left bar to obtain a reinforcement. Subsequently, the animals were trained to make longer strings of alternated responses on the two bars in order to obtain a reinforcement (i.e., R–L–R–L, etc.). These authors found that the animals with hippocampal lesions could learn the alternation of lever presses more readily than normal animals. Using a discrete trial procedure, Means, Walker, and Isaacson (1970) found the same type of result. However, Buerger (1970) did not have success in training cats on an alternation problem in an operant chamber, unless these animals had had preoperative training in the task. However, his animals suffered relatively small lesions in the extreme ventral portions of the hippocampus. The damaged area included the entorhinal cortex as well as some portions of the amygdala.

Relations with the Autonomic Nervous System

Kaada (1951), in his classic study of the effects produced by limbic system stimulation, failed to find any effect produced by hippocampal stimulation on respiration or blood pressure in cat, dog, or monkey. These initial results of Kaada have been frequently supported (e.g., Koikegami, Dodo, Mochida, & Takahashi, 1957; Koikegami & Fuse, 1952; Pampiglione & Falconer, 1956). On the other hand, some contrary observations were made by Votaw and Lauer (1963), who found that stimulation of the hippocampus in the anterior portions of the temporal lobe reduced respiration and heart rate. This initial depressive response was followed by increases in both measures. Kaada (1972) investigated the effects of hippocampal stimulation on heart rate and respiration in both awake and anesthetized rabbits. Some small and transient effects were found when the hippocampus was first stimulated, but these quickly habituated and further stimulation was ineffective. The stimulation did not influence responses to a conditioned stimulus that signaled shock nor did it modify the decrease in heart rate and respiration normally found when smoke was blown into the rabbit's nose. In addition, hippocampal afterdischarges failed to alter heart rate or respiration. The conclusions of these authors supported the original results obtained by Kaada (1951) in that the hippocampus remained one of the few "autonomically silent" regions of the limbic system.

On the other hand, some changes in heart rate responses to stimulation have been found after septal or hippocampal lesions. For example, Sanwald, Porzio, Deane, and Donovick (1970) found that heart rate habituation to a series of tones was decreased following septal or hippocampal lesions. Somewhat contrary to this result, Jarrard and Korn (1969) reported habituation of the heart rate in animals with hippocampal damage while they were engaged in a locomotor exploratory task even though their activity did not habituate. In another aspect of this study, the heart rate of animals with hippocampal lesions increased after a single shock experience in a passive-avoidance training task where the heart rate of animals with neocortical lesions and of normal animals decreased after shock. The heart rate effect found in the animals with hippocampal lesions was short-lived, however. By the second trial after the shock, identical heart rates were found in the animals in all groups, although the hippocampal-lesioned animals still exhibited impaired passive avoidance. Thus, heart rate and behavior were not closely related in this study. Nevertheless, the heart rate response of the animals with hippocampal lesions on the first postshock trial was not only different in magnitude from that of the control animals, but also different in nature.

Ely, Greene, and Henry (1977) found increased blood pressure and a reflex bradycardia in mice with hippocampal lesions when they had to interact with other animals, but not when they were individually caged. In large colonies, the lesioned animals had lower heart weights, indicating that the bradycardia may have been a chronic condition.

Hecht, Hai, Garibyan, Hecht, and Treptow (1978) reported that after repeated stress experiences over the course of 3 weeks, there is a rise in blood pressure and a reduction in heart rate of intact rats. Hippocampal damage was reported to eliminate these alterations.

The effect of hippocampal lesions on gastric activities has been inconsistent (e.g., Anand & Dua, 1956; Sen & Anand, 1957). The effect of hippocampal activity, however, may be quite indirect. For example, Feldman, Wajsbort, and Birnbaum (1967) reported that while dorsal hippocampal stimulation had no effect on gastric secretion, it abolished the facilitation of secretion produced by posterior hypothalamic stimulation. Kim, Choi, Kim, Kim, Park, Ahn, and Kang (1976) report that large hippocampal lesions increased the number of gastric ulcers found in restrained rats. Sectioning the vagus nerve eliminated the ulcer-enhancing effects of the lesion.

Neuroendocrine Regulation

A large number of studies have tried to determine relationships between the pituitary-adrenal hormones and the hippocampus, but the results of such studies have not always been successful. Nevertheless, there is a close association among the neuroendocrine systems, the hippocampus, and behavior. Reviews of the literature on this topic related to pituitary, adrenal, and sexual hormones have been provided by Bohus (1975); McEwen, Gerlach, and Micco (1975); McGowan-Sass and Timiras (1975); and Van Hartesveldt (1975). In recent years, the relations of the hippocampus to other neuroendocrine systems has been explored, specifically the endogenous opiate systems.

Surprisingly, the role of the hippocampus in modulating the circadian rhythms found in a variety of hormonal systems remains uncertain. This uncertainty is due, partly, to the use of different procedures and to the different times at which steroid measurements are made. Neither large lesions of the hippocampus nor lesions restricted to its dorsal or ventral regions influence circadian rhythms reflected in corticosteroid levels. The studies that have reported results that seem to indicate circadian changes after hippocampal lesions may actually have been measuring modest but differential changes related to the stressful aspects of the procedure. The evidence that does indicate a relationship between the hippocampus and corticosteroid levels, however, suggests that the ventral hippocampal area is more important than the dorsal (Knigge, 1961; Bohus, 1975). Supporting this view is the observation that steroid implantation in the ventral hippocampus flattened out the diurnal curves of plasma corticosteroids (Slusher, 1966); that is, both the peaks and the valleys were reduced in size.

As emphasized before, the amount of time between the lesion and the subsequent observations is critical for understanding the effects of lesions. Lengvári and Halász (1973) found decreased circadian corticosteroid levels in rats at 1 and 2 weeks after section of the fornix, but not 3 weeks postoperatively. Many studies that have reported lesion effects on corticosteroid activities tested the animals after less than a 3-week recovery period. Nyakas, de Kloet, and Bohus (1979) also found a transient rise in corticosteroids after medial or lateral septal lesions, which disappeared by 30 days after surgery.

The large amount of research that has tried to relate hippocampal function to the pituitary adrenal system is motivated by the fact that the hippocampus binds more corticosterone than any other brain region, including the hypothalamus (McEwen, Weiss, & Schwartz, 1969). The accumulation of radioactively labeled corticosterone is substantial in the CA_1 and CA_2 regions, as well as in the dentate region, and this pattern of accumulation seems to be uniform along the septotemporal axis (Stumpf, 1970; McEwen *et al.*, 1975). The lateral septal area also shows substantial corticosterone binding. In this connection, it may be of interest that lateral septal lesions, but not medial septal lesions, increased the number of coticosterone receptors in the hippocampus 30 days after surgery (Nyakas *et al.*, 1979). No effect on receptor numbers was found 10 days postoperatively.

Osborne, Sivakumaran, and Black (1979) found that animals with lesions of the fornix evaluated after a 3-week recovery period failed to show normal corticosteroid elevations during the extinction of an operant response (see also Coover, Goldman, & Levine, 1971), as well as elevations due to handling and transport to a novel environment, but they were not different from controls under baseline conditions. Iuvone and Van Hartesveldt (1976) found elevated corticosterone levels when animals were placed in open fields. Woodruff and Kantor (1980) found that plasma ACTH levels were more elevated in animals with lesions of the fornix than in controls 1 hr after reaching criterion performance in an avoidance task. Immediately after reaching the criterion performance, the ACTH levels in all experimental and control groups were extremely high, about 5 times the levels found after ether stress. At 1 hr afterward, when the fornix-lesioned animals were still at 3 times the level of the ether-stress animals, the controls had returned to the level of the ether-stress conditions. This finding suggests a normal ACTH responsiveness but a prolonged time of release.

While the binding of corticosterone in the hippocampus has been well documented, neither its biochemical nor its behavioral consequences are well understood. Meyer, Luine, Khylchevskaya, and McEwen (1979) were unable to find neuron-specific enzymatic changes in hippocampus related to corticosteroid levels. Using a hippocampal slice preparation, Etgen, Lee, and Lynch (1979) provided evidence of an increased synthesis of a protein with an apparent molecular weight of 54,000 when the slice was incubated with corticosteroids. Influences of the corticosteroids have also been shown by means of electrophysiological measures at the single-cell level (Pfaff, Silva, & Weiss, 1971) and by means of the measurement of changes in more general electrical rhythms, including the threshold for the elicitation of seizure activity (Endröczi, 1972). Despite this evidence for steroid-induced changes in hippocampal activity, the functional significance of these actions remains obscure.

The confusion may be due, in part, to the fact that the role played by the hippocampus in neuroendocrine function depends on other conditions in the internal or external environment of the animals. The results of Slusher (1966) after corticosteroid implantation in the ventral hippocampus suggest that the actions of the hippocampus depend on the state of the organism. Kawakami, Seto, Terasawa, Yoshida, Miyamoto, Sekiguchi, and Hattori (1968) have also shown that under stressful conditions, hippocampal stimulation inhibits corticosterone secretion, but that under nonstressful conditions, it increases secretion. The presumed stress of social interaction has been shown to produce an exaggerated corticosterone release in mice with hippocampal lesions (Ely et al., 1977).

Since adrenalectomy results in the more rapid extinction of an appetitive runway response and hippocampal lesions make this response more resistant to extinction, it is possible that the two treatments act at some common level. If so, it might be possible to produce more rapid extinction after hippocampal damage by the administration of corticosterone. This experiment was attempted by Micco, McEwen, and Shein (1979). They found that the increased resistance to extinction in the lesioned animals was not altered by the administration of the steroids.

McGowan-Sass and Timiris (1975) found that the corticosteroids influence the evoked potentials recorded from the hippocampus after sensory stimulation. The evoked potentials induced by somatosensory stimulation were most altered in the dorsal hippocampus, while those induced by visual stimulation were most affected in the ventral hippocampus.

Lovely (1975) found that the enhancement of active-avoidance behavior often found after hippocampal damage does not occur in hypophysectomized animals. The facilitation induced by septal lesions was unaffected by the loss of the pituitary gland. The fact that the endocrine changes induced by loss of the pituitary failed to influence animals with septal lesions may be related to the role of this area in mediating the effects of short ACTH fragments (Verhoef, Witter, & de Wied, 1977).

Corticotropin (ACTH) has direct effects on the activity of the hippocampus as evidenced by its effects on single-cell activities (Pfaff et al., 1971) and by the effects of rhythmic slow activities (Kawakami, Koshino, & Hattori, 1966), although the effects may be observed only during some aspects of a learning situation (Urban, Lopes Da Silva, Storm van Leeuwen, & de Wied, 1974). ACTH shifts the rhythmic slow activities to a bit higher frequency during reticular formation stimulation, an effect that can be duplicated by increasing the intensity of the stimulation (Urban & de Wied, 1975). Therefore, it appears that the activities of the hippocampus are susceptible to modification by ACTH.

While some of the short N-terminal fragments of ACTH (e.g., $ACTH_{4-10}$) have selective, although subtle, effects on the learning and the extinction of certain avoidance and appetitive tasks (de Wied, 1974), the longer ACTH fragments (such as $ACTH_{1-16}$ and $ACTH_{1-24}$) induce prolonged excessive grooming when placed in the rat ventricular system (see Gispen & Isaacson, 1981, for a review). Destruction of the hippocampus, but not the septal area, reduces the sensitivity of the animal to this neuropeptide effect (Elstein, Hannigan, & Isaacson, 1981). It seems that the neuropeptide effects related to learning and extinction are more closely associated with the septal region than with the hippocampus, while those related to excessive grooming have the opposite relationship.

The sex-related steroid hormones bind to hippocampal cell receptors, although to a lesser extent than in the hippocampus. The affinity of hippocampal receptors for the gonadal steroids is less than for the corticosteroids. There are changes in hippocampal electrical excitability associated with the estrous cycle (Terasawa & Timiras, 1968). Adult female rats with hippocampal lesions show increased levels of luteinizing hormone and follicle-stimulating hormone. Stimulation of the hippocampus has been reported to enhance progesterone formation (Kawakami, Seto, Terasawa, & Yoshida, 1967) and to inhibit ovulation (Velasco & Taleisnik, 1969). There are reasons to suspect that both of these effects are mediated by fibers of the medial corticohypothalamic tract that project from the hippocampal formation to the arcuate nucleus of the hypothalamus. Electrical potentials recorded in hippocampal slices showed sex-based differences in response to estradiol and testosterone when these hormones were added to the incubation medium (Teyler, Vardaris, Lewis, & Rawitch, 1980).

The hippocampus appears to contain relatively few opiate receptors (e.g., Atweh & Kuhar, 1977; Le Motte, Snowman, Pert, & Snyder, 1978). Sar *et al.* (1978) have found some immunoreactive staining fibers and processes in the hippocampus. These seem to be clustered in a dense fashion only around cells in the CA_2 region. Despite the relative paucity of endogenous opiate systems in the hippocampus, some effects of the endogenous opiates have been established on electrical activities recorded in this tissue. β-Endorphin, but not met-enkephalin, produces a shift toward higher-frequency rhythmic activities in the hippocampus. The effect is similar to that of ACTH (Urban & de

Wied, 1976). Destruction of the hippocampus also eliminates the excessive grooming induced by the injection of β-endorphin into the ventricular system (Gispen & Isaacson, 1981).

The iontophoretic application of most hippocampal neurons seems unaffected by morphine or the enkephalins, although some cells showed excitatory or inhibitory responses. A proportion of the inhibitory effects were stereospecific to opiate agonists and were reduced by naloxone (Fry, Zieglgänsberger, & Herz, 1979). The relatively small proportion of excitatory responses found by Fry *et al.* relative to those reported by others (e.g., Nicoll, Alger, & Jahr, 1980a) may be due to their construction of the microelectrode. It was made so as to affect dendrites more than cell bodies. Elazar, Motles, Ely, and Simantov (1979) have found that the microinjection of leu-enkephalin into the hippocampus can induce electrical seizure activities that are blocked by naloxone. Evidence of a synchronizing effect of enkephalins on hippocampal activity has also been reported by Martinez, Jensen, Creager, Veliquette, Messing, McGaugh, and Lynch (1979). This effect may be due to a disinhibitory effect produced by the peptide on interneurons (Nicoll, Alger, & Jahr, 1980b). Bär, Schotman, and Gispen (1980) have found that the enkephalins can induce alterations in the phosphorylation of a specific protein band in the hippocampus. These observations all suggest that the endogenous opiate systems may exert potent influences on the electrical and chemical activities of the hippocampus, but their functional importance in behavior remains to be discovered.

STUDIES OF LEARNING AND MEMORY

Avoidance Conditioning

A facilitation of two-way active-avoidance conditioning and an impairment in the two-way active-avoidance conditioning and passive-avoidance problems after hippocampal damage are now reasonably well documented in several species.

Isaacson, Douglas, and Moore (1961) were the first to document the more rapid acquisition of two-way active-avoidance tasks in rats. However, 20 years earlier, Allen (1941) had shown that dogs with bilateral hippocampal destruction could acquire an olfactory discrimination, and many of his lesioned animals acquired the task more rapidly than the control animals. The study by Isaacson *et al.* (1961) actually stemmed from unpublished observations by Dr. Corneliu Giurgea and me to the effect that dogs with bilateral hippocampal destruction acquired a leg-lift avoidance response faster than normal animals.

The guinea pig learns two-way active-avoidance behavior rather poorly, if at all, because of a tendency to be inactive after foot shock. Ireland *et al.* (1969) found that hippocampal lesions enhanced this form of active-avoidance learning. Weiss and Hertzler (1973) replicated these results with procaine injections into the hippocampus.

Attempts to fractionate the effects of hippocampal lesions on behavior (see Jarrard, 1980) have indicated that facilitated two-way active-avoidance learning arises from damage to the fimbria, the part of the fornix system containing most of the fibers connecting the hippocampus with the septal area (Jarrard, 1976). Damage to CA_1 or the outer covering of the alveus through which many axons from CA_1 cells reach the subiculum does not produce this facilitation (Jarrard, 1976; Myhrer, 1976). Myhrer (1975) also found that complete fimbria lesions produced a facilitation of two-way active avoidance and that small lesions made in the inner portion of the fimbria produced impaired active-avoidance learning. Damage to the perforant pathway made with a lesion involving the entorhinal cortex also impaired active-avoidance learning. The poor performance of the animals in the active-avoidance situation found by Myhrer may have been due to an increased amount of immobility during training. While CA_1 lesions fail to influence the acquisition of two-way active-avoidance problems, this damage may alter the animals' tendency to respond to the buzzer used as the conditioned stimulus in most studies (e.g., Filho, Moschovakis, & Izquierdo, 1977).

A problem with this approach is that the fimbria lesions undoubtedly disrupt a variety of fibers of diverse origins that travel in this fiber system. These include efferents from subicular and entorhinal cortical areas that reach telencephalic and diencephalic locations. Even lesions of the perforant pathway as used by Myhrer may interrupt the entorhinal efferent system on the way to its various forebrain targets. In general, it seems unlikely that these various pathway-lesion approaches will reveal a great deal about the roles of various CA fields in behavior.

A more rapid acquisition of a number of different types of problems has been found subsequent to hippocampal damage. Duncan and Duncan (1971) found that hippocampal destruction facilitated the learning of an operant avoidance task but impaired the learning of a visual dicrimination problem in a T-maze based on the avoidance of foot shock. The failure to find a facilitation of learning in the T-maze avoidance task could be due to an impairment in the ability of the animal to use the brightness cues because of inadequate saliency, to a difficulty with the spatial aspects of the T-maze, or to both. By means of other techniques, faster acquisition of a nictitating membrane response has been found in rabbits (Schmaltz & Theios, 1972). Rabbits have also been shown to exhibit faster acquisition of the two-way active-avoidance response and impaired passive-avoidance behavior following hippocampal lesions (Papsdorf & Woodruff, 1970).

A deficit in passive-avoidance tests subsequent to hippocampal destruction has been found in several species (e.g., Isaacson & Wickelgren, 1962; Nonneman & Isaacson, 1973; Papsdorf & Woodruff, 1970). However, the effect depends on the location and the size of the lesion within the hippocampus, the specific requirements of the task (Snyder & Isaacson, 1965), the strength of the tendency of the animal to make the approach response that is punished, the strength and the amount of foot shock, and the intertrial interval.

The strength of the approach response is difficult to specify with precision. The tendency to make a response depends on the training given the animal in the task, the motivational circumstances (usually the amount of deprivation), and the value of the incentives provided. In 1966, Kimble, Kirkby, and Stein reported that animals with hippocampal lesions had to receive specific training in the to-be-punished approach response if a deficit was going to be found. This suggestion was given further support in an experiment by Stein and Kirkby (1967). However, Isaacson et al. (1966) did not find specific training to be necessary, provided that sufficient motivation was used to induce the response. The important factor is the total behavioral tendency to make the approach response, and not the training per se (Isaacson, 1967). The strength of the approach response can be manipulated through training or through adjustments in the motivation of the animals or the incentives used. Wishart and Mogenson (1970a) found that if experiences with passive-avoidance procedures were given before surgery, hippocampal lesions did not produce animals with a passive-avoidance deficit. This result provides general support of the view that the effect of the hippocampal lesion somehow fixates the predominant behavioral dispositions of the animals.

In experiments by Cogan and Reeves (1979), animals with large hippocampal lesions were shown to be able to perform well in passive-avoidance tasks, provided multiple shock experiences were given or high levels of foot shock were used in a single trial. If a 60-min intertrial interval was used with high foot shock, no deficit was observed, whereas an intermediate deficit occurred with high foot shock and a 60-sec intertrial interval. The authors believe that their results are best interpreted on the basis of lesion-induced alterations of attentional mechanisms.

Investigations of dorsal-ventral hippocampal differences in regard to passive-avoidance abilities seem to indicate the ventral region, along with adjacent subicular and entorhinal cortex, as most important (Kimura, 1958; Nadel, 1968; Ross, Walsh, & Grossman, 1973; Van Hoesen et al., 1972; Entingh, 1971). When atropine was injected into the ventral hippocampal-entorhinal area of young animals, a passive-avoidance deficit was observed. Injections into the dorsal hippocampus were without effect (Blozovski, 1979).

The tendency to avoid or to incorporate less of a food or liquid adulterated with a specific taste when the taste had been experienced prior to becoming ill is referred to as *bait shyness*, or *taste aversion learning*. It is of theoretical interest because the taste associated with the illness precedes the sickness by hours. Presumably, the memory of the taste must be maintained over this period for the association to be formed. Because some investigators had thought that the hippocampus was the basis of at least some form of memory, and because the experimental model resembles a passive-avoidance paradigm, animals with hippocampal lesions were expected to be impaired in this task. However, this expectation has not been fulfilled by the data from most studies. For example, bilateral hippocampal lesions did not affect the acquisition or the resistance to extinction of an aversion to the taste of sucrose after it had been paired with lithium-induced sickness (Murphy & Brown, 1974). Animals with ventral hippocampal lesions showed normal, or better-than-normal, acquisition of a taste aversion based on sickness induced by apomorphine while exhibiting impairments in both passive avoidance and conditioned suppression of drinking (Best & Orr, 1973). Facilitated taste-aversion learning after ventral, but not dorsal, hippocampal lesions has also been found by McGowan *et al.* (1972). After electrical stimulation of the hippocampus, no effect was found on the presumed recovery from a fear of novel places or from a learned taste aversion (Kesner & Berman, 1977).

Most often, exposing animals to a stimulus before training has been shown to decrease the ability of that stimulus to serve as a signal once training is started. This phenomenon is now called *latent inhibition* and has been viewed as learning to ignore some aspects of the environment (MacKintosh, 1975). Ackil, Mellgren, Halgren, and Frommer (1969) studied the effects of presenting a tone to animals before it was used as the conditioned stimulus (CS) in a two-way active-avoidance task. Giving 30 exposures to the tone before conditioning retarded the learning of both normal animals and animals with neocortical lesions. Not only was the acquisition of the task impaired, but the number of responses made during extinction was also reduced. In other words, preexposure to the signal seemed to make learning more difficult and more fragile. The learning of the animals with hippocampal lesions was unchanged by the preexposure to the CS. They learned the task quickly and were more resistant to extinction, whether or not they had received the pretraining exposure to the CS. The preexposure to the tone before training did affect other behaviors of the animals with hippocampal destruction, however. For example, Ackil *et al.* found that the activity of animals with hippocampal damage placed in the apparatus and given the 30-tone presentations was the same as that found in the control groups. Animals without this experience were hyperactive.

Using the rabbit nictitating-membrane response, Solomon and Moore (1975) found that dorsal hippocampal lesions impair latent inhibition. Septal lesions impair this phenomenon in a two-way active-avoidance task (Weiss, Friedman, & McGregor, 1974), and a similar effect was found in a one-way avoidance task by Olton and Isaacson (1969). Lesions in the medial raphe complex that selectively deplete serotonin in the septohippocampal complex also eliminate the latent inhibition effect measured by the nictitating membrane paradigm (Solomon, Nichols, Kiernan, Kamer, & Kaplan, 1980). It should be noted that hippocampal destruction does not impede the conditioning of the eye-retraction–nictitating-membrane response (Schmaltz & Theios, 1972; Solomon, 1977).

Olton (1973) pointed out that it is necessary to understand the cues used by subjects of different species in establishing avoidance responses. Spatial cues are likely to be important to rats in learning this problem. If rats with hippocampal destruction are deficient in the use of spatial cues in learning, this deficiency could help to explain the effect of the hippocampal destruction on these problems. For example, the intact animal may associate the locations of both sides of the two-way active-avoidance chamber with painful shocks and therefore may hesitate to approach either place. The hippocampal-lesioned animal, if it suffers from an inability to utilize information about the spatial locations of the goal boxes in an optimal fashion, is less likely to be able to make an association of a spatial area with the electrical shock. Consequently, the animal should experience less conflict about returning to a location in which shocks had been received and should establish the shuttlebox behavior more rapidly. The deficit in the one-way avoidance task should be due to the fact that the animal is less likely to establish an association between the location of the box in which it is placed and the punishing shocks. The location of the other "safe" compartment should also be less well established. A similar explanation for passive avoidance deficits could be adopted.

Also, as mentioned earlier, the reduced ability to utilize information about spatial location could make the lesioned animal learn a different response than that of the intact animals. Animals with hippocampal damage may learn "to run" at the sound of the warning signal rather than to run to a particular place. The CS would act as a "trigger."

Appetitive Tasks

The performance of animals with hippocampal lesions engaged in acquiring tasks based on obtaining incentives like food or water, when hungry or thirsty, is sometimes different and sometimes the same as that of intact animals. One of the main goals of researchers is, therefore, to determine in which tasks the lesioned animals exhibit changed behavioral patterns. Animals with hippocampal damage are not greatly different from normal animals in learning to press levers in operant chambers for food or water when the rewards are provided after each lever press (continuous reinforcement). Their behavior does becomes unusual when certain types of reinforcement schedules are used by the experimenter, especially those in which the animal must wait between bar presses to obtain rewards, that is, the DRL (differential reward of low rates of responding) schedule. This reinforcement schedule was first used with animals with hippocampal lesions to test their ability to withhold responses by Clark (Van Hartesveldt) and Isaacson (1965). It was felt that if the lesioned animals suffered from a general inability to inhibit responses they would perform poorly on the task.

The DRL Impairment

The impairment of animals with hippocampal lesions on DRL schedules has now been established in several species, including the nonhuman primate (Jackson & Gergen, 1970). The DRL impairment occurs in animals with two-stage lesions in which one hippocampal formation on one side of the brain is destroyed first and then the other at a later time, even when specific DRL training is given between the two operations (Curtis & Nonneman, 1977). Damage to the fimbria and the fornix, but not to the dorsal alveus, can produce impaired DRL performance (Jarrard & Becker, 1977; Johnson, Olton, Gage, & Jenko, 1977). The impaired performance can be seen even on short-delay DRL schedules, that is, DRL-2 (on which a 2-sec delay is required). In a study by Boitano et al. (1980), the animals were trained to criterion performance on the DRL-2 schedule and then advanced to longer delay schedules. Impairments were found on all delays. The DRL deficit has two aspects: a greatly exaggerated rate of response and a reduction in the ratio of reinforced responses to total responses (efficiency). Obviously, these two characteristics are not entirely independent. High rates of response will almost certainly produce low efficiency scores, but there is some reason to doubt that the complete explanation of the deficit shown by animals with hippocampal damage is their higher rate of response. For example, certain drugs can alter the animals' rates of response without changing efficiency scores (Van Hartesveldt, 1974). Extending this line of work, Fish (1976, described in Isaacson, 1980a) found that low doses of haloperidol would reduce the excessive number of operant responses made by animals with hippocampal damage, but the drug failed to improve the overall efficiency of performance.

The DRL impairment is an example of a deficit that occurs when the lesioned animals are trained with one schedule of reinforcement and then transferred to another. This transfer produces an uncertainty about the reinforcement contingencies in their training environment. When animals with hippocampal lesions are changed from one set of training contingencies to another, their behavior becomes greatly activated relative to that of normal animals. This effect has been found both for DRL schedules and for variable-interval schedules (Jarrard, 1965). This conclusion is based in part on the results obtained by Schmaltz and Isaacson (1966), who demonstrated that it was the *change* from the continuous reinforcement conditions to a partial or intermittent reinforcement schedule that was debilitating. Animals with hippocampal lesions trained entirely under DRL reinforcement contingencies, including those procedures used to establish the bar-press response in the first place, were not impaired. Similar results have been reported by others (Ellen & Aitken, 1970; Ellen, Aitken, & Walker, 1973). Pretraining factors may not play as large a role after septal lesions (Ellen, Aitken, & Stahl, 1973). The DRL impairment is an example of a more general behavioral anomaly that is found when the animals are subjected to alterations in the environment.

When training animals on a DRL schedule, usually no cue is given to signal the end of the delay period. Animals must depend on internal cues of some kind to determine the appropriate delay between responses. Pellegrino and Clapp (1971) found that when an external cue is provided to signal the end of the delay period, subjects with hippocampus or with amygdala lesions can perform adequately on the task. This result has been replicated by Van Hartesveldt and Walker (1974). In addition, these latter authors determined whether some extraneous behaviors could be used by the lesioned animals to help "time" their responses. They gave animals objects to manipulate, such as blocks of wood to gnaw during the delay period. These added objects did not help the rats with hippocampal lesions gauge the appropriate waiting interval on a DRL-20 task. The animals with hippocampal damage chewed the blocks of wood more than did the control animals, but they did so while maintaining extremely high response rates on the DRL task. Improvements were found when a specific signal was given to indicate the end of the delay period.

The impaired DRL performance exhibited by animals with hippocampal destruction might be due to a heightened level of motivation. This hypothesis was investigated by Carey (1969). He compared the performance of animals with hippocampal lesions tested under a 23.5-hr water deprivation with those of normal animals at the same level of deprivation, or at 1 or 2 additional days of deprivation. He found that the response rates of the animals with hippocampal lesions were greater than those of the normal animals under all deprivation regimes.

Studying cats with hippocampal damage, Nonneman and Isaacson (1973) found that the rate of response under continuous reinforcement conditions was diagnostic for the degree of impairment suffered when the lesioned animals were shifted to the DRL schedule. Animals with hippocampal lesions having high response rates under continuous reinforcement (CRF) showed exaggerated response rates, rates well beyond those of normal animals when shifted to the intermittent schedule. Animals with lower response rates under CRF did not have as large increases when the schedule requirements were changed. On the other hand, the response rate under CRF was not a determinant of effective performance for normal cats. Regardless of their response rates under CRF, intact animals could adjust them downward to create the appropriate-length pauses required to obtain reinforcement.

Kearley, Van Hartesveldt, and Woodruff (1974) investigated possible sex differences in DRL performance after hippocampal destruction. They found that the amount of weight lost on the deprivation schedule was correlated with the poor performance on the DRL schedules and that male animals were farther below their target weights than the females. However, lesions produced pronounced impairments in animals of either sex and made them resistant to extinction. The females were more resistant to extinction than the lesioned males. DRL performance was unaffected by either corticosterone or ACTH (peripheral) administration.

Discrimination Learning

In most experiments, animals with hippocampal damage have been reported to have little trouble with the learning of visual discrimination problems. Many studies used animals trained in a two-choice maze fashioned as a T or a Y. As is reported below, it is now clear that animals with hippocampal damage do not behave as do normal animals on such problems. Whether or not a substantial difference between normal and lesioned animals is found depends on several characteristics of the training situation. In addition, however, there is evidence that hippocampal lesions can affect visual discrimination learning even when tested in operant situations.

Woodruff and Isaacson (1972) found that bilateral destruction of the hippocampus greatly impaired the learning of a visual discrimination in an operant paradigm. Rats were trained to respond to the lever over which a small light was illuminated in a two-lever operant chamber. In this original study and a subsequent replication using a slightly modified procedure (Woodruff, Schneiderman, & Isaacson, 1972), the animals with hippocampal damage failed to show any signs of learning the discrimination problem over 10–20 days of training. These results were surprising in light of the older data, especially those from maze studies, which had revealed relatively rapid learning of visual discriminations by the animals with hippocampal damage. For example, Kimble (1961, 1963) studied the acquisition of simultaneous and successive brightness-discrimination problems using a Y-maze. These names of the discrimination tasks refer to two conditions in which black and white cardboard inserts were placed in the two arms of the maze. In the simultaneous discrimination, the animals were confronted with a gray starting arm (the base of the Y) and, at the choice point, with one black arm and one white arm. These arms formed the top arms of the Y. A food reward was given at the end of either the black or the white arm, depending on the arbitrary designation of which was to be considered "correct" for a particular animal. The location of the white or black insert in the right or left arm of the Y was predetermined according to a quasi-random schedule. In the successive discrimination task, the animals were faced with a situation in which the starting stem was gray and both upper arms were either black or white. The animal had to learn to enter the right arm of the Y when both arms were white (to follow the rule "right if both white") and to enter the left arm of the Y when both arms were black (to follow the rule "left if both black") or vice versa. The stimulus situation as it might appear to an animal on two different trials is shown in Figure 17.

As a group, animals with hippocampal damage were impaired, relative to normal animals and to animals with brain damage restricted to the posterolateral neocortex, in the acquisition of the successive discrimination. These same subjects, however, were not impaired in learning the simultaneous discrimination.

SIMULTANEOUS DISCRIMINATION

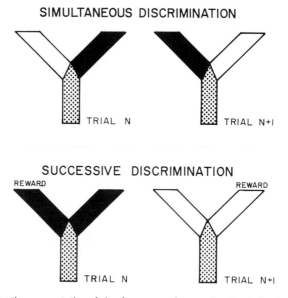

SUCCESSIVE DISCRIMINATION

Figure 17. Schematic representation of simultaneous and successive discrimination tasks. In the simultaneous discrimination task, the situation faced by the animals on two different trials is shown (trial n and trial n + 1). The start arm is gray. A black or a white insert is placed in the right or left arm on different trials on a nonsystematic basis. The animal is rewarded for approaching one of the colors. The successive discrimination is shown as it could appear on two successive trials. On any given trial, the two cross-arms are either black or white. The animal must turn right or left depending on the color present in the two arms. From Isaacson and Kimble (1972).

Complete understanding of Kimble's results depends on a more complete analysis of the data, and there is one additional factor of the experimental design to consider. All the animals in this study were trained on both the simultaneous discrimination and the successive discrimination problems. This training was done in a balanced fashion: some subjects learned the simultaneous discrimination as their first task, while the other subjects learned the successive discrimination first. Considering animals that learned the simultaneous problem first, there was little difference among the three experimental groups. All animals learned to approach the black arm more readily than they learned to approach the white arm. This result suggests that all rats, whether lesioned or not, found the hypothesis "approach the darker arm" more compatible with their predispositions than the alternative hypothesis, "approach the lighter arm." This result is not surprising, since rats tend to approach the darker parts of new environments (Munn, 1950). The point is that rats enter a learning situation with predispositions that help or hinder them in solving the new task.

When the simultaneous discrimination was learned as the second task (i.e., after the animals had already learned the successive discrimination), there was a substantial difference between the normal animals and those with either neocortical or hippocampal damage.

Training on the successive discrimination task served to provide the normal animals with an effective orientation toward the simultaneous problem. Indeed, four of the five normal subjects started with the correct hypothesis, and, more importantly, *all* normal subjects attacked the problem while operating on a "brightness hypothesis." The previous training had served to disconfirm a "place (spatial) hypothesis." As a consequence, normal animals no longer needed to test the "food on the right" or "food on the left" hypothesis. They acted on hypotheses related to the brightness of the arms of the maze.

The animals with hippocampal damage that performed poorly were acting in accordance with a position hypothesis that the normal animals had eliminated during their previous training, despite the fact that the lesioned animals had given up this strategy while solving the previous task. When starting their second problem, they returned to the place hypothesis and did so with vigor. Such behavior would be difficult to reconcile with the view that the lesioned animals cannot process spatial information.

For all animals, the successive discrimination problem is more difficult than simultaneous problems. Why the successive problem is more difficult can best be understood in terms of the type of hypothesis that must be held for the correct solution. The animals must learn "if both arms are white, go right," and "if both arms are black, go left," or vice versa. In addition, the animals must learn to suppress all forms of spatial and brightness hypotheses.

The successive discrimination task can be viewed in several ways. One way is to assume that the animal compares the two situations with which it is confronted on various trials. It may compare the effects of responses to the left and right arms of the Y, given on subsequent trials, when the arms of the maze are both white or both black. According to this view, the animal learns one complex problem. Another way of looking at this task, however, is to think of the problem as two separate tasks: a "white maze" and a "black maze."

In this view, it would be anticipated that the animal could master one of these problems without doing very well on the other. This seems to be the case. Normal animals can perform quite well on one of the two problems (e.g., the white maze task) while performing at almost chance levels on the other (e.g., the black maze task). Furthermore, if the successive discrimination is analyzed as if it were two tasks, the performance of animals is "nonincremental" in each. That is, the animals make as many errors in the last half of the presolution trials as in the first half. This sort of nonincremental learning is found in the successive discrimination task *unless* the data are considered on the basis of the black-maze–white-maze subdivisions.

If the two-task orientation is adopted for learning the successive discrimination problem, it is possible to determine the ease with which each task is acquired. Animals in all experimental groups learned one of the two tasks (i.e., white maze, black maze) with about the same number of correct and incorrect responses. The difference among the groups came about in the number of responses required to master the second task. Normal animals were only slightly slower in acquiring the second subproblem than the first. They did so while maintaining an adequate performance level on the first subproblem. For the subjects with hippocampal damage, however, the lesion limited their capacities. *They were able to learn one of the two subproblems as rapidly as the normal animals but were seriously impaired in learning the second.* A similar impairment was found to result from neocortical destruction alone. Impairments in difficult brightness-discrimination problems after posterior neocortical damage in the rat have been reported in several studies (Bauer, 1974; Lewellyn, Lowes, & Isaacson, 1969; Woodruff et al., 1972), and these may be related to the type of difficulty described above.

In an experiment reported by Kimble and Kimble (1970), rats were trained for a water reward in a brightness discrimination task to criterion performance. Each rat was given 1 additional day of training after the day it reached criterion performance. Extinction testing began the next day. The animals again received 10 trials each day with a 10-min intertrial interval.

When a traditional measure of learning (trials to the learning criterion) was used, there were no differences among the groups of normal animals, the animals with neocortical lesions, and the animals with hippocampal and neocortical lesions. In fact, both brain-damaged groups took somewhat fewer trials to reach the acquisition criterion than did the normal animals. However, the tendency to exhibit "hypothesis behavior" (Krechevsky, 1935) was different among the groups. Kimble and Kimble defined two kinds of hypotheses. A *spatial hypothesis* was defined as a sequence of three or more consecutive responses to either the light or the dark arm of the maze, provided that the response sequence included responses to both the left and the right arms.

The hypothesis behavior of the normal animals was characterized as consisting of many short series of trials in accord with one or the other hypothesis. The individual performances of the subjects can be seen in Figure 18. They are similar to the performances of the animals

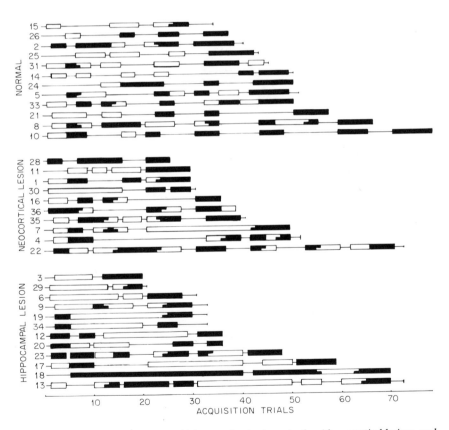

Figure 18. The number of trials on which normal animals, animals with neocortical lesions, and those with hippocampal lesions exhibited behaviors consistent with a spatial hypothesis (open rectangles), a brightness hypothesis (filled rectangles), or an undefined strategy (straight line only) while learning a brightness discrimination task. From Isaacson and Kimble (1972).

with lesions restricted to the neocortex. The hippocampally lesioned animals, however, could be characterized as evidencing fewer but longer hypotheses. These animals with hippocampal damage tended to stay with a particular hypothesis almost 50% longer than the other animals. As can be observed in Figure 19, the longer sequences of hypothesis-based responses occurred only when the subjects were

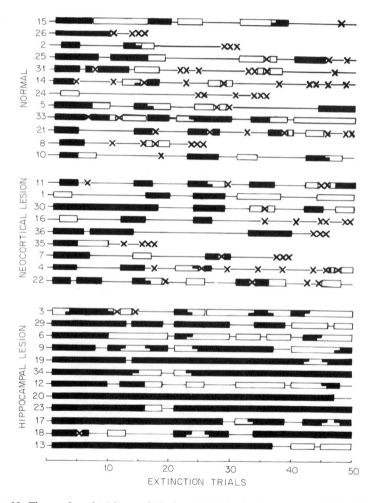

Figure 19. *The number of trials on which the animals in the three groups exhibited behavior consistent with a spatial, brightness, or undefined hypothesis during extinction of the brightness discrimination. Hypotheses as designated in Figure 18. The symbol X designates no response. From Isaacson and Kimble (1972).*

acting on a place hypothesis and not when they were acting on a brightness hypothesis. Not all of the animals with hippocampal damage evidenced this pattern, but the majority did: 8 out of 12 of them produced hypothesis runs of 10 or more trials during acquisition, whereas only 1 animal with neocortical damage and no normal animal did.

Another measure that distinguished among the groups was the percentage of total trials during acquisition that could be included in either a spatial or a brightness hypothesis. For the normal rats, about half (53.8%) of the trials were "hypothesis trials." The animals with only neocortical damage responded on the basis of one of the hypotheses on about two-thirds of their trials. Animals with hippocampal lesions exhibited hypothesis-based behavior on over four-fifths (81.3%) of the trials. A simple descriptive generalization seems to follow from these data: the normal animals and, to a slightly smaller extent, those with neocortical lesions were more variable in their hypothesis behavior during acquisition training than were animals with hippocampal damage.

During extinction, two basic behavioral events were monitored: (1) whether or not the animal continued to make any response or choice at all, as defined by an entry into either goal arm; and (2) the choice of the goal arm (if one was made).

The willingness to continue approaching and entering the goal arms was evaluated both by the number of trials necessary to attain the extinction criterion of three consecutive nonentries into a goal arm and by the approach latencies on those trials in which the animal entered one of the two goal arms within the 60 sec allowed. While the median approach latencies for the normal animals and for those with neocortical damage increased during the 50 extinction trials, the median approach latency for the rats with hippocampal lesions remained virtually unchanged. None of the rats with hippocampal lesions reached the extinction criterion, as contrasted with 42% of the normal and 44% of the neocortically damaged animals.

Since all the animals were trained to approach the brighter arm of the Y-maze during acquisition, it might have been expected that a preponderant number of responses of all animals would be toward that arm during extinction. Actually, the hippocampally lesioned animals exhibited this tendency far more than did animals in either of the other two groups. The point is that while the choice behavior for

both normal animals and those with neocortical lesions rapidly became more variable during extinction, that of the animals with hippocampal lesions was characterized by long strings of responses in
accord with a brightness hypothesis, usually (but not always) consisting of approach responses to the brigher arm. Further analysis of
these data has been published (Kimble & Kimble, 1970).

Of special significance is the fact that at the end of acquisition,
the animals with hippocampal lesions were now responding extensively in accordance with the brightness hypothesis. The special at-
tractiveness of the place hypothesis had been supplanted by the
brightness hypothesis. During extinction, this acquired hypothesis
was given up only with great reluctance. This finding suggests that
the predominant hypothesis was held beyond normal limits of dis-
confirmation by animals with hippocampal damage and that the status
of a "predominant hypothesis" can be achieved either through preex-
perimental, and possible genetic, influences or through the results of
specific training. However, it should be remembered that animals
with hippocampal damage returned to a previously rejected place
hypothesis when being trained in the simultaneous discrimination as
their second task (Isaacson & Kimble, 1972). This result leads to the
conclusion that the perseveration of the acquired hypothesis is maintained during nonreinforcement in the same experimental environment, but that the initially predominant (spatial) hypothesis can be
reactivated when the testing procedures are changed. The animals
with hippocampal lesions may suffer from both a perseveration of a
hypothesis during conditions of nonreward and a decreased ability
to transfer experiences between two different, yet similar, training
paradigms.

Olton (1972) has extended our knowledge of the behavioral deficits following hippocampal destruction in discrimination tasks by
pointing out that the ability to suppress a preferred response, as
measured by the latency of the response, is less affected than is the
ability to make the correct choice from two possible responses. In
Olton's study, animals had to make a choice between two stimulus
positions, and most animals initially responded to one or the other
position (i.e., acted on a place hypothesis). Both normal and brain-
lesioned animals evidenced differential latencies of response to the
positive and negative stimuli before they gave up consistently responding to their favorite place. The animals with hippocampal dam-

age continued to respond to the preferred place for many days after the differential latencies to the positive and negative places had first become evident. After the onset of differential latencies, control animals quickly began to respond to the side where the positive stimulus was presented. These results are an example of a dissociation of the overt, expressed behavior and presumptive knowledge about the environment held by the animals with hippocampal damage. The differential latencies to the two stimuli must reflect the fact that the animals know that the response to a particular place is less likely to produce a reward when the negative stimulus is there than when the positive stimulus is there. Despite this information, the animals with hippocampal damage perseverate the spatial hypothesis. Can the failure to use, misuse, or overuse spatial information account for the deficiencies found in discrimination or other learning tasks? Becker and Olton (1980) trained rats to choose between two stimulus objects in conditions in which neither the absolute location of the objects nor their relative position could predict the correct response. Either frontal neocortical lesions or fimbria–fornix lesions impaired postoperative performance and a reversal of the object discrimination. This finding suggests that the impairments found on reversal and other tasks cannot be due entirely to the spatial characteristics of the task. Retention of a maze problem in which the animals had to select straight-ahead paths or ones that went up a ladder was impaired by dorsal hippocampal lesions (Thompson, 1979). Thus, the behavioral impairments found were not dependent on either the usual spatial or right–left turn requirements of the task.

An important determinant of the ability of animals with hippocampal lesions to acquire a maze problem is the length of the arms of the maze (Strong, 1978). However, the length of the arm is also related to how long the animal can observe the cues associated with the appropriate response. The duration of stimulus exposure and the time between choices are confounded with the length of the maze arms.

By the use of selective lesions, Livesey and Meyer (1979) have found that lesions of the CA_1 area of the dorsal hippocampus produced a deficit in the learning and reversal of a "go–no-go" discrimination in the rat. Lesions of the dentate gyrus produced impairments in the reversal of the task. Similar results had been observed when these regions were electrically stimulated so as to produce a blockade of normal neuronal activities (Livesey & Bayliss, 1975; Livesey & Meyer, 1975). The data from the experiments with the "blocking" electrical stimulation indicate that the animals failed to learn that the S^Δ was a signal for the occurrence of nonreward. However, animals with nonfunctional CA_1 areas reduced responding quite readily when rewards were no longer delivered; yet they always required several responses to become aware of the nonreward condition. Control animals came to predict the nonreward condition on the basis of the S^Δ signal. A similar type of explanation of the effects of the behavior of animals with hippocampal lesions was given by Henke (1979). These effects are found not only with small hippocampal lesions but can be found after large lesions as well (e.g., Woodruff & Isaacson, 1972; Bauer, 1974).

Douglas and Pribram (1969) proposed that destruction of the hippocampus reduced a monkey's ability to learn about signals that signal nonreinforcement. Lesions of the amygdala were proposed to interfere with the animal's ability to learn about signals with positive significance, a so-called reward-register system. As far as the hippocampus is concerned, several of the studies mentioned above would fit into such a model. Han and Livesey (1977) found in a brightness discrimination task that prolonging the duration of the signal that preceded nonreinforcement aided animals with hippocampal lesions, while prolonging the signal preceding reinforcement assisted animals with amygdala lesions. Both lesions were small, and those of the hippocampus involved the CA_1 area, primarily.

The ability of animals with hippocampal lesions to learn or to retain the memory of discrimination problems depends on a number of factors, some of which are relevant to possible interpretations of the nature of the behavioral deficits produced. Retention of a visual discrimination problem was impaired by hippocampal lesions when the context of the behavioral choice was altered (Winocur & Olds, 1978), a result supporting the idea that the hippocampus is especially important in the use of contextual information (Hirsh, 1974, 1980; Hirsch & Krajden, in press). Jarrard (1975) has reported evidence of the especially disruptive effects of interfering activities given before the testing of animals with hippocampal lesions, a point supported by Winocur (1979) and by Thomas (1978). The memory of patients with hippocampal formation damage seems especially susceptible to disruption by interfering events (Weiskrantz & Warrington, 1975).

However, in the study of Winocur, the interpolated activity that served as the interfering event was training in an insoluble problem during which position habits were established. The impairments found were at least partly the result of a perseveration of these position responses. The prolonged exhibition of inappropriate responses served as the foundation of Kimble's (1968) theory that hippocampal lesions reduce the ability of animals to inhibit responses to cues no longer having behavioral relevance. However, it must be emphasized again that the perseveration of responses cannot account, by itself, for all of the deficits reported in reversal learning by animals with hippocampal lesions (e.g., Harley, 1979).

A number of studies have found electrical evidence indicating changes in the neuronal activity of the dentate gyrus that are more-or-less associated with behavioral discrimination performance (e.g., Berger, Alger, & Thompson, 1976; Segal, Disterhoft, & Olds, 1972; Segal, 1973). Deadwyler, West, and Lynch (1979) found that while the significance of auditory stimulation was correlated with the prolonged discharge of dentate gyrus cells, the input to the region over the perforant path was not. This finding was thought to provide evidence that the reward value of the sensory events was added in the dentate gyrus and was probably relayed by septal afferents (Deadwyler, West, & Robinson, 1981). In the study of electrical charges in the hippocampus during the learning of the rabbit nictitating-membrane response, a correlation between the discharge rates of cells and the acquisition of the response has been reported (Berger & Thompson, 1978). In this study, no differences in cellular responsiveness related to the response were observed among the CA_1, CA_3, and dentate areas. The results of these studies may be related to changes in overall excitability in the hippocampus, which may be due to alterations in the catecholaminergic input (Segal, 1977). It is possible that similar changes could be observed in many brain regions and thus may not be specific to the hippocampus. Thompson and his co-workers have found that the greater the number of slow waves in the hippocampal EEG before training, the more rapid the acquisition of the nictitating response (Berry, Rinaldi, Thompson, & Verzeano, 1978; Berry & Thompson, 1978, 1979). The association is especially strong between the slow-wave domination and the number of trials required for the first few conditioned responses to occur. Gabriel and Saltwick (1980) have found that a burst of rhythmic activity in the theta range can be observed in the second or so preceding conditioned avoidance responses in rabbits.

As summarized by Berger, Clark, and Thompson (1980) and Thompson, Berger, Berry, Hoehler, Kettner, and Weisz (1980), the discharge of many neurons in the rabbit hippocampus shows a strong, time-locked relationship to the learning and performance of the nictitating-membrane response. Furthermore, the changes in unit activity precede the actual execution of the response. These changes may be due to alterations in the activities of monoaminergic innervation of the hippocampus, as mentioned above, or to some other influence (see also Disterhoft & Segal, 1978). A pressing need in this line of research is the determination of the nature of changes found in other limbic and nonlimbic areas during such conditioning. The possible roles played by diffusely projecting systems also need to be elaborated. Another question of importance relates to the significance of such changes for the learning and the retention of the conditioned response. As mentioned earlier, rabbits without the hippocampus acquire the nictitating-membrane response at least as rapidly as control animals. Whatever else can be said, this finding indicates that the hippocampus is not an essential region for the formation of the memory on which that behavior is based. The important changes observed by Thompson, Berger, and their associates may reflect changes related to the memory processes but certainly are not the only memory processing occurring in the brain.

Best and Best (1976) presented data supporting the idea that the cellular discharges occurring in the hippocampus following sensory stimulation are dependent on the state of the animal (awake or asleep) at the time of stimulation and the meaning of the stimulation. These authors assumed that input from other regions must mediate "state effects" and that the hippocampus probably receives information about stimulus saliency from other cortical regions. They interpreted their results as being consistent with the idea that the structure could act to attenuate the effects of irrelevant stimulation that are competing for some form of mental or neuronal registration, an idea clearly in line with data from lesion studies, for example, the failure of animals with hippocampal lesions to show stimulus "overshadowing" (Rickert et al., 1979). Solomon (1977) demonstrated that the conditioning of a nictitating-membrane response to a tone accomplished before the conditioning of the response to the compound stimulus *tone plus light* would block the association usually made to the light when tested by itself. This blocking did not occur in animals with hippocampal lesions. A similar result has been found in rats by means of an operant paradigm (Rickert *et al.*, 1978). These results would also indicate the difficulty the lesioned animals had in tuning out irrelevant or redundant information.

Recordings made from cells in the CA_1-subicular region of the hippocampal formation of rabbits learning a discriminated avoidance response have revealed different types of responses in cells with different firing characteristics. Some cells show accentuated bursts in the second or so before a response is made after training is well established but burst throughout the time that the conditioned stimuli are presented early in training (Gabriel & Saltwick, 1980). Analysis of the responding of nonbursting cells indicates excitatory discharges early in conditioning to both the CS^+ and CS^-. The same occurred during the initial training, with the significance of the conditioned stimuli reversed. In later stages of training, no responses were seen after either CS (Saltwick & Gabriel, 1980). In general, the hippocampus is seen as a behavioral gating mechanism that releases a behavior for expression, depending on the acquired significance of the stimulus and other factors (Gabriel, Foster, Orona, Saltwick, & Stanton, 1980). The gate is open for behavior to occur when rhythmic activities predominate in the bursting cells.

FRUSTRATION

In 1972, Kimble and I (Isaacson & Kimble, 1972) alluded to the possible usefulness of Maier's description of frustration-induced behavior (Maier, 1949) in describing and explaining the effects of hippocampal destruction. We felt that since animals with hippocampal damage could give us some hypotheses as readily as intact animals, even though their selection of new hypotheses might be limited, their behavior could not be explained as a simple perseveration of learned responses or hypotheses. Animals with hippocampal damage seem to have sufficient flexibility in behavior under many circumstances but lose it when the environment becomes uncertain or rewards are not obtained with accustomed regularity.

The behavior exhibited in the frustration-inducing situations was viewed as *not* being based on normal motivational considerations. It was the result of a fixation of a response (or hypothesis) when the animal or person was forced to make some response (see Maier, 1964). It is important to recognize that Maier first observed fixated, perseverative behaviors when animals were presented with insoluble problems. The frustrated animals continued to exhibit the fixated behavior even when the problem was made soluble. Maier also recognized that there were considerable individual differences in the tolerance of animals to frustrating circumstances; some animals quickly adopted fixated, non-goal-directed behavior patterns, whereas others required much longer exposure to the insoluble problems.

Are there points of similarity between frustration-instigated behaviors and the behaviors often exhibited by animals with hippocampal lesions? Many animals with hippocampal damage exhibit long strings of inappropriate behaviors during the learning and reversal of discrimination problems. Not all the lesioned animals exhibit these behaviors, partly because of the nature of the hypothesis being tested by the animals, but also because of the tendencies of the individual animals to respond with fixated behaviors to the frustrations of the testing situation. The hippocampal lesion may tend to lower the threshold for frustration-induced effects, but in animals constitutionally resistant to frustration, this lower threshold would mean that the effects produced by the lesions would be reflected in the proportion of animals affected. The effect would be all-or-none for any particular animal, but some animals might not be influenced in a particular task. This result is exactly what was found by Nonneman and Isaacson (1973) in their study of task-dependent behavioral changes induced by hippocampal lesions made early or late in life. In our study, the earliness of the lesion determined the proportion of animals affected on a particular task.

Maier (1949) also pointed out that the response that becomes fixated is not predictable from the responses learned in the past. This same result has been found in studies accomplished in my laboratory. We have been unable to predict the response to be fixated by a particular animal with hippocampal lesions during reversal training on the basis of the number of past responses or the number of reinforced responses made in accordance with a particular hypothesis. This finding suggests that at some point, the animal changes its pattern of behavior from one that is goal-oriented or hypothesis-directed to one that is not goal-oriented. The perseverated response may not be the one to which the animal has been trained or the first one exhibited in the training situation.

In some experimental situations, including training on brightness discrimination problems, the effects of posterior neocortical lesions seem to resemble the effects of hippocampal destruction. While the neocortex of the rat (and maybe of other species) may not be essential for learning visual discriminations, it may be presumed to be of some value or use to the animal (e.g., Bauer & Cooper, 1964). When it is destroyed, the animal should be handicapped and the problem less easily solved. To the extent that this handicap occurs, the probability is increased that frustration-induced perseverative acts will occur in a group of animals. The reduction in threshold for the frustration response produced by the additional destruction of the hippocampus would potentiate this tendency. In some discrimination experiments, a maximal effect could be found after the neocortical participation.

Perseverative responding due to frustration or to brain damage does not develop immediately in those problems in which the lesioned animals show abnormal patterns of behavior (e.g., during reversals and extinction). It develops more-or-less slowly over the course of time and after the animals have found that successful performance is not quickly reached. This finding suggests that animals with hippocampal lesions develop a perseverative mode of responding secondary to the inability to solve the problem.

The surprising aspect is that while perseverative responding may be secondary to an inability to solve a particular problem, this inability could stem from a reduced ability to give up an inappropriate hypothesis or to focus attention properly. Hirsh (1970) found that the changes observed in the behavior of the animals with hippocampal lesions were not identical. Some animals exhibited an enhanced alternation of responses, while others showed perseveration of responses. The point is that all of the animals studied by Hirsh did not perform in the same sort of perseverative fashion, even though they all perseverated in some way. Pribram et al. (1969) suggested that monkeys with hippocampal lesions were faced with an inability to retain hypotheses pertaining to the problem before them in the face of interfering tendencies.

Douglas and Pribram (1969) found that monkeys with hippocampal damage trained on a discrimination problem had more difficulty

when there was one positive cue presented along with several negative cues than when one positive cue and one negative cue were
presented. The more negative cues there were available, the greater
was the impairment. However, the addition of negative (nonrewarded) stimuli to the task produces another effect that could be the
cause of the behavioral deficit. With only two stimuli available (i.e.,
a rewarded stimulus and a nonrewarded stimulus), the animals obtain
a reward on about one-half of the training trials before the problem
is learned. With four negative stimuli and one positive stimulus, the
animal receives a reward on only about 20% of its prelearning trials.
Pigareva (1974) found that the frequency of rewards was of importance
to the animals with hippocampal damage. When reinforcement probabilities were low (33% or 25% of reinforced responses), no learning
of a conditioned response based on food reward was observed.

Altered responses to frustrating events can be measured in many
ways. One of these is the measurement of changes in responding in
the face of a change in rewards. Using a double alley paradigm,
Swanson and Isaacson (1969) found a typical frustration effect in animals with hippocampal lesions. The running speed in the second
alley increased when the reward was withheld at the end of the first
alley. Franchina and Brown (1971) failed to find a significant decrease
in response latencies when the size of the rewards was reduced in
a runway situation (a "negative contrast effect"). Van Hartesveldt
(1973) found that rats with hippocampal lesions acquired a bar-press
response equally rapidly for large and small water rewards, whereas
control animals learned more slowly when the small reinforcements
were provided. When animals trained for large rewards were
switched to smaller ones, there were increases in *responding*, presumably an attempt to incorporate more water during a testing session.
As a result, Van Hartesveldt's data cannot be seen as providing a
basis for the evaluation of reward contrast effects as has sometimes
been claimed. Mikulka, Freeman, and Hughes (1981) have reported
that hungry animals with amygdala or hippocampal lesions trained
on high- or low-sucrose concentration solutions show either positive
or negative contrast effects when the solutions are switched, depending on whether the animals are shifted from low to high or from
high to low concentrations. Using a straight runway, P. N. Strong
(personal communication, 1981) has found that hippocampally lesioned animals demonstrate a normal increase in running speed and

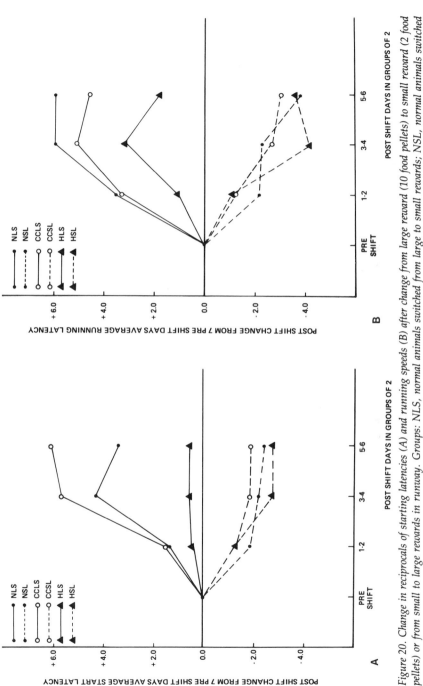
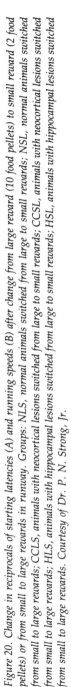

Figure 20. Change in reciprocals of starting latencies (A) and running speeds (B) after change from large reward (10 food pellets) to small reward (2 food pellets) or from small to large reward in runway. Groups: NLS, normal animals switched from large to small rewards; NSL, normal animals switched from small to large rewards; CCLS, animals with neocortical lesions switched from large to small rewards; CCSL, animals with neocortical lesions switched from small to large rewards; HLS, animals with hippocampal lesions switched from large to small rewards; HSL, animals with hippocampal lesions switched from small to large rewards. Courtesy of Dr. P. N. Strong, Jr.

a reduction in the time required to leave the start box when shifted from small to large rewards. However, when shifted from large to small rewards, they fail to slow down as much as controls. This effect is illustrated in Figure 20. This finding would indicate a normal positive contrast effect but an impaired negative effect.

It would appear that animals with hippocampal damage can show a reduced negative contrast effect when measures of acquired performances are used, such as by Strong, but not when consumatory responses are employed.

The lesioned animals are, however, generally less sensitive to the size of the rewards provided during the learning of a response, and this fact could provide difficulties for the interpretation of such studies.

By and large, animals with hippocampal or fornix damage seem to exhibit fewer signs of frustration than controls (e.g., Gray, 1970). Animals with lesions of the fornix bite the lever less frequently when extinction training is begun after performing on a continuous reinforcement schedule for food rewards (Osborne & Black, 1978). Therefore, it appears that, while in some situations hippocampal formation damage may induce behavioral patterns that resemble the "non-goal-oriented" behaviors of animals subjected to insoluble problems, many of the actions of these animals would suggest a decreased sensitivity to the experience of frustration induced by the omission or the reduction of rewards.

ELECTRICAL RHYTHMS OF THE HIPPOCAMPUS

The electrical rhythms of the hippocampal formation have been attractive for neurophysiological researchers because of the relatively well-known and simple anatomy of the system and because of the large potential rhythmic activities (the rhythmic, slow potentials) that can be easily recorded from various portions of it (Jung & Kornmüller, 1938). Summaries of research on these rhythmic potentials as they relate to behavior are available as chapters by Bennett, by Vanderwolf et al., by Black, by Winson, by Vinogradova, by Ranck, by Crowne, and by Radcliffe in Isaacson and Pribram (1975). More recent reviews include those of Robinson (1980), Vanderwolf and Robinson (1981),

Buzsáki *et al.* (1980), Komisaruk (1977), and Lopes Da Silva and Arnolds (1979).

Before considering this topic further, it is important to remember that the Greek letters used to name the electrical activities of the brain refer to the frequency of electrical rhythms and not to the brain areas from which the records are obtained. In common usage, delta rhythms are those of frequencies of 3 Hz and below. Theta rhythms are those of frequencies between 4 and 8 Hz, while alpha frequencies are those between 8 and 12 Hz. All of these rhythms can be found in recordings made from the structures of the limbic system, from the neocortex, and even from the midbrain and the brain stem. Some confusion has been created in the recent literature because of the description of rhythmic activities as "theta rhythms," when the frequencies are not in the appropriate range. At times, recordings of 8 Hz and faster obtained from the hippocampus have been called "hippocampal theta" because of their mathematical and aesthetic purity. To reduce confusion, it would be better to describe them simply as *rhythmic activities* and to designate the predominant frequency as closely as possible.

Investigations of the rhythmic electrical activities of the hippocampus have generally tried to associate such activities with movements (Vanderwolf, 1969, 1971), attention or orienting (Grastyán, Lissák, Madarász, & Donhoffer, 1959; Bennett, 1971), memory processing (Adey, 1964; Elazar & Adey, 1967), or the activation of special muscle groups (Klemm, 1970; Komisaruk, 1968, 1970).

The rhythmic slow potentials probably reflect nonpropagated electronic changes in synaptic potentials (e.g., Green, Maxwell, Schindler, & Stumpf, 1960; Green & Petsche, 1961). The fluctuations of the rhythmic potentials are related to the excitability of hippocampal pyramidal cells (Rudell, Fox, & Ranck, 1980), and some cells do fire in close association with rhythmic slow potentials. Such cells have been called *theta cells* (Ranck, 1975). Other cells do not fire in close relationship to the slow potentials. It is possible that theta cells are a set of interneurons within the hippocampus. Although the afferent fibers from the septal area thought to be responsible for normal rhythmic slow activities (RSA) seem to reach diffuse regions of the hippocampus, two RSA-generating zones seem to exist: one in the CA_1 field, and the other in the dentate (Winson, 1974; Bland, Andersen, &

Ganes, 1975). The phase relations of the electrical rhythms of the two generators depend on the state of the animal. These rhythms are in phase during slow-wave sleep but are phase-reversed during paradoxical sleep and when the animals are awake (Buzsáki, Grastyán, Kellényi, & Czopf, 1979). The generators seem to be located in areas of relatively low cell density: the outer molecular layer of the dentate and the stratum oriens of the hippocampus. Since the electrical rhythms recorded depend on the distances of the electrodes from the two generators and the relationship between multiple electrodes and the generator sites, differences among the results obtained by different groups of investigators are not surprising.

Vanderwolf and his associates (e.g., Vanderwolf & Robinson, 1981) have attempted to relate RSA to the behavior of the rat. They found that RSA occurs when "voluntary" movements are initiated by the animals, including the grabbing and holding of food. High-voltage irregular activity is found when the animals are motionless, chewing, licking, vocalization, scratching, or engaged in sexual activities—in short, in almost all reflexive acts, some of which are clearly consumatory in nature. Voluntary acts are called *Type 1 behaviors*. The more reflexive acts are called *Type 2*. Other behaviors associated with RSA (Type 1) include swimming, jumping, digging, object manipulation, and postural changes.

However, RSA can occur when the animals are motionless, especially in some species (Kramis, Vanderwolf, & Bland, 1975; Winson, 1972). This finding has led to the differentiation of RSA into subtypes based primarily on pharmacological factors. Neither atropine nor scopolamine eliminates the RSA associated with "voluntary" movements, but both cholinergic drugs eliminate non-movement-related RSA. On the other hand, movement-associated RSA is decreased by volatile anesthetics, such as ether (Vanderwolf et al., 1978; Whishaw, 1976). The atropine-insensitive RSA is usually made up of somewhat higher frequencies (7–12 cps) than the atropine-sensitive type (4–7 cps).

It should be noted that even though atropine does not block or eliminate the RSA associated with voluntary movements, the electrical activities of the hippocampus may be influenced by the drug. The predominant frequencies of RSA found during swimming or running for a water reward, or found during REM sleep are altered after the administration of atropine (Buzsáki et al., 1980; Usui & Iwahara, 1977).

Therefore, the term *atropine-insensitive* seems too strong. The nature of the RSA recorded is altered by the drug—it is not just eliminated by it.

When rats are lesioned in the posterior hypothalamus or are given reserpine, alcohol, or urethane, long trains of RSA can be observed during immobility (De Ryck & Teitelbaum, 1978; Kolb & Whishaw, 1977; Robinson & Whishaw, 1974). Electrical stimulation of the reticular formation or strong, stressful environmental stimulation may also elicit RSA without movement (Whishaw, 1972; Robinson & Vanderwolf, 1978). Both anatomical locations seem to be able to generate the movement-related and immobility-related RSA which, as mentioned, has pharmacological distinctiveness.

There is general agreement on the fact that locomotion is accompanied by RSA in rats, guinea pigs, cats, rabbits, and dogs. Positive correlations have been found between the speed of movement and the predominant frequency of the RSA (Teitelbaum & McFarland, 1971; Arnolds, Lopes Da Silva, Aitink, & Kamp, 1979a,b,c). However, there is substantial evidence that the association of RSA with movements is not the entire story of RSA.

Studying the electrical rhythms of the cat hippocampus in an operant paradigm, Buzsáki, Grastyán, Haubenreiser, Czopf, and Kellényi (1981) found that RSA in the 5–6 cps range accompanied orienting behaviors to the CS, but desynchronized activity occurred during lever pressing. In a signaled shock paradigm, the cats showed increases in frequencies of RSA after the CS even though movements during this period decreased. Rats also showed similar changes in RSA even though they increased rather than decreased their motor actions. Bennett, French, and Burnett (1978) have found that providing an external cue for the solution of a DRL problem increased the amount of RSA recorded from the dorsal (but not the ventral) hippocampus of rats. These authors view this result as reflecting an increase in the attention being paid to the occurrence of the external cue.

Buzsáki *et al.* (1981) and Bennett *et al.* (1978) believe that RSA from hippocampal recordings is closely associated with the direction of the animal's attention to environmental stimuli. The relationship of RSA to movement, these authors believe, is that movements are usually directed toward or away from certain aspects of the environment. Yet, awareness or evaluation of the environment can occur without movement, and in such conditions, RSA can be detected without overt movement.

It should be noted that through the use of hippocampal or septal area stimulation, the electrical recordings made from the hippocampus could be changed without altering behavior. Hippocampal synchrony could be induced that did not disrupt the performance of the behaviors usually associated with hippocampal desynchrony. The elicitation of desynchrony did not affect the behaviors usually associated with hippocampal RSA (Kramis & Routtenberg, 1977). This finding implies that a particular form of hippocampal activity is not essential to the execution of particular behaviors. The rhythms may be a by-product of activity in other regions related to movement and possibly to other uses of information about movements or their consequences.

Not only do the amount and duration of rhythmic activity in the hippocampus change with alterations in the animal's environment, but its frequency is altered as well. Lopes Da Silva and Kamp (1969) found a change in theta frequency ranges from 4–5 Hz to 5–6 Hz when a dog that was pressing a pedal in an operant situation backed away from the pedal after a reinforcement. In a subsequent article, Kamp, Lopes Da Silva, and Storm Van Leeuwen (1971) found the same increase in hippocampal frequencies when a dog changed its behavior from turning around looking for a thrown stick to actually running after it. In a series of studies, Arnolds *et al.* (1979a,b,c) made strong correlations of movements with the amplitude, rhythmicity, and frequency of hippocampal electrical rhythms. They believe that the hippocampal EEG reflects the intensity of motor behaviors and that the records should not be regarded as either showing or not showing RSA. These authors see the EEG as a continuum of activity without cutoff point between states. They argued that when different hippocampal recordings are found during similar behaviors, closer examination will reveal that the behaviors are also different, perhaps in a subtle way and perhaps varying somewhat from one species to another. For example, RSA occurs while eating and drinking in the dog but not in the rat. Furthermore, head movements were associated with small head movements in the dog but not in the cat (Kemp & Kaada, 1975).

The arrest of ongoing behavior patterns has been found to be associated with a desynchronization of electrical activities recorded from the hippocampus, while the initiation of behaviors has been associated with RSA. In a task presumed to require the inhibition of movement, Bennett and Gottfried (1970) found that the EEG from the cat hippocampus was dominated by desynchronized activity.

Pond, Lidsky, Levine, and Schwartzbaum (1970) recorded electrical rhythms from the hippocampus in free-roving animals. These authors found that normal eating produced irregular and desynchronized activity in the hippocampus. On the other hand, if feeding behavior was elicited by direct hypothalamic stimulation, RSA was produced in the hippocampus. Pond *et al.* found that stimulation of the hypothalamus without an appropriate goal object present produced RSA in the hippocampus, but the frequency was 1–2 Hz below that found when stimulation occurred with the appropriate goal object present. This finding is important since it shows that even though the hippocampus may be inhibited by the stimulation of the hypothalamus, as measured by changes in electrical rhythms, its activity can still be subject to modification by the environment.

In 1965, Stumpf suggested that the theta frequency recorded from the hippocampus might be useful as an indicator of reticular formation arousal. It may be a better indicator of arousal mediated by the posterior hypothalamus. Stimulation in this region is more likely to produce RSA in the hippocampus than is stimulation of the reticular formation, although both areas can produce these activities when electrically stimulated. The RSA is of a "purer" nature when produced by hypothalamic stimulation than when produced by reticular formation stimulation. Only the stimulation of the posterior hypothalamus produced RSA in the hippocampus. Stimulation of the anterior hypothalamus produces a desynchronization of the hippocampus and, in addition, a high-frequency rhythmic response in the amygdala and the olfactory bulb (Kawamura, Nakamura, & Tokizane, 1961).

There is little doubt that there are multiple systems through which other brain regions regulate electrical rhythms of the hippocampus. Torii (1961) identified two systems, each of which stood in a particular relationship to both hippocampal activity and regulation of the autonomic nervous system. The first was a system including the ventromedial tegmentum, the lateral hypothalamus, and the medial septal area. Electrical stimulation applied at 100 Hz to the structures of this system produced desynchronized activity in the hippocampus and parasympathetic effects in the autonomic nervous system. The second system involved the dorsolateral central gray and the periventricular hypothalamus. Stimulation in these areas produced rhythmic activities in the hippocampus and sympathetic responses in the autonomic nervous system. Similar indices of sympathetic arousal were found associated with hippocampal RSA by Kemp and Kaada (1975). The basic distinction between lateral desynchronizing and medial synchronizing systems of the hypothalamus relative to hippocampal rhythms has been supported by the study of Anchel and Lindsley (1972). They also were able to confirm the suggestion of Torii that the synchronizing influences reaching the medial (paraventricular) regions of the hypothalamus from the tegmentum are carried over the dorsal bundle of Schütz. The desynchronizing influences were thought by Torii to be reaching the hypothalamus over the mammillary peduncle.

Anchel and Lindsley reported that the rhythmic slow activities elicited by medial hypothalamic stimulation can be blocked by lesions of the dorsal fornix, but that the desynchronization response is not affected by these lesions. Anchel and Lindsley suggested that input from the fibers of tegmental origin that pass through the dorsal bundle of Schütz and the medial hypothalamus reach both the septal area regions presumably containing the pacemakers for hippocampal RSA and the intralaminar nuclei of the thalamus. The two branches of this ascending system could have opposite effects in their regions of termination, such as producing slow rhythmic activities in the hippocampus and desynchronization in the neocortex. Lindsley and his colleagues (Lindsley & Wilson, 1975; Macadar, Chalupa, & Lindsley, 1974) have found that high-frequency stimulation of the raphe complex produces hippocampal desynchronization and has been associated with an ascending serotonergic system. Lesions of the median raphe allow low-frequency RSA to be found during immobility in the rat, something not usually observed (Maru, Takahashi, & Iwahara, 1979). It is possible that the serotonergic systems have an inhibitory effect on RSA-generating systems of the forebrain. In urethane-anesthetized animals, repetitive stimulation of the median raphe complex disrupted the bursting discharges of a population of cells in the medial septal area whose discharges were related to RSA in the hippocampus. As the burst discharges of these cells were reduced, the hippocampus evidenced a desynchronized state (Assaf & Miller, 1978). However, urethane and other general anesthetics seem to block the atropine-resistant form of hippocampal RSA (Robinson & Vanderwolf, 1978), and the results of studies with such preparations must be interpreted with this limitation in mind.

Although stimulation of the lateral aspects of the posterior hypothalamus can produce a desynchronized hippocampal state, the electrical rhythms recorded from the hippocampus do not seem to stand in any particular or necessary relationship to the rewarding effects produced by electrical stimulation of the same hypothalamic area or of the septal area. Pond and Schwartzbaum (1970) found no difference between the types of hippocampal EEG patterns found after rewarding or aversive stimulation of the hypothalamus or the midbrain. RSA in the hippocampus was produced by both types of stimulation and was related to the intensity of the stimulation rather than to its affective qualities. Ball and Gray (1971) stimulated the septal area and could get either RSA or desynchronization from the hippocampus by using different frequencies of stimulation. The different frequencies of stimulation were not related to the behavioral effects produced by the stimulation, since the animal would depress a lever to obtain stimulation at all frequencies used. Ito and Olds (1971) found that stimulation in a rewarding area of the lateral hypothalamus produced inhibitory effects on the activity of single cells in the hippocampus (but an excitatory effect on the activity of cells in the cingulate cortex). The increase in excitability found after the rewarding stimulation in the cingulate region could be related to the enhanced responsiveness to sensory signals found in that region during conditioning (Gabriel & Saltwick, 1980; Gabriel, Foster, & Orona, 1980).

The electrical rhythms of the hippocampus influence the excitability of cells in the structure and their response to stimulation over normal afferent pathways. The average evoked potentials in the hippocampus are influenced by the EEG patterns and the behavior of the animals (Leung, 1980). Under most conditions, the EEG and behavior are closely associated and can be viewed as indicating a state of the animal. Transmission of impulses through the hippocampal formation depends on this state. Winson and Abzug (1977) stimulated the cortical afferent pathway in the angular bundle and recorded the induced activity in the dentate gyrus and the CA_1 field. Monosynaptic responses in the dentate were greater during sleep than during wakefulness. In the CA_1 field, the trisynaptic response was greatest in slow-wave sleep and less substantial during either paradoxical sleep or when the animal was awake. This work was extended to the study of two forms of the awake state: (1) during a quiet awake period and (2) during the performance of voluntary movements (Winson & Abzug, 1978). Again, the results indicated that the pathway through the hippocampus to the CA_1 cells was more efficient in slow-wave sleep than in other states. The primary decrease found in these other conditions seems to be due to a release from tonic inhibition being exerted at the dentate gyrus during slow-wave sleep. The tonic inhibition may be due to the activities of ascending monoamine systems. During periods of bodily movement, the response of some CA_3 cells can be correlated with rhythmic slow potentials. This correlation could mean that RSA affects the excitability of a class of CA_3 cells, but probably not those that project to the CA_1 region over the Schäffer collateral system.

In training an animal in a discrimination paradigm, Deadwyler *et al.* (1981) found that the evoked response in the outer portion of the molecular layer of the dentate gyrus changed as the animal learned that the auditory signal predicted water availability. One component of the response appears to be a sensory-based negative potential mediated by the perforant pathway. A second negative-potential component was related to the acquired significance of the sensory signal. The development of this second response was related to input derived from the septal region. Buzsáki *et al.* (1981) have also reported evoked-potential studies in which the response to the CS habituated over trials in the outer molecular layer of the dentate gyrus, that is, when the meaning of the signal became more predictable.

Black and his associates were successful in conditioning RSA (4–7 Hz) and a desynchronized state in the same dogs by using both food and brain stimulation as rewards. Black, Young, and Batenchuk (1970) demonstrated RSA conditioning in curarized dogs as well, an indication that the conditioning of the RSA of the hippocampus need not be mediated via bodily activities. These authors found that desynchronization of the neocortex can be associated with any type of electrical activity in the hippocampus. The main behavioral correlate of hippocampal slow activity discovered was locomotor movement. When the hippocampus evidenced a desynchronized state, the animals were likely to be standing still (Black, 1972). When the animals were taught to make an active conditioned response, there were increases in RSA. When the animals were trained to inhibit overt responses, a much decreased level of RSA was obtained. In a related experiment, Holmes and Beckman (1969) found that RSA was a good indicator of whether a cat would run a simple runway for a food reward when signaled to do so.

Movements are not necessary for the occurrence of RSA from the hippocampus, since RSA can be conditioned in animals immobilized under curare. Using a related approach, Black has tried to make animals be immobile and yet produce RSA in the hippocampus. The animals had to do both in order to be rewarded. This response was possible for lower frequencies but not for the higher frequencies in the "slow range" (Black & DeToledo, 1971).

MEMORY

One of the major reasons for the intensive research that has been conducted on the hippocampal formation for the past 30 years has been the reports of amnesiac effects following bilateral damage, or presumed bilateral damage, to the medial temporal lobes in people (Scoville, 1954; Scoville & Milner, 1957; Penfield & Milner, 1958). The amnestic syndrome is characterized by a loss of recent memory, in particular from the time of the surgery to almost the present time. Material seems to be maintained in memory for short periods, ranging in minutes, but once the situation is altered or the patient is distracted, the information is quickly lost and cannot be retrieved. The deficit is sometimes called a *deficit in recent memory*.

The deficit is not absolute, as patients show dim awareness of events that have happened after surgery. The most famous patient studied, case H.M., could remember President John Kennedy and his assassination when shown a Kennedy half-dollar (Milner, Corkin, & Teuber, 1968). There is also compelling evidence that H.M. and other patients with similar conditions have residual memory abilities that can be revealed by the use of appropriate retrieval cues or hints, or by the use of nonverbal prompting (e.g., Weiskrantz & Warrington, 1975). It should also be emphasized that many of the patients in whom the lesions produced memory disorders were ones who had long-standing and severe epileptic disorders or who had signs of epileptiform activity postoperatively. This fact led me to consider the possibility that the seizure activity, coupled with the surgery of the temporal lobe, produced the amnesia, which would not be found after the surgery without the epileptic disorder (Isaacson, 1972a).

Electrical Seizures

The hippocampus is thought of as an area of the brain especially prone to seizure activity. Almost any physical or chemical disturbance will lead to a series of epileptiform afterdischarges. The afterdischarges may spread beyond the hippocampus to involve other regions of the limbic system or may remain confined to the hippocampus. The propagation of these seizures to other structures, if it does occur, is quite different, depending on whether the seizure focus is in the dorsal or the ventral hippocampus.

Woodruff, Gage, and Isaacson (1973a) have found that the seizure-prone nature of the hippocampus is dependent on projections to it from the pontine portions of the brain stem. In rabbits, a section through the brain stem ahead of the pons makes the hippocampus no more prone to seizure activity than the posterior neocortex. The hippocampus is most seizure-prone when large-amplitude slow waves can be recorded from it. Since the serotonergic input to the hippocampus tends to desynchronize the hippocampus, as reviewed earlier in this chapter, the sections made by Woodruff *et al.* may have produced their effects by eliminating this source of input.

An *epileptogenic focus* is a group of cells thought to be responsible for the production of abnormal electrical patterns recorded from brain tissue. The cells in an epileptogenic focus are more excitable than normal cells and have the capability of generating autonomous paroxysmal discharges.

Epileptogenic foci can be artificially created by the direct application of many different compounds and procedures, including the application of aluminum hydroxide gel, penicillin, other antibiotics, cobalt powder, conjugated estrogens, and pentylenetetrazol (Metrazol) and by local freezing. The mechanism by which penicillin acts to create an epileptogenic focus is not entirely established, but the affected cells show a depolarizing shift in membrane potentials that trigger bursts of discharges. In the interictal state, each burst initiates an inhibitory potassium potential. Full-blown seizures occur when this inhibitory potential disappears (Alger & Nicoll, 1980). When recording from the hippocampus at prolonged times after penicillin injection, epileptiform activity can frequently be observed (Schmaltz, 1971) in anesthetized animals. Spike discharges occur singly, in bursts, or in trains that last over periods of 10–20 sec or longer. In about half of the animals studied, spiking was not observed, but bursts of high-voltage fast activity could be recorded against a relatively normal background. However, Woodruff, Fish, and Alderman (1977) found that the interictal epileptiform discharges could not be found as early as 4 days after the intrahippocampal administration of sodium penicillin-G in freely moving, awake animals. It is likely that the nature and the amount of the penicillin used to induce the epileptiform activity are of importance for the length of time it will take for its electrical effects to be noticed (Van Hartesveldt, Petit, & Isaacson, 1975; Woodruff, Kearley, & Isaacson, 1974). It is also possible that the presence of epileptiform discharges may not be closely related to the neuronal abnormalities induced by the drug responsible for the behavioral changes.

From several studies, it is clear that penicillin injected into the hippocampus can produce profound behavioral effects that are quite different from those found after the surgical destruction of the same areas.

Probably the most dramatic results were those obtained by Schmaltz (1971). In his work, a two-way active-avoidance task was used. This shuttlebox task is one in which the performance of animals with bilateral destruction of the hippocampus by aspiration is enhanced. Schmaltz found that penicillin injected unilaterally into the rat hippocampus greatly impaired the animals in learning the task.

Equally interesting was the observation that animals with the impaired performance due to penicillin injection showed better performance during the last five trials each day than during the first five. The animals apparently were able to learn something about the problem within each day's training session but started the next day's training as if this previous training had not taken place. This inability to carry over the effects of training from one day to the next suggested an inability to incorporate the memories from the past into a form useful on subsequent days. Significant impairments were obtained with unilateral injections of penicillin into the hippocampus; however, the effect is much more pronounced when a unilateral injection of penicillin is combined with ablation of the contralateral hippocampus.

Nakajima (1969) has found impairment in the learning and re-learning of a shock-motivated spatial discrimination in a T-maze following the injection of actinomycin D into the hippocampus. The learning impairment is similar to that produced by electrolytic lesions of the hippocampus, but the electrolytic lesion fails to influence retention as measured by relearning on the following day. The actinomycin-injected animals, on the other hand, showed impaired retention of the problem when tested by relearning. This deficit is suggestive of a memory impairment of events occurring beyond the training period.

Olton (1970) confirmed the observations of Schmaltz and extended them by considering the effects of penicillin injections into different brain regions in otherwise intact animals and in animals with bilateral aspirative destruction of the hippocampus. He used an avoidance-training paradigm similar to that used by Schmaltz. Penicillin injections into the septal area or into the entorhinal cortex failed to produce the same debilitating effects as did injections into the hippocampus. In animals with bilateral destruction of the hippocampus, the rate of active-avoidance learning was improved and was not altered by penicillin introduced into the septal area. Penicillin injections into the entorhinal cortex, on the other hand, offset the improvement in performance produced by hippocampal destruction. This finding was interpreted as suggesting that the interaction between the hippocampus and the adjacent entorhinal cortex is of greater significance than the hippocampus–septal-area interaction.

Hamilton and Isaacson (1970) studied the effect of penicillin implantation in a variety of brain-stem locations. When behavior on the two-way active-avoidance tasks was studied, locations in the ventral tegmental area were especially effective in disrupting learning. Drug implantation sites in the reticular formation produced slight, if any, debilitating effects. Penicillin application to many other regions (e.g., the mammillary bodies, the caudate nucleus, the midline thalamus, and the dorsomedial thalamic nucleus) failed to disrupt the avoidance behavior. After the avoidance training had been completed, the animals were tested on a visual discrimination task for food reward. All of the animals were able to learn this visual discrimination problem. Therefore, the debilitation was specific to the avoidance task and did not carry over to the visual discrimination problem. Animals with penicillin implanted in one hippocampus with the contralateral hippocampus surgically removed (the most impaired preparation studied by Schmaltz and Olton) were also studied on this task. No deficit in their behavior was observed.

The results obtained by Hamilton and Isaacson (1970) in testing animals on the visual discrimination task have been confirmed by Woodruff and Isaacson (1972). Woodruff *et al.* (1974) made daily injections of penicillin into the hippocampus and found an impairment of acquisition of the visual discrimination performance.

However, Woodruff *et al.* (1977) failed to replicate the results of Schmaltz and Olton described above. Statistically insignificant impairments in two-way active-avoidance performance were found after the application of sodium G penicillin into the hippocampus when the animals were tested 4 months after the injection of the drug. The bilateral injection of aluminum hydroxide into the hippocampus facilitated the acquisition of the active-avoidance task rather than impairing it. The failure to find penicillin-induced effects could be due to the time allowed after injection before testing, the type of penicillin used, or other factors.

This line of research has led us to several possible conclusions. One is that the epileptic condition induced in the hippocampus, coupled with a unilateral lesion, produces behavioral alterations that are interpretable as deficits in recent memory. The nature of the change in behavior probably depends on the nature of the abnormal neural activity, its location, and the time allowed between the creation of the focus and the testing. For example, aluminum hydroxide and penicillin implantations may have quite different effects on behavior. The effects will probably vary as a function of brain location and the subsequent spread of aberrant activity to different associated regions. The occurrence of spike discharges in the EEG is probably not necessary for the behavioral impairment. The possibility that an interaction occurs between an epileptic condition in temporal lobe structures or associated regions and subsequent surgical intervention remains a viable hypothesis.

Lesion Location

The reason that the hippocampal formation was identified as the region essential for the recent memory deficit was that removal of the anterior medial temporal lobes failed to produce the behavioral changes in similar patients. Only when the lesion went deeper to include the hippocampus did a memory deficit emerge. This interpretation has been strengthened by the fact that damage found in areas related to the hippocampal formation also produces memory disorders (e.g., Korsakoff's syndrome).

Horel (1978) has argued that the lesion that is responsible for the amnesiac effect after medial temporal lobe lesion is the "temporal stem" of the temporal lobe. This is the white matter region that is the bridge between the temporal lobe and the rest of the forebrain. The area consists of fibers that go between temporal lobe cortical regions as well as between the amygdala and other subcortical areas of the brain. The lesions made in the human patients with a memory loss must have damaged this area, and studies in animals with behavioral changes that could be related to impaired memory processes also involve this region. Lesions confined to the hippocampus rarely, if ever, induce behavior deficits that are based on memory impairments. However, Mair, Warrington, and Weiskrantz (1979) reported on two alcoholic patients with severe memory impairment suffering from Korsakoff's psychosis without involvement of the temporal stem, the hippocampus, or the amygdala. Marked gliosis, shrinkage, and other signs of abnormality were found in the mammillary bodies and an area nearby the medial dorsal nucleus of the thalamus. Quite similar results were reported by Victor, Adams, and Collins (1971).

Mishkin (1978) has presented evidence that lesions that involve both the amygdala and the hippocampus produce impairments that closely resemble a short-term memory deficit. Animals with combined lesions had difficulty remembering whether objects had been seen before and performed worst at the longer delay times. In another experimental paradigm, the lesioned animals performed poorly on a task that was similar to the human's learning a list of objects or words. While the combined lesions impaired these memory tasks, lesions of either the amydala or the hippocampus did not.

Cognitive Approaches

Correlated with the relatively recent blossoming of "cognitive theories" in psychology is the proliferation of cognitive theories of hippocampal function, especially in regard to memory. These range from theories relating the hippocampal formation to the evaluations of conditioned operations in memory (e.g., Hirsh, 1980; Hirsh & Krajden, in press; Kesner, 1980) to those related to reductions in the saliency of stimuli (e.g., Moore, 1979; Moore & Stickney, 1980), in the temporal processing of stimuli (Solomon, 1979, 1980), and in cognitive mapping (O'Keefe & Nadel, 1978) and working memories (Olton, Becker, & Handelmann, 1980). The work of Solomon, Moore, and their associates has been discussed earlier in the chapter and is not reviewed again here.

O'Keefe and Nadel (1978, 1979) proposed that rats generate cognitive maps about their environment and prefer to use them whenever possible. Experimentally, the use of cognitive maps is most often studied in elevated mazes with multiple arms and diverse stimuli surrounding them. The use of cognitive maps is thought to be different from the learning of routes or pathways through enclosed mazes. Evidence supporting the cognitive map approach has been based primarily on behavioral studies of animals with experimental disruption of the hippocampal system (the septal area, the fornix–fimbria, the hippocampus, and the entorhinal regions), although other evidence comes from the study of response patterns of single cells in the hippocampus in animals in different portions of their test environments.

Some neurons of the hippocampus show enhanced discharges when the animal is in a particular place (O'Keefe, 1976; O'Keefe & Dostrovsky, 1971). When the discharges of cells correlate with a "place," many of the discharges are closely related to the edges of the apparatus. Fewer cell response correlates are related to areas in the center of the test environment. The cues used to determine a place include cues such as lights, sound, and touch but do not seem to be dependent on prior turns required to get to the place (O'Keefe & Conway, 1978).

Ranck (1973) found cells that respond selectively to an animal's behavior in a maze and its behaviors following reward or nonreward. Miller and Best (1980) found that lesions of either the fornix or the entorhinal area disrupted the correlation of "place units" with their response to preferred locations. After such lesions, hippocampal cells responded primarily to the cues of the maze rather than to the "place" in the more general environment. These results indicate that the hippocampal formation receives information that is related to the environment of the animal, but how many other regions in the brain also receive similar information?

Perhaps the strongest evidence supporting a cognitive map theory was derived from studies in which lesioned animals failed to perform well on a multiple-arm elevated maze. In such situations, hungry animals are given the opportunity to obtain food pellets at the end of each arm. An optimal performance would be to choose each arm once, gaining the pellet located at the end of each arm. Animals with hippocampal damage do this poorly, making multiple visits to previously visited areas (e.g., Olton, 1978; Olton & Samuelson, 1976). Since the arms of the mazes are similar to each other except in spatial location, it could be thought that the animals were essentially "lost" in their spatial worlds.

However, Olton and his colleagues have proposed a different explanation of these results and one that can be tested against the cognitive map theory in a number of ways. Their idea is that the hippocampal formation is necessary to "working memory" (see Olton, Becker, & Handelmann, 1979). This form of memory is viewed as that used in "holding" information for a relatively brief period of time. This form of memory can be distinguished from "reference memory," a form of memory that is longer-lasting. These two forms of memory are inferred from the experimental procedures with which the animals are tested (Olton *et al.*, 1979, p. 314). Two procedures are used. In one, the information given the animal to solve a problem is useful for only the subsequent trial (working memory) and then is useless. In the other, the information given is of use throughout a prolonged series of trials or tests (reference memory). It is thought that working memory differs from reference memory because of its greater flexibility in the stimulus–response associations required to perform the task, its greater susceptibility to interference produced by prior testing, and its need to keep track of the temporal order of the stimuli being presented. The effect of hippocampal damage could be to alter one or more of these behavioral characteristics.

By means of tests involving the use of working-memory procedures, it has become clear that animals with hippocampal lesions can use extramaze cues to determine their location and also that they can be severely impaired in performance in situations in which only intramaze cues are needed for successful performance. For example,

Olton and Papas (1979) studied the effects of fornix–fimbria lesions on performance in a 17-arm radial maze in which 8 of the arms were baited (had food at the end of the arm) and 9 were not. Different arrangements of placing the baited and unbaited arms were used, but the results were similar in that the lesioned animals were able to avoid the unbaited arms (reference memory) but unable to remember the baited arms from which they had previously removed and eaten the food (working memory). They could not remember the previously chosen arms, a result found also by Jarrard (1978).

In regard to the use of intramaze cues, Olton and Feustle (1981) moved the positions of four arms of a + maze between trials. They did this each time an animal had made a response to one of the arms and had removed the food pellet(s) at the end. Each of the four arms had distinctive stimuli associated with it. In this procedure, a correct performance could be achieved on the basis of the cues associated with each arm, and a cognitive or spatial map was not required. However, the animal had to remember which arm it had previously responded to, so that empty arms would not be selected. This presumably required working memory. After fimbria–fornix lesions, animals were greatly impaired on this task. Buzsáki *et al.* (1981) have shown that on some tasks in which an impairment of working memory is found, an alternative explanation of the poor behavior may exist. These authors found that animals with fimbria lesions exhibited strings of behavioral responses quite different from chance (and therefore dependent on memory), but most easily explicable on the basis of excessive perseveration of a hypothesis readily abandoned by controls (see Hirsh, 1970; Olton, 1972; Isaacson & Kimble, 1972; Grastyán & Buzsáki, 1979).

Kesner (1980) prefers a formulation in which the hippocampus is seen as mediating the temporal and spatial attributes of the memories required in a learning task. This mediation is considered separate from a system involving the brain-stem reticular formation and the frontal neocortex (in the rat). Memories are thought to be stored on the basis of the attributes of stimuli in the environment. Only those related to space and time are processed by the hippocampus. Other attributes are presumed to be processed by other brain regions. Therefore, the learning and the memories affected by hippocampal dysfunction, induced by the electrical stimulation of the dorsal hippocampus in Kesner's studies, should be specific to those tasks in which space and time are essential attributes, but normal performance would be expected on others not requiring the use of these particular attributes.

Hirsh and his associates (Hirsh, 1980; Hirsh & Krajden, in press) have proposed an alternative formulation in which the hippocampus is an essential component of the brain's mechanisms that are responsible for conditional operations. Conditional operations are logical operations of the form, "If X, go right; if Y, go left." In other words, the appropriate response depends on the presence of a limited number of cues, whether internal or external, that dictate the correct response. Other cues in the situation remain constant during the test. Hirsh, Davis, and Holt (1979) found that animals with damage to the fornix or to the dentate gyrus (Hirsh, Holt, & Mosseri, 1978) have difficulty in responding differentially when hungry or thirsty in a T-maze where water is found at the end of one cross arm and food at the other. Normal animals made their choices on the basis of their motivational state. The lesioned animals did not. Similar results had been found after nearly complete hippocampal ablation (Hsaio & Isaacson, 1971). Hirsh believes that animals with hippocampal damage cannot use a "conditional" learning process and have only a more rudimentary stimulus–response associational learning mechanism available. They behave only as "Hullian" rats (Hull, 1952). They do not act on stimuli in a conditional fashion.

In all of these theories, some singular functional characteristic of mind or behavior is being sought. The authors have tried to associate a functional attribute(s) to an anatomical region. To some, this is a hopeless undertaking: "It is predictable that, for higher nervous functions, one can localize a lesion but not a function" (Mountcastle, 1978, p. 26). I have provided a different type of approach for understanding the significance of the hippocampus relative to behavior (Isaacson, 1980b).

Long-Term Potentiation

Electrophysiological observation of long-term changes in the excitability of hippocampal neurons following repetitive stimulation has also spurred speculation concerning the structure's role in memory. Typically, short bursts of tetanic stimulation (10–50 Hz applied for

10–15 sec) result in the potentiation of synaptic transmission through both the intact hippocampus (Bliss & Lømo, 1973) and the hippocampal slice preparation (Schwartzkroin & Wester, 1975). The potentiation may last for several hours, or even days (Buzsáki, 1980). Andersen, Sundberg, Sveen, and Wigström (1977) found that the long-term potentiation was specific to the input system activated by the tetanizing burst and was probably due to enhanced transmitter release. Long-term potentiation depends on the presence of extracellular calcium (Wigström, Swann, & Andersen, 1979). Frequency-specific alterations in membrane phosphorylation have also been reported (Bär, Schotman, Gispen, Tielen, & Lopes Da Silva, 1980). Dunwiddie and Lynch (1978) have found the long-term facilitation to be superimposed on a more general depression of responsiveness that can be found in all or many of the cell's processes. The maximal suppressive effect occurred when stimulating frequencies were in the theta range (5 Hz). Stimulation frequencies greater than 10 Hz are required to obtain the potentiation effect.

Long-term potentiation has been found in the hippocampus by stimulation over a variety of afferent pathways, suggesting that it is not unique to a particular afferent system (Bliss, 1979).

These exciting findings may have importance for naturally occurring changes that are related to learning or performance. The stimulation used to induce the long-term potentiation is somewhat unusual in its high-frequency, intense character, but other types of stimulation may also induce such effects. It is also quite possible that similar types of long-term effects will be found in other brain regions. Indeed, it would be surprising if the hippocampus had long-term potentiation as a unique characteristic. Most likely, it will be found in other systems as well.

REFLECTIONS AND SUMMARY

The hippocampal formation seems to exert less influence over the autonomic system than do the other regions of the limbic system. It appears to be less closely associated with alterations in moods and emotions than the amygdala or the septal area and to be more aligned with the evaluation of, and the response to, events in the external world. The dissociation from the body's internal affairs is not absolute, however. The hippocampus seems closely tied to the neuropeptides and corticosteroids, influencing their release and being influenced by circulating levels of the hormones. As with most limbic influences, the behavioral effects are subtle and are found only in conditions in which the limbic influences on mental or behavioral acts are important.

As judged by the effects of lesion or stimulation studies, the hippocampal formation influences are revealed only under certain conditions. Many behaviors seem to be affected by these procedures. It is only when special demands are placed on the individual that the effects of hippocampal destruction become apparent. These demands include times of environmental uncertainty, changes in reward schedules, and the presence of limited opportunities for the evaluation of environmental cues. These effects are due, possibly, to the reductions found in the amount of time spent on individual acts related to observation of the environment (e.g., Isaacson, 1981). As with damage to other limbic system regions, many types of behavioral episodes become shortened in duration.

In the interpretation of the effects of lesions, attention must be given to the animal's genetics, histories, and testing environment, as well as to the amount of time that has elapsed after surgery. Many of the changes that are found after surgery are very likely due to secondary changes induced in other structures, and the nature of these alterations changes over time. These changes produce alterations in the behavioral consequences of the damage. Many of the usual consequences of hippocampal damage are due to secondary alterations in the basal ganglia, particularly in the nucleus accumbens.

The hippocampus seems well designed to act as a gatekeeper for both sensory and motor activities. Information, or at least nerve impulses, passes more-or-less readily through the system, depending on the state of the organism as reflected in its hormonal conditions, its activity, and its direction of attention. Because of the system's strong input from the biogenic amine systems, it could also act as a forebrain transducer of their effects on many forms of behavior.

Because of its close ties to the neocortical, the basal gangliar, and the limbic systems, the hippocampus stands as a neuromodulator of activities in many brain regions, and it is not surprising that its dysfunction should produce abnormalities in the "higher" capacities of the brain, those represented in conditional reactions or requiring the flexible components of memory, that is, those temporary rules on which some behaviors must be based. Nevertheless, the actual impairments are best thought of as the consequence of disruptions in many systems, not just as a result of an imperfect hippocampus.

6

The Graven Image, Lethe, and the Guru

In this final chapter, I suggest a way of looking at the limbic system as it may function with other portions of the central nervous system to influence behavior. The limbic system does not do its work independently of other "systems" of the brain. Therefore, *no reasonable theory of the activity of the limbic system can be developed until a more general framework for the brain's activities has been achieved*. This accomplishment is not likely in the foreseeable future.

Yet, the human mind seeks a theoretical structure for understanding the diverse facts of nature and of science. Most people need some conceptual framework for thinking about the brain and its parts. It is because of such a need that telephone switchboard theories, computer-analogy theories, and holographic models have been advocated. All are only metaphors taken from other contexts and applied to brain activities. There is nothing wrong with metaphors as long as they are not confused with fact.

THE TRIUNE BRAIN

Paul MacLean (1970) has suggested that neural and behavioral distinctions can be made among three types of systems found in the brains of mammals. This differentiation is based in part on comparative anatomy, neurochemistry, and evolutionary theory. MacLean's basic divisions of the brain are a protoreptilian brain (or R-complex), a paleomammalian brain, and a neomammalian brain. The protoreptilian brain is thought to represent a fundamental core of the nervous system, consisting of systems in the upper spinal cord and parts of the midbrain, the diencephalon, and the basal ganglia. The paleomammalian brain is, in essence, the limbic system. The neomammalian brain refers to the neocortical developments, so prominent in primates.

MacLean believes that what is the R-complex in the brains of existing mammals derives from a form of mammal-like reptiles that once populated the earth in large numbers. These creatures apparently disappeared in the Triassic period, having once ranged widely on the earth. Although many skeletal remains have been found in South Africa, evidence of their presence has been found on all continents. It is from these mammal-like reptiles that modern mammals may have developed (MacLean, 1978). The R-complex structures of the mammalian brain are quite different from the neural organization of the brains of living reptiles. An illustration of portions of the R-complex of a primate brain is given in Figure 21. In general, modern reptiles have neural tissue that is similar to the core structure of the R-complex, to limbic structures, and to "neocortical" tissue, as well. In their state of evolution, they probably bear only a vague resemblance to the reptile–mammals of the Permian and Triassic periods. The significance of the triune brain approach relates to the usefulness of describing behavioral functions in terms of the actions and interactions of more-or-less specific anatomical systems. In this sense, the triune brain model deserves serious consideration as a metaphor for the hierarchical structures of the brain as they relate to behavior.

MacLean regards the protoreptilian brain as responsible for stereotyped behaviors based on "ancestral learning and ancestral memories"; it plays a crucial role in the establishment of home territories, the finding of shelter and food, breeding, social dominance, and other primal behavior patterns. The paleomammalian or limbic brain is thought to be nature's tentative first step toward providing self-awareness, especially awareness of the internal conditions of the body. To MacLean, it is a "visceral brain" (see MacLean, 1949), but it also has some role related to neocortical formations more generally. It is thought to be able to override the ancestral basis of behavior found in the protoreptilian brain, the R-complex. The elaboration of infor-

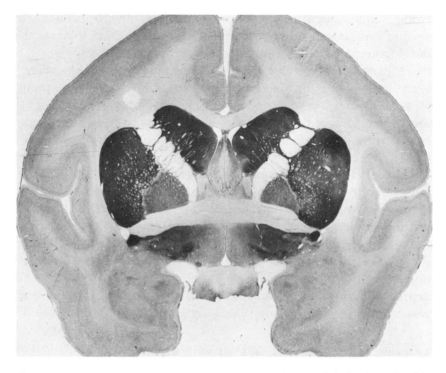

Figure 21. A cross-section of a squirrel monkey brain stained to reveal the basal ganglia of the forebrain through the use of a procedure in which regions high in cholinesterase appear black. The dark areas in the photograph are those of the R-complex. From "Cerebral Evolution and Emotional Processes: New Findings on the Striatal Complex" by P. D. MacLean, Annals of the New York Academy of Sciences, 1972, 193, 137–149. Copyright 1972 by the New York Academy of Sciences. Reprinted by permission.

mation arising from inside the person or the animal is thought to provide a necessary component of, or context for, significant memories. All memories, according to MacLean's view, depend on a mixture of information from the inner and outer worlds. The hippocampus is thought to be an especially good place for such mixtures to occur. It receives "internal information" from the septal area and "external information" from sensory systems projecting to nearby transitional cortical areas (MacLean, 1972).

The neocortex is "mother of invention and father of abstract thought" (MacLean, 1978, p. 332). It is viewed as being responsible for the cold (nonemotional) analysis of the external environment. It operates "unhindered by signals and noise generated in the internal

world." It is thought to have a predilection for dividing things into smaller and smaller units, to perform abstractions, and to allow the development of reading, writing, and arithmetic.

My own thoughts about the function of the "three brains in one" agree fairly well with MacLean's analysis as it relates to the proto-reptilian brain. I consider the limbic system a strong modulator of the R-complex. One of the more interesting questions in neuroanatomy has been how this modulation is achieved. This subject will be dis-cussed in more detail later in the chapter. In general, the roles played the neocortex also need further elaboration. It must have more in-teresting duties than the fine-grain analysis of the external world. It is responsible for the generation of expectancies about the future. If the limbic system does indeed act to modulate the ancient tendencies of the protoreptilian brain, including memories, then it also acts to produce forgetfulness. It is acting as the river (or goddess) of forget-ting: Lethe. If the neocortex does look to the future, it is acting as a neural guru. From these considerations, the title of the chapter came about.

Learning and Memory in Animals with Limited Brains

Living animals with a variety of types of nervous systems exhibit remarkable adjustments to their environments. For that matter, sin-gle-celled animals have extraordinary adjustive capacities. They sur-vive and propagate, often doing so in the context of environmental changes that require structural or behavioral modifications. The nerv-ous system develops to make these same types of adjustments pos-sible for animals made up of many diverse kinds of cells. The devel-opment of the nervous system seems to add no unique quality to basic animal life, but it does allow larger populations of highly spe-cialized cells to operate synergistically to achieve ends advantageous to the entire group of cells that is the individual.

Learning and memory are possible for animals made up of rel-atively few cells (see McConnell & Jacobson, 1973). These animals make adjustments suited to their specialized patterns of behavior and their ecological circumstances. It might be argued, however, that an-imals with no nervous system or a meager one would be less intel-ligent than those with more elaborate coordinating systems. This dif-ference in intelligence could be reflected in the ability to learn new

tasks; however, it is doubtful that comparisons in learning abilities can be made among animals of different species. Historically, the comparative study of differences in the intelligence of animals came to naught because the behavioral capabilities of animals of various species cannot readily be compared, owing to the specialized character of species-typical behaviors. Furthermore, each species has its own way of analyzing the world in which its members live through its specialized sensory systems. The comparison of intellectual abilities among existing species cannot reveal evolutionary trends, since all living forms are highly specialized and, by definition, successful.

If it is true that animals with the most meager of nervous systems are capable of complex adjustments to the world and of modifying their behavioral patterns according to the demands of the environment, it is likely that these fundamental aspects of animal behavior could easily be served by relatively modest accounts of neural tissue. According to such a view, the basic operations necessary for life *and* for many of the adjustments required by changes in the environment, including learning and memory, could be accomplished by the neural apparatus of brain regions that represent homologues of the basal ganglia, the hypothalamus, the brain stem, and the spinal cord in mammals.

If there is some universality in the abilities of animals relative to adjustments to a changing environment, these should be found in the behavior of many species. Consider the learning of simple behaviors in the fish as a point of departure. Conditioned responses of different sorts have been readily formed to visual and auditory stimuli (Froloff, 1925), water temperature, small changes in the salinity of the water (Bull, 1928), and water currents (Sears, 1934). Discriminations among stimuli can also be made by some fish, and Reeves (1919) was able to train them to discriminate between blue and red-orange lights. Higher-order conditioning can also be established, at least by goldfish. For example, fish trained to approach a disk for food can be trained to approach the disk only when a chemical is added to the water (Sanders, 1940). Active avoidance learning is rapidly acquired by fish and toads (Behrend & Bitterman, 1963; Crawford & Langdon, 1966).

Not only can fish learn many types of problems readily, but their learning is also often marked by *sudden* improvements in performance. In a study using sharks, Aronson, Aronson, and Clark (1967) found a rapid reduction in errors over the first few trials in their learning

to strike targets for food reward. Invertebrates (Morrow & Smithson, 1969) can learn simple problems quite readily with their relatively limited neurological apparatus, and their learning, also, is often characterized by abrupt, steplike reductions in the number of errors made.

Lesions of the forebrain of fish are without drastic effects on their performance in learning various problems; for example, such lesions do not disrupt learning to discriminate one colored patch of paper from others. Sears (1934) found that goldfish were able to acquire a conditioned response to light after a large part of the optic lobes had been damaged and, in addition, that these lesions did not disturb the retention of the discrimination when the fish were tested 3 days postoperatively.

The neural mechanisms responsible for rapid learning and long-term memory are not limited to whatever forebrain tissue exists in fish. Nevertheless, there are some differences in the performance of fish relative to that of mammals. These differences include observations that fish extinguish learned responses more quickly if small food rewards are used in training than if large rewards are used (Gonzales & Bitterman, 1967). Just the opposite is true of mammals with intact brains. Fish also extinguish partially reinforced responses more rapidly than continuously reinforced responses, again a result opposite to that found in mammals (Wodinsky & Bitterman, 1959, 1960). This finding suggests that the learning mechanisms of the fish brain are associated with the number, the frequency, and the magnitude of primary rewards. Thus, fish seem to be perfect representatives of stimulus–response association models of learning. They are little affected by the variables often thought to be associated with "expectations" held about the environment. It is commonly held that mammals extinguish more rapidly after training with large rather than with small rewards because of the greater disruptive effects produced when the expected reward is no longer furnished. The effectiveness of partial reward schedules during extinction is also related to changes in what the animals have come to expect in previous training sessions.

Surprisingly little work has been done on the permanence of memory in animals with meager forebrain tissue. They would be expected to have strong and stable forms of memory, since fish and amphibians tend to live in environments that change more slowly than do those above the water. However, the apparent stability of the sea environment may be more apparent than real—especially to the

species that populate the ocean. The permanence of memory in any animal is an empirical question to be resolved by observation and experimentation.

Beritoff (1971) believed that over the course of brain evolution, there was little change in the permanency of "memories" for conditioned reflexes, but a large change in the ability of animals to hold "images" of rewards and punishments for short periods of time. The ability to hold images in a short-term or working memory would be associated with the development of the limbic and the neocortical systems.

These tentative conclusions drawn from studies of neurally simpler organisms need not apply to the functions of the R-complex brain of advanced animals. In all likelihood, there are substantial functional differences in the R-complex of mammals and the rather different neural cores in fish, living reptiles, and amphibians.

Huston and Borbély (1973) investigated the learning capacities of rats that had most of the forebrain destroyed by aspiration. The lesions included all of the neocortex, most of the limbic system, and much of the striatum. The thalamus and the hypothalamus were left more-or-less intact. Behaviors were trained by the use of rewarding electrical stimulation of the hypothalamus. These authors were able to condition simple movements of the head or the tail by operant procedures; that is, the movements became more frequent when they were followed by the stimulation of the hypothalamus. Most of the "thalamic animals," those without damage to the diencephalon, were able to demonstrate conditioning but were unaffected by extinction procedures. Once they had been conditioned, they persisted in the learned movements even in the absence of rewards. The researchers could induce the animals to stop making the acquired movements, however, by training them to make a different, competing response. Animals which have had much of the forebrain tissue related to the neomammalian and paleomammalian brain removed exhibit a strong persistence of behavior. Responses can be acquired but there is a diminished potential to terminate them. The animals are creatures limited in their behavior by stimulus–response associations. Furthermore, it is likely that the stimuli to which associations can be formed are the most prominent in a situation because of their intensity or their central location.

However, the R-complex is involved with the execution of behaviors that represent species-typical acts. For example, destruction of the pallidal portions of the R-complex in squirrel monkeys eliminates "display behaviors" exhibited to stranger monkeys (MacLean, 1975, 1979). When the above-described work is coupled with work in other species, the R-complex is necessary for ritualistic displays and the averbal communication associated with them. At the human level, MacLean believes that certain behavioral tendencies are due to an inheritance of dispositions mediated by this same, primal brain region. These include certain violent reactions, the preference for routine or "ritualistic" actions, and some forms of displacement activities. Deception is another type of behavior that is native to the R-complex, one that is independent of intelligence.

THE PALEOMAMMALIAN BRAIN

The paleomammalian brain, or the limbic system, represents an advance in neural tissue because it represents a device for providing the animals that have this tissue with better means of coping with the environment. Parts of the limbic system are concerned with primal activities related to food and sex; others are related to emotions and feelings; and still others combine messages from the external world with those from inside. Disruption of the usual activities of the limbic system by epileptic activities or interictal episodes can produce a host of experiences and feelings, some of the most interesting being those associated with knowledge of fundamental truths, feelings of depersonalization, hallucinations, and paranoid feelings (MacLean, 1970). Mandell (1980) attributed many "other worldly" experiences occurring after certain psychoactive drugs to the deregulation of limbic system activities, producing the functional equivalent of a seizure state.

Another way to conceptualize the limbic system may be to see it as a regulator of the R-complex. On the basis of behavioral analysis, this regulation seems to be inhibitory in nature. Stimulation of the limbic system often produces a suppression of ongoing behaviors, and lesions made within it often seem to "release" various activities. Each limbic system structure may be sensitive to the characteristic conditions under which its regulation of the R-complex becomes manifest. Thus, each of the limbic system structures would be highly specialized, and is tuned to specific changes of the internal or external environment. The hypothesis is that however specialized the structures of the limbic system may be, their end product is the regulation of activities in the R-complex.

The effects of destruction of the hippocampus and the septal area are difficult to characterize in general terms and, consequently, interpretations have been varied. Among the characteristics shared by animals suffering destruction of either the septal or the hippocampal areas is an overly energetic responsiveness under some environmental conditions. The damage need not be to the hippocampus proper but can be to the adjacent transitional cortical areas (Engelhardt & Steward, 1980). This result indicates that damage to areas that send neural input to limbic system areas can produce behavioral reactions similar to those produced by damage to the limbic region itself. The effects of lesions of the amygdala are equally varied but include a potentiation of behaviors guided by positive incentives.

One of the behavioral characteristics that marks limbic system damage is an unusual transfer of experiences. Schmaltz and Isaacson (1968), for example, demonstrated that animals with hippocampal lesions were impaired on the acquisition of a DRL-20 schedule if it was presented after the animals had been trained on a continuous reinforcement schedule. The animals that were trained on a DRL-20 schedule without prior continuous reinforcement experience were not impaired on the acquisition of a DRL-20 schedule.

This type of deficit found after limbic damage can be interpreted as a "failure of forgetting," since the effects of the continuous reinforcement schedule carry over and interfere with performance on the new task. The animals with hippocampal damage are unable to overthrow the habitual way of responding.

If the limbic system plays a critical role in the suppression of "proreptilian habits" then limbic system destruction should interfere with the development of learning sets. Learning sets represent an acquired way to approach a problem. Large lesions of the temporal lobe (including the associated limbic structures) in primates do interfere with object-discrimination learning sets (Riopelle, Alper, Strong, & Ades, 1953). Schwartzbaum and Poulos (1965) have found that lesions of the amygdala produce impaired formation of learning sets as measured by repeated reversals of a discrimination problem.

Gabriel, Foster, Orona, Saltwick, and Stanton (1980) have presented evidence from the analysis of multielectrode recordings that discriminations between two stimuli differentially related to rewards appear first in the deeper layers of the cingulate cortex and then appear later in the anteroventral nucleus (AV) of the thalamus and in the superficial cingulate layers. Both the thalamic changes are thought to represent a process of "relegation" in which the neural codes of the discrimination become subcortical following an original cortical location. The projections from the AV back to the cingulate may act to alter normal processing in the lower layers where the original neuronal discrimination occurred, "short-circuiting" these mechanisms. The lower layers of the cingulate cortex appear to be related to the initial formation of discrimination performance but not its continued performance.

In the model of Gabriel *et al.*, the hippocampus is seen to function in several ways, including the association of different sensory discriminations with their behavioral consequences and the releasing of the appropriate behavioral responses themselves. The relative inactivity of the hippocampus, as judged by the rhythmic activity in hippocampal theta cells, is a prelude to the execution of the learned response. The activation of the hippocampus is thought to inhibit the performance of the response. When cue–reward circumstances change, such as during reversal or extinction conditions, it is the hippocampus that acts to produce the change in behavior. It is of special interest in this regard that the neuronal discrimination between stimuli persist in the deep cingulate cortex after behavioral reversal has occurred.

The results of Gabriel and his co-workers are generally in accord with the idea that the neocortex and the associated transitional cortex look toward the future and that the limbic system, acting through suppressive mechanisms, tends to allow new directions in behavior to occur.

In many experiments, animals with hippocampal damage are impaired by what has been learned previously. In this case, the prior learning of one aspect of a problem interferes with learning another aspect of the same problem.

The more general conclusion seems to be that specific training in a particular situation produces changes in the animals that are difficult to overcome and that persist into the future, disturbing the acquisition of new behaviors and the alteration of hypotheses in the light of changed environmental circumstances. This carry-over from the past is a type of negative transfer of training and may also be considered a case of abnormally strong proactive interference.

Warrington and Weiskrantz (1973; see also Weiskrantz & Warrington, 1975) demonstrated that amnesic patients with recent memory problems could be greatly improved by giving them additional information when they were being tested for the retention of verbal information. One technique involved giving the subjects the first two letters of the to-be-remembered words. The improvements that were found suggested that the patients were able to store the information and that their problem was in the retrieval of the words. Warrington and Weiskrantz also found that the patients had many more words from lists learned previously intruding on their tests for retention. Taken together, the implication is that the patients had difficulty with the retrieval of acquired information because of a failure to suppress adequately the words learned under similar circumstances in the past.

INFERRED CHARACTERISTICS OF THE R-COMPLEX

One of my basic assumptions is that lesions of the limbic system act to remove the mechanisms of the R-complex components of the brain from certain regulatory influences normally supplied by the damaged regions. The lesion technique does not reveal the activities of the pure R-complex, of course, since regulation can still occur through the remaining limbic system structures and from the neocortex. What the lesion techniques may reveal is the nature of those circumstances under which a particular region of the limbic system does exert its influences.

The circumstances under which the hippocampus acts to regulate the activities of other brain regions seem to be conditions of uncertainty. Life becomes uncertain when old patterns of responding fail to produce the anticipated rewards, when old habits fail to pay off. By turning things around, the hippocampus can be seen as a mechanism that suppresses the activity in the R-complex when the unexpected happens. This suppression prevents the animal from continuing in its old ways of responding and from overreacting in general.

An animal with damage to the amygdala, on the other hand, reveals quite a different sort of behavioral syndrome. It is slow to initiate new responses and seems characterized by a reduction in reactive quality. Both the joys and the disasters of life seem reduced. This finding suggests that the role of the amygdala under normal conditions is to accentuate the arousal and activation of the hypothalamic systems when external conditions are appropriate. In some ways, the amygdalar contributions seem opposed to those of the hippocampus. However, because of the diversity of function found within the amygdalar system, this observation is at best a description of the contributions of certain portions of the amygdala and not of "the amygdala" as an entity. Lesions in some portions of the amygdala produce behavioral effects quite similar to those of the hippocampus.

Regarding the hippocampus, the septal area, and the cingulate region as "entities" is no more justifiable than regarding the amygdala as a unified structure or system. Each of the limbic structures, including the hypothalamus itself, is a complex set of subsystems in terms of anatomical relationships with other brain regions and in terms of behavioral functions. We should talk about limbic systems, not a limbic system. Different portions of each of the limbic areas act synergistically with each other and in a similar fashion on the hypothalamus and the protoreptilian brain. Other portions act in different, and sometimes opposing, ways. The ultimate aim of each, however, can be regarded as changing the activities or the character of activities in the R-complex.

Lesions or stimulation of the limbic system can produce an intensification or a reduction of activities in systems representative of activities of the core brain. Accordingly, most or all of the activities of the hypothalamus should be capable of modification by manipulations of the limbic system.

If we return to the characteristics of the R-complex brain inferred from studies of the limbic system, a picture emerges of a neural system that reacts to changes in the environment by increasing or decreasing the intensity of the predominant response sequence. Modifications of behavior are possible, of course, but these tend to be made on the basis of the establishment of new responses. Suppression of response on the basis of nonreward or punishment is difficult. Some subportions of the limbic system act to suppress established responses, while others intensify them. In the intact animal, the net effect of all of these systems on behavior is probably the result (at the R-complex level) of the total amount of facilitating and inhibiting influences.

The greatest change that occurs as a correlate of increased forebrain tissue is the ease with which rapid and, perhaps, temporary associations can be achieved. Earlier in this chapter we noted the proposal of Beritoff that the temporary "image" of the place of food or of punishment could be held only briefly by fish and for an even briefer period by fish with forebrain damage. The limbic system makes possible the suppression of the traditional ways of responding in order to allow behavioral modifications based on information from the internal environment as directed by the neocortical tissue. Both the limbic system and the neocortex become elaborated in mammals and usually work in concert.

These observations would be compatible with the view that the limbic system is responsible for the suppression of previously learned behavioral sequences. Therefore, it can be viewed as the mechanism that is directed toward the elimination of influences from the past, that is, from the stored memories of the protoreptilian brain. The limbic brain thus fulfills the role of Lethe. It provides the basis of forgetting chronic memories, the graven images of the protoreptilian brain, and opens the way for new, temporary associations. It does so in collaboration with the neocortical systems, which have their own role to play in behavior.

THE NEOCORTEX: THE GURU

While it is presumptuous to suggest that the functions of any brain region are understood at all well, it is especially so in connection with the systems of the neocortex. The neocortex presents neuroscientists with a great challenge.

It may be best to consider first the behaviors for which the neocortex is not essential. In many species, lesions of the primary sensory areas of the neocortical surface do not eliminate the capacity to use sensory information in the performance of either learned or unlearned tasks. Lesions of the primary auditory neocortex do not alter auditory thresholds for frequency or intensity (e.g., Diamond & Neff, 1957). Destruction of the primary visual areas does not eliminate some forms of pattern-discriminative capacities, even in primates (Humphrey & Weiskrantz, 1967; Weiskrantz, 1980). Similar results have been found in the somatosensory system.

From the point of view of motor activities, the primary motor areas of the neocortex impose a rapidly conducting system controlling fine-grain movements of the extremities by means of a reasonably effective motor apparatus largely based in the subcortical and the brain stem regions. A comparable development can be seen on the sensory side, with the neocortical systems adding capacity for the higher resolution of sensory stimulation (e.g., Bauer & Cooper, 1964).

The neocortex, then, seems to be especially capable of the quick and efficient processing of information that has too many fine details to be easily handled by the mechanisms in the lower brain regions. Its adjustive contributions are those that require a delicacy beyond the capabilities of the lower centers.

Portions of the neocortex may speed up the processing of information, at least of some types of information. Gerbrandt, Spinelli, and Pribram (1970) have shown that stimulation of the inferior temporal neocortex can alter the activity in the visual areas of the neocortex of a bored and disinterested monkey to the extent that the neural reactions are comparable to those obtained from the animal when it is paying keen attention. By implication, this inferior temporal neocortex can be thought of as regulating the excitability and the processing time of the primary sensory systems.

Whether an animal pays attention to visual stimulation depends on the possibility that the stimulation will influence its life in important ways. Wilson, Kaufman, Zieler, and Lieb (1972) have shown that the inferior temporal neocortex is involved in making this determination. Lesions in the anterior portions of the inferior temporal neocortex changed monkeys so that they responded based on the number of past rewards associated with a stimulus instead of on the most recent association with a reward. It was as if some ability to hold recent reward associations in mind was decreased in favor of a more habitual association of a stimulus with reward. The association of rewards with stimuli interferes with learning to respond to the stimuli currently being rewarded in changed reinforcement conditions. This reliance on the more established way of responding found after inferior temporal lesions may pose a handicap, a proactive interference, on problems in which new adjustments to the visual environment are required. With the neocortical lesion, reliance on the past can interfere with the flexibility of behavior required in circumstances of change.

But surely, it might be said, the great neocortical mantle does more than provide additional speed and precision in information processing. Surely, it must be involved in those aspects of behavior valued most by educators: knowledge, learning, and memory. Since these are the "highest" attributes of humans, they should be subserved by the "highest" neural machinery of the brain.

Unfortunately, there is precious little evidence for such a view. What evidence there is shows a remarkable retention of previously learned information after neocortical damage. The search for the location of the engram has not been successful. The memory engrams of the brain are everywhere or nowhere.

Karl Lashley (1929) developed his theories of "mass action" and "equipotentiality" because of failures to find specific locations within the brain that, when destroyed, eliminated the memories of previously learned problems. In maze studies, he found the greater the amount of neocortex destroyed, the greater the loss in retention in rats. The location of the lesions *per se* was not critical, a finding that indicated that the information was diffusely stored.

The storage of any information at neocortical sites can be questioned (see Isaacson, 1976; Meyer & Meyer, in press). The amount of the deficit in the retention of a preoperatively learned problem following neocortical insult depends on the length of the postoperative recovery period and the treatments given the animals in this period. Treatments that produce greater "arousal," whether they be environmental or chemical, tend to reduce the usual deficits and to facilitate recovery. Moreover, if steps are taken to control for the "distortions" of the sensory world produced by damage to the primary sensory areas, often no loss in retention is found at all after surgery (Bauer & Cooper, 1964). This suggests that memories may *not* be localized uniquely in the neocortex at all. Furthermore, there is a strong possibility that the real problem faced by animals after destruction of the visual neocortex is the retrieval of previously learned information.

The one well-established characteristic that separates humans from other animals is the use of language. This capability is closely related to certain neocortical areas, especially regions of the left hemisphere. Damage to this neocortical area in humans produces one or more of the several speech and language abnormalities that have been documented in the clinical literature. With language and the messages communicated by language, humans become free from domination by their environment.

Of the many benefits given to us by the ability to use language, one may be of special significance. This is the ability to institute changes in perspective, beliefs, and activities quickly on a permanent or a temporary basis. Information can be received and stored in the twinkling of an eye, and its influence can be brief or lasting, depending on a number of factors. Spoken or written language conveys information in a very rapid manner. Indeed, through their own implicit verbal abilities, it would appear that people can originate new organizations of the knowledge that has been acquired in the past.

With language, humans can override the demands both of their internal environment and of the outer world. They can reject the feelings of thirst and hunger in favor of abstract goals, sometimes goals of their own creation. Thus, we have martyrs who starve to death to further their own "salvation" or the "salvation" of others. Human beings can reject the directions provided by the world and the people around them. They can, in short, be free of internal and external factors that shape the destinies of those animals without language.[1]

To exercise this freedom, humans must override and suppress the well-learned or genetically determined behaviors that are presumed to be properties of the R-complex. Therefore, the neocortical mechanisms must overcome the habits and memories of the past, either indirectly by activating some portions of the paleomammalian brain, or by a more direct control process. In short, the neocortex, too, is profoundly concerned with suppressing the past.

The neocortical systems use the paleomammalian brain mechanisms to accomplish this suppression of previously learned behaviors as required to alter behavior. For the neocortical systems to "gain control" of the organism, the past must give up its domination of behavior.

The R-complex is concerned with the past. It learns and remembers but is poor at forgetting. The neocortical brain looks to the future, either to tomorrow, next week, next year, or to heavenly rewards. The neocortex is the brain of anticipation. It prepares for, anticipates, and predicts the future. All religious leaders, the gurus, have pleaded

---

[1] Before his death, the great humanistic psychologist, Sidney M. Jourard, speculated on the significance of a person listening to and obeying voices and commands from significant others in the past. Some of these speculations are reported by me in *Somatics*, 1981, 3(3), 3–6.

with people to give up their old ways and images of the past. The sin of excessive "attachment" to things, places, and even roles is excoriated in the wisdom of East and West alike. In the triune brain metaphor, this means that the graven images of the protoreptilian brain must be overcome.

It is paradoxical that this most delicate and yet dominating neocortical brain is the one responsible for our longest and most elaborate memories, memories even longer than those subserved by the R-complex. By the use of language, we can store the memories of the past. We build libraries and repositories of information that can extend our knowledge of the past for thousands of years, far beyond the life span of the protoreptilian brain. The neocortical contribution of language enables us to forecast the future and to anticipate conditions hours, weeks, years, and centuries from the present. It is this extension of time, both forward and backward, that represents the singular advance produced by the neocortex.

But what about those human qualities that are generated by our brains? The neocortex as described to this point would seem merely to be a prognosticator of the future, a computer with programs designed to predict future events without pity, empathy, or love. It is not computing power that makes the human being; rather, it is the application of this power for the benefit of others.

MacLean (1978) suggested that the valued characteristics of humanness come from the brain's ability to look within and to evaluate its own emotions and feelings. These, then, are projected onto others so that we can feel their joys or sorrows, pain or happiness, along with them. This ability, MacLean believes, arises from the development of the prefrontal neocortex. It is able to sample the limbic regions that signal the internal activities representative of the emotions and, combining the results with calculations about the future, to generate human understanding. Mogenson, Jones, and Yim (1980) have suggested that the frontal cortical areas may play a role in coordinating the signals from the limbic system that are to be integrated with the activities of the "cognitive brain," that is, the majority of the neocortical surface.

Douglas and Marcellus (1975) examined the evolution of the primate brain using a factor-analytic method. They found two factors that seem to account for most of the differences found among the data from the 63 species for whom appropriate data were available.

The first factor was related to increasing encephalization; the stuctures whose size was reflected on this factor were the neocortex, cerebellum, diencephalon, and midbrain. The second factor was related to the size of the limbic system, as reflected by the amygdala and the hippocampus. Interestingly, the striatum was a special area, one whose size was associated with the size of the structures associated with both factors.

Looking at the position of the human on both factors provides an unusual conclusion: What makes the human brain unique is a high level of development on both factors. That is, not only may people differ from other primates in their ability to look into themselves to generate feelings about others, but the feelings themselves may be more intense or elaborate as well.

Perhaps the most puzzling feature of brain organization, especially as it relates to the three brains of MacLean, is the ways in which interactions may occur between the three brains, especially in the relationship between the limbic system and motor systems, since the anatomical relationships between the limbic system and the basal ganglia are sparse. Recently, however, work on the projections from the limbic system to the nucleus accumbens and the ventral tegmental area, closely associated with the nucleus accumbens, has made the limbic–basal ganglia association clearer. Furthermore, the fact that appropriate dopaminergic stimulation of the nucleus accumbens can normalize some behaviors after hippocampal destruction indicates that the association is functional (Reinstein *et al.*, in press). In fact, the nucleus accumbens can be thought of as a limbic striatum. However, the limbic system exerts influences, probably secondary or indirect, on the caudate nucleus as well (e.g., Bär *et al.*, 1980). By means of the limbic–striatal connection, the association of the neocortical and the limbic systems and the paleomammalian and R-complex brain systems come together. Indeed, with the strong neocortical input into the striatal regions, all three brains converge at this site. Dysfunctions of the nucleus accumbens are thought to be a possible basis for schizophrenia, probably because of the resulting disconnection of the input from the various neural systems (e.g., Stevens, 1979). With such a disconnection, the behaviors based on each system would become independent and would be dissociated from each other. This is the definition of schizophrenia: behavior dissociated from reality.

If we return to the question of what a human is, the answer

seems to be an organism in which the three major systems of MacLean act together and in harmony. We need to know the world, to appreciate and sympathize with others, and to be able to use abstractions to help realize our individual potential without reducing that of others. When brain regions become impaired and no longer serve us properly, a variety of symptoms result, but it is impossible to make statements about *the* region responsible for a particular change, except in trivial instances. It is harmony of the systems working together that is of critical importance, and to understand the brain, we must someday learn the secrets of its composition.

References

Aaron, M., & Thorne, B. M. Omission training and extinction in rats with septal damage. *Physiology and Behavior*, 1975, *15*, 149–154.

Ackil, J. E., Mellgren, R. L., Halgren, C., & Frommer, G. P. Effects of CS preexposures on avoidance learning in rats with hippocampal lesions. *Journal of Comparative and Physiological Psychology*, 1969, *69*, 739–747.

Adey, W. R. Neurophysiological correlates of information transaction and storage in the brain. In E. Stellar & J. M. Sprague (Eds.), *Progress in physiological psychology* (Vol. 1). New York: Academic Press, 1964.

Adey, W. R., & Meyer, M. An experimental study of hippocampal afferent pathways from prefrontal and cingulate areas in the monkey. *Journal of Anatomy*, 1952, *86*, 58–74.

Aghajanian, G. K., Bloom, F. E., & Sheard, M. H. Electron microscopy of degeneration within the serotonin pathway of rat brain. *Brain Research*, 1969, *13*, 266–273.

Ahlskog, J. E. Food intake and amphetamine anorexia after selective forebrain norepinephrine loss. *Brain Research*, 1974, *82*, 211–240.

Ahlskog, J. E. Feeding response to regulatory challenges after 6-hydroxydopamine injection into the brain noradrenergic pathways. *Physiology and Behavior*, 1976, *17*, 407–411.

Ahlskog, J. E., & Hoebel, G. B. Overeating and obesity from damage to a noradrenergic system in brain. *Science*, 1973, *182*, 166–169.

Ahlskog, J. E., Randall, P. K., & Hoebel, B. G. Hypothalamic hyperphagia: Dissociation from noradrenergic depletion hyperphagia. *Science*, 1975, *190*, 399–401.

Ahmad, S. S., & Harvey, J. A. Long-term effects of septal lesions and social experience on shock-elicited fighting in rats. *Journal of Comparative and Physiological Psychology*, 1968, *66*, 596–602.

Akil, H., & Liebeskind, J. C. Monoaminergic mechanisms of stimulation-produced analgesia. *Brain Research*, 1975, *94*, 279–296.

Akil, H., & Mayer, D. J. Antagonism of stimulation-produced analgesia by p-CPA, a serotonin synthesis inhibitor. *Brain Research*, 1972, *44*, 692–697.

Albert, D. J., & Chew, G. L. The septal forebrain and the inhibitory modulation of attack and defense in the rat: A review. *Behavioral and Neural Biology*, 1980, *30*, 357–388.

Albert, D. J., & Richmond, S. E. Septal hyperreactivity: A comparison of lesions within and adjacent to the septum. *Physiology and Behavior*, 1975, *15*, 339–347.

Albert, D. J., & Richmond, S. E. Reactivity and aggression in the rat: Induction by α-adrenergic blocking agents injected ventral to anterior septum but not into lateral septum. *Journal of Comparative and Physiological Psychology*, 1977, *91*, 886–896.

Albert, D. J., & Wong, R. C. K. Hyperreactivity, muricide, and intraspecific aggression in the rat produced by infusion of local anesthetic into the lateral septum or surrounding areas. *Journal of Comparative and Physiological Psychology*, 1978, *92*, 1062–1073b.

Alger, B. E., & Nicoll, R. A. Epileptiform burst after hyperpolarization: Calcium-dependent potassium potential in hippocampal CA1 pyramidal cells. *Science*, 1980, *210*, 1122–1124.

Alheid, G. F., McDermott, L., Kelly, J., Halaris, A., & Grossman, S. P. Deficits in food and water intake after knife cuts that deplete striatal DA or hypothalamic DA or hypothalamic NE in rats. *Pharmacology, Biochemistry and Behavior*, 1977, *6*, 273–287.

Allen, W. F. Effect of ablating the pyriform–amygdaloid areas and hippocampi on positive and negative olfactory conditioned reflexes and on conditioned olfactory differentiation. *American Journal of Physiology*, 1941, *132*, 81–92.

Altman, J., Brunner, R. L., & Bayer, S. A. The hippocampus and behavioral maturation. *Behavioral Biology*, 1973, *8*, 557–596.

Amaral, D. G., & Routtenberg, A. Locus coeruleus and intra-cranial self-stimulation: A cautionary note. *Behavioral Biology*, 1975, *13*, 331–338.

Anand, B. K., & Dua, S. Effect of electrical stimulation of the limbic system ('visceral brain") on gastric secretion and motility. *Indian Journal of Medical Research*, 1956, *44*, 125–130.

Anchel, H., & Lindsley, D. B. Differentiation of two reticulohypothalamic systems regulating hippocampal activity. *Electroencephalography and Clinical Neurophysiology*, 1972, *32*, 209–226.

Andersen, P., Bland, B. H., & Dudar, J. D. Organization of the hippocampal output. *Experimental Brain Research*, 1973, *17*, 152–168.

Andersen, P., Sundberg, S. H., Sveen, O., & Wigström, H. Specific long-lasting potentiation of synaptic transmission in hippocampal slices. *Nature*, 1977, *266*, 736–737.

Arnolds, D. E. A. T., Lopes Da Silva, F. H., Aitink, J. W., & Kamp, A. Hippocampal EEG and behavior in dog: I. Hippocampal EEG correlates of gross motor behaviour. *Electroencephalography and Clinical Neurophysiology*, 1979, *46*, 552–570. (a)

Arnolds, D. E. A. T., Lopes Da Silva, F. H., Aitink, J. W., & Kamp, A. Hippocampal EEG and behaviour in dog: II. Hippocampal EEG correlates with elementary motor acts. *Electroencephalography and Clinical Neurophysiology*, 1979, *46*, 571–580. (b)

Arnolds, D. E. A. T., Lopes Da Silva, F. H., Aitink, J. W., & Kamp, A. Hippocampal EEG and behaviour in dog: III. Hippocampal EEG correlates of stimulus-response tasks and of sexual behaviour. *Electroencephalography and Clinical Neurophysiology*, 1979, *46*, 581–591. (c)

Aronson, L. R., Aronson, F. R., & Clark, E. Instrumental conditioning and light–dark discrimination in young nurse sharks. *Bulletin of Marine Science*, 1967, *17*, 249–256.

Asdourian, D., Dark, J. G., Chiodo, L., & Papich, P. S. Active avoidance in rats with unilateral hypothalamic and optic nerve lesions. *Physiology and Behavior*, 1977, *19*, 209–212.

Assaf, S. Y., & Miller, J. J. The role of a raphe serotonin system in the control of septal unit activity and hippocampal desynchronization. *Neuroscience*, 1978, *3*, 539–550.

Atnip, G., & Hothersall, D. Response suppression in normal and septal rats. *Physiology and Behavior*, 1975, *15*, 417–421.

Atrens, D. M., Ljungberg, T., & Ungerstedt, U. Modulation of reward and aversion processes in the rat diencephalon by neuroleptics: Differential effects of clozapine and haloperidol. *Psychopharmacology*, 1976, *49*, 97–100.

Atweh, S. F., & Kuhar, M. J. Autoradiographic localization of opiate receptors in rat brain: II. Telencephalon. *Brain Research*, 1977, *134*, 393–405.

Bachus, S. E., & Valenstein, E. S. Individual behavioral responses to hypothalamic stimulation persist despite destruction of tissue surrounding electrode tip. *Physiology and Behavior*, 1979, *23*, 421–426.

Baez, L. A., Ahlskog, J. E., & Randall, P. K. Body weight and regulatory deficits following unilateral nigrostriatal lesions. *Brain Research*, 1977, *132*, 467–476.

Bagshaw, M. H., & Benzies, S. Multiple measures of the orienting reaction and their dissociation after amygdalectomy in monkeys. *Experimental Neurology*, 1968, *20*, 175–187.

Bagshaw, M. H., & Pribram, K. H. Effect of amygdalectomy on transfer of training in monkeys. *Journal of Comparative and Physiological Psychology*, 1965, *59*, 118–121.

Bagshaw, M. H., Pribram, J. D. Effect of amygdalectomy on stimulus threshold of the monkey. *Experimental Neurology*, 1968, *20*, 197–202.

Bagshaw, M. H., Kimble, D. P., & Pribram, K. H. The GSR of monkeys during orienting and habituation and after ablation of the amygdala, hippocampus, and inferotemporal cortex. *Neuropsychologia*, 1965, *3*, 111–119.

Bagshaw, M. H., Mackworth, N. H., & Pribram, K. H. The effect of resections of the inferotemporal cortex or the amygdala on visual orienting and habituation. *Neuropsychologia*, 1972, *10*, 153–162.

Baisden, R. H., Isaacson, R. L., Woodruff, M. L., & Van Hartesveldt, C. The effect of physostigmine on spontaneous alternation in infant rabbits. *Psychonomic Science*, 1972, *26*, 287–288.

Ball, G. G., & Gray, J. A. Septal self-stimulation and hippocampal activity. *Physiology and Behavior*, 1971, *6*, 547–549.

Bandler, R., & Fatouris, D. Centrally elicited attack behavior in cats: Post-stimulus excitability and mid-brain-hypothalamic inter-relationships. *Brain Research*, 1978, *153*, 427–433.

Bär, P. R., Schotman, P., & Gispen, W. H. Enkephalins affect hippocampal membrane phosphorylation. *European Journal of Pharmacology*, 1980, *65*, 165–174.

Bär, P. R., Gispen, W. H., & Isaacson, R. L. Behavioral and regional neurochemical sequelae of hippocampal destruction in the rat. *Pharmacology, Biochemistry and Behavior*, 1981, *14*, 305–312.

Bär, P. R., Schotman, P., Gispen, W. H., Tielen, W. H., & Lopes Da Silva, F. H. Changes in synaptic membrane phosphorylation after tetanic stimulation in the dentate area of the rat hippocampal slice. *Brain Research*, 1980, *198*, 478–484.

Barker, D. J. Alterations in sequential behavior of rats following ablation of midline limbic cortex. *Journal of Comparative and Physiological Psychology*, 1967, *64*, 453–460.

Barker, D. J., & Thomas, G. J. Ablation of cingulate cortex in rats impairs alternation learning and retention. *Journal of Comparative and Physiological Psychology*, 1965, *60*, 353–359.

Barker, D. J., & Thomas, G. J. Effects of regional ablation of midline cortex in alternation learning by rats. *Physiology and Behavior*, 1966, *1*, 313–317.

Barrett, T. W. Studies of the function of the amygdaloid complex in *Macaca mulatta*. *Neuropsychologia*, 1969, *7*, 1–12.

Bauer, R. H. Brightness discrimination of pretrained and nonpretrained hippocampal rats reinforced for choosing brighter or dimmer alternatives. *Journal of Comparative and Physiological Psychology*, 1974, *87*, 987–996.

Bauer, R. H., & Cooper, R. M. Effects of posterior cortical lesions on performance of a brightness discrimination task. *Journal of Comparative and Physiological Psychology*, 1964, *58*, 84–92.

Beatty, W. W., & Schwartzbaum, J. S. Enhanced reactivity to quinine and saccharin solutions following septal lesions in the rat. *Psychonomic Science*, 1967, *8*, 483–484.

Beatty, W. W., & Schwartzbaum, J. S. Commonality and specificity of behavioral dysfunctions following septal and hippocampal lesions in rats. *Journal of Comparative and Physiological Psychology*, 1968, *66*, 60–68.

Becker, J. T., & Olton, D. S. Object discrimination by rats: The role of frontal and hippocampal systems in retention and reversal. *Physiology and Behavior*, 1980, *24*, 33–38.

Beckstead, R. M. An autoradiographic examination of corticocortical and subcortical projections of the mediodorsal-projection (prefrontal) cortex in the rat. *The Journal of Comparative Neurology*, 1979, *184*, 43–62.

Behrend, E. R., & Bitterman, M. E. Sidman avoidance in the fish. *Journal of the Experimental Analysis of Behavior*, 1963, *54*, 700–703.

Ben-Ari, Y., Zigmond, R. E., Shute, C. C. D., & Lewis, P. R. Regional distribution of choline acetyltransferase and acetylcholinesterase within the amygdaloid complex and stria terminalis system. *Brain Research*, 1977, *120*, 435–445.

Bengelloun, W. A. Elimination of the septal deficit in one-way active avoidance. *Physiology and Behavior*, 1979, *22*, 615–619.

Bengelloun, W. A., Burright, R. G., & Donovick, P. J. Nutritional experience and spacing of shock opportunities alter the effects of septal lesions on passive avoidance acquisition by male rats. *Physiology and Behavior*, 1976, *16*, 583–587.

Bengelloun, W. A., Burright, R. G., & Donovick, P. J. Septal lesions, cue availability, and passive avoidance acquisition by hooded male rats of two ages. *Physiology and Behavior*, 1977, *18*, 1033–1037.

Bengelloun, W. A., Finklestein, J., Burright, R. G., & Donovick, P. J. Presurgical handling and exploratory behavior of rats with septal lesions. *Bulletin of the Psychonomic Society*, 1977, *10*, 503–505.

Bengelloun, W. A., Baddouri, K., & El Hilali, M. *Effects of septal lesions on the renal sodium gradient.* Paper presented at the 8th Annual Meeting, Society for Neuroscience, St. Louis, November 5–9, 1978.

Bennett, T. L. Hippocampal theta activity and behavior: A review. *Communications in Behavioral Biology*, 1971, *6*, 37–48.

Bennett, T. L., & Gottfried, J. Hippocampal theta activity and response inhibition. *Electroencephalography and Clinical Neurophysiology*, 1970, *29*, 196–200.

Bennett, T. L., French, J., & Burnett, K. N. Species differences in the behavior correlates of hippocampal RSA. *Behavioral Biology*, 1978, *22*, 161–177.

Berger, B. D., Wise, C. D., & Stein, L. Norepinephrine: Reversal of anorexia in rats with lateral hypothalamic damage. *Science*, 1971, *172*, 281–284.

Berger, T. W., & Thompson, R. F. Neuronal plasticity in the limbic system during classical conditioning of the rabbit nictitating membrane response: I. The hippocampus. *Brain Research*, 1978, *145*, 323–346.

Berger, T. W., Alger, B., & Thompson, R. F. Neural substrate of classical conditioning in the hippocampus. *Science*, 1976, *192*, 483–485.

Berger, T. W., Clark, G. A., & Thompson, R. F. Learning-dependent neuronal responses recorded from limbic system brain structures during classical conditioning. *Physiological Psychology*, 1980, *8*, 155–167.

Beritoff, J. S. *Vertebrate memory: Characteristics and origin.* New York: Plenum Press, 1971.

Bernard, B. K., Berchek, J. R., & Yutzey, D. A. Alterations in brain monoaminergic functioning associated with septal lesion induced hyperreactivity. *Pharmacology, Biochemistry and Behavior*, 1975, *3*, 121–126.

Bernardis, L. L., & Skelton, F. R. Growth and obesity following ventromedial hypothalamic lesions placed in female rats at four different ages. *Neuroendocrinology*, 1966/1967, *1*, 265–275.

Berry, S. D., & Thompson, R. F. Prediction of learning rate from the hippocampal EEG. *Science*, 1978, *200*, 1298–1300.

Berry, S. D., & Thompson, R. F. Medial septal lesions retard classical conditioning of the nictitating membrane response in rabbits. *Science*, 1979, *205*, 209–211.

Berry, S. D., Rinaldi, P. C., Thompson, R. F., & Verzeano, M. Analysis of temporal relations among units and slow waves in rabbit hippocampus. *Brain Research Bulletin*, 1978, *3*, 509–518.

Best, M. R., & Best, P. J. The effects of state of consciousness and latent inhibition on hippocampal unit activity in the rat during conditioning. *Experimental Neurology*, 1976, *51*, 564–573.

Best, P. J., & Orr, J. Effects of hippocampal lesions on passive avoidance and taste aversion conditioning. *Physiology and Behavior*, 1973, *10*, 193–196.

Bishop, M. P., Elder, S. T., & Heath, R. G. Intracranial self-stimulation in man. *Science*, 1963, *140*, 394–396.

Black, A. H. The operant conditioning of central nervous system electrical activity. In G. H. Bower (Ed.), *The psychology of learning and motivation* (Vol. 6). New York: Academic Press, 1972.

Black, A. H., & DeToledo, L. The relationship among classically conditioned responses: Heart rate and skeletal behavior. In A. H. Black & W. F. Prokasy (Eds.), *Classical conditioning* (Vol. 2): *Current research and theory*, New York: Appleton-Century-Crofts, 1971.

Black, A. H., Young, G. A., & Batenchuk, C. The avoidance training of hippocampal theta waves and its relation to skeletal movement. *Journal of Comparative and Physiological Psychology*, 1970, *70*, 15–24.

Black, S. L., & Mogenson, G. J. The regulation of serum sodium in septal lesioned rats: A test of two hypotheses. *Physiology and Behavior*, 1973, *10*, 379–384.

Blackstad, T. W. Commissural connections of the hippocampal region in the rat, with special reference to their mode of termination. *Journal of Comparative Neurology*, 1956, *105*, 417–538.

Blackstad, T. W. On the termination of some afferents to the hippocampus and fascia dentata. An experimental study in the rat. *Acta Anatomica*, 1958, *35*, 202–214.

Blanchard, D. C., Blanchard, R. J., Lee, E. M. C., & Nakamura, S. Defensive behaviors in rats following septal and septal-amygdala lesions. *Journal of Comparative and Physiological Psychology*, 1979, *93*, 378–390.

Blanchard, R. J., & Blanchard, D. C. Effects of hippocampal lesions on the rat's reaction to a cat. *Journal of Comparative and Physiological Psychology*, 1972, *78*, 77–82.

Blanchard, R. J., & Blanchard, D. C. Aggressive behavior in the rat. *Behavioral Biology*, 1977, *21*, 197–224.

Blanchard, R. J., & Fial, R. A. Effects of limbic lesions on passive avoidance and reactivity to shock. *Journal of Comparative and Physiological Psychology*, 1968, *66*, 606–612.

Bland, B. H., Andersen, P., & Ganes, T. Two generators of hippocampal activity in rabbits. *Brain Research*, 1975, *94*, 199–218.

Blass, E. M., & Hanson, D. G. Primary hyperdipsia in the rat following septal lesions. *Journal of Comparative and Physiological Psychology*, 1970, *70*, 87–93.

Blass, E. M., Nussbaum, A. L., & Hanson, D. G. Septal hyperdipsia: Specific enhancement of drinking to angiotensin in rats. *Journal of Comparative and Physiological Psychology*, 1974, *87*, 422–439.

Bliss, T. V. P. Synaptic plasticity in the hippocampus. *Trends in Neurosciences*, February 1979, pp. 1–4.

Bliss, T. V. P., & Lømo, T. Long-lasting potentiation of synaptic transmission on the dentate area of the anaesthetized rabbit following stimulation of the perforant path. *Journal of Physiology*, 1973, *232*, 331–356.

Blozovski, D. PA-learning in young rats with dorsal hippocampal- and hippocampoentorhinal atropine. *Pharmacology, Biochemistry and Behavior*, 1979, *10*, 369–372.

Boast, C. A., & McIntyre, P. C. Bilateral kindled amygdala foci and inhibitory avoidance behavior in rats. *Physiology and Behavior*, 1977, *18*, 25–28.

Bohus, B. The hippocampus and the pituitary-adrenal system hormones. In R. L. Isaacson & K. H. Pribram (Eds.), *The hippocampus* (Vol. 1): *Structure and development*. New York: Plenum Press, 1975, pp. 323–355.

Boitano, J. J., Dokla, C. P. J., Mulinski, P., Misikonis, S., & Kaluzynski, T. Effects of hippocampectomy in an incremental-step DRL paradigm. *Physiology and Behavior*, 1980, *25*, 273–278.

Bonin, G. von, & Bailey, P. The neocortex of *Macaca mulatta*. Urbana, Ill.: Illinois Monographs in Medical Sciences, 1947.

Bonvallet, M., & Bobo, E. G. Changes in phrenic activity and heart rate elicited by localized stimulation of amygdala and adjacent structures. *Electroencephalography and Clinical Neurophysiology*, 1972, *32*, 1–16.

Bower, G. H., & Miller, N. E. Rewarding and punishing effects from stimulating the same place in the rat's brain. *Journal of Comparative and Physiological Psychology*, 1958, *51*, 669–674.

Boyd, E. S., & Gardner, L. C. Effect of some brain lesions on intracranial self-stimulation in the rat. *American Journal of Physiology*, 1967, *213*, 1044–1052.

Brady, J. V., & Nauta, W. J. H. Subcortical mechanisms in emotional behavior: Affective changes following septal forebrain lesions in the albino rat. *Journal of Comparative and Physiological Psychology*, 1953, *46*, 339–346.

Brady, J. V., & Nauta, W. J. Subcortical mechanisms in control of behavior. *Journal of Comparative and Physiological Psychology*, 1955, *48*, 412–420.

Breglio, V., Anderson, C., & Merrill, H. K. Alteration in footshock threshold by low-level septal brain stimulation. *Physiology and Behavior*, 1970, *5*, 715–719.

Brick, J., Burright, R. G., & Donovick, P. J. Stress responses of rats with septal lesions. *Pharmacology, Biochemistry and Behavior*, 1979, *11*, 695–700.

Brodal, A. The amygdaloid nucleus in the rat. *Journal of Comparative Neurology*, 1947, *87*, 1–16.

Brodal, A. *Neurological anatomy*. New York: Oxford University Press, 1969.

Brown, G. E., & Remley, N. R. The effects of septal and olfactory bulb lesions in stimulus reactivity. *Physiology and Behavior*, 1971, *6*, 497–501.

Brown, G. E., Harrell, E., & Remley, N. R. Passive avoidance in septal and anosmic rats using quinine as the aversive stimulus. *Physiology and Behavior*, 1971, *6*, 543–546.

Brown-Grant, K., & Raisman, G. Abnormalities in reproductive function associated with the destruction of the suprachiasmatic nuclei in female rats. *Proceedings of the Royal Society London, Biological Sciences*, 1977, *198*, 279–296.

Brutkowski, S., & Mempel, E. Disinhibition of inhibitory conditioned responses following selective brain lesions in dogs. *Science*, 1961, *134*, 2040–2041.

Buddington, R. W., King, F. A., & Roberts, L. Emotionality and conditioned avoidance responding in the squirrel monkey following septal injury. *Psychonomic Science*, 1967, *8*, 195–196.

Buerger, A. A. Effects of preoperative training on relearning a successive discrimination by cats with hippocampal lesions. *Journal of Comparative and Physiological Psychology*, 1970, *72*, 462–466.

Bugnon, C., Block, B., Lenys, D., Gouget, A., & Fellman, D. Comparative study of the neuronal populations containing β-endorphin, corticotropin and dopamine in the arcuate nucleus of the rat hypothalamus. *Neuroscience Letters*, 1979, *14*, 43–48.

Bull, H. Studies on conditioned responses in fish. *Journal of the Marine Biological Association*, 1928, *15*, 485–533.

Bunnell, B. N. Amygdaloid lesions and social dominance in the hooded rat. *Psychonomic Science*, 1966, *6*, 93–94.

Burkett, E. E., & Bunnell, B. N. Septal lesions and the retention of DRL performance in the rat. *Journal of Comparative and Physiological Psychology*, 1966, *62*, 468–472.

Bush, D. F., Lovely, R. H., & Pagano, R. R. Injection of ACTH induces recovery from shuttle-box avoidance deficits in rats with amygdaloid lesions. *Journal of Comparative and Physiological Psychology*, 1973, *83*, 168–172.

Butter, C. M., Mishkin, M., & Rosvold, H. E. Conditioning and extinction of a food-rewarded response after selective ablations of frontal cortex in rhesus monkeys. *Experimental Neurology*, 1963, *7*, 65–75.

Butters, N., & Rosvold, H. E. Effect of septal lesions on resistance to extinction and delayed alternation in monkeys. *Journal of Comparative and Physiological Psychology*, 1968, *66*, 389–395.

Buzsáki, G. Long-term potentiation of the commissural path-CA1 pyramidal cell synapse in the hippocampus of the freely moving rat. *Neuroscience Letters*, 1980, *19*, 293–296.

Buzsáki, G., Grastyán, E., Kellenyi, L., & Czopf, J. Dynamic phase-shifts between theta generators in the rat hippocampus. *Acta Physiologica Academiae Scientarum Hungaricae*, 1979, *53*, 41–45.

Buzsáki, G., Grastyán, E., Mód, L., & Winiczai, Z. Importance of cue location for intact and fimbria-fornix-lesioned rats. *Behavioral and Neural Biology*, 1980, *29*, 176–189.

Buzsáki, G., Grastyán, E., Haubenreiser, J., Czopf, J., & Kellényi, L. Hippocampal slow wave activity: Sources of controversy. In H. Matthies (Ed.), *IBRO* (Vol. 7). Magdeburg, GDR: Symposium on Learning and Memory, 1981.

Campbell, C. B. G., & Hodos, W. The concept of homology and the evolution of the nervous system. *Brain, Behavior, and Evolution*, 1970, *3*, 353–367.

Campenot, R. B. Effect of amygdaloid lesions upon active avoidance acquisition and anticipatory responding in rats. *Journal of Comparative and Physiological Psychology*, 1969, *69*, 492–497.

Caplan, M., & Stamm, J. DRL acquisition in rats with septal lesions. *Psychonomic Science*, 1967, *8*, 5–6.

Carder, B. Effects of septal stimulation on active avoidance in rats. *Physiology and Behavior*, 1971, *6*, 503–506.

Cardo, B. Action de lesions thalamiques et hypothalamiques sur le conditionnement de fruite et la differenciation tonale chez le rat. *Journale de Physiologie (Paris)*, 1960, *52*, 537–553.

Carey, R. J. Motivational and reinforcement scheduling factors in the effect of hippocampal injury on operant behavior. *Physiology and Behavior*, 1969, *4*, 959–961.

Carey, R. J. Quinine and saccharin preference–aversion threshold determinations in rats with septal ablations. *Journal of Comparative and Physiological Psychology*, 1971, *76*, 316–326.

Carlson, N. R. Two-way avoidance behavior of mice with limbic lesions. *Journal of Comparative and Physiological Psychology*, 1970, *70*, 73–78.

Carlson, N. R., & Cole, J. R. Enhanced alternation performance following septal lesions in mice. *Journal of Comparative and Physiological Psychology*, 1970, *73*, 157–161.

Carlson, N. R., & Norman, R. J. Enhanced go, no-go single-lever alternation of mice with septal lesions. *Journal of Comparative and Physiological Psychology*, 1971, *75*, 508–512.

Carlson, N. R., & Vallante, M. A. Enhanced cue function of olfactory stimulation in mice with septal lesions. *Journal of Comparative and Physiological Psychology*, 1974, *87*, 237–248.

Carlson, N. R., Carter, E. N., & Vallante, M. Runway alternation and discrimination of mice with limbic lesions. *Journal of Comparative and Physiological Psychology*, 1972, *78*, 91–101.

Carlton, P. L. Brain-acetylcholine and inhibition. In J. T. Tapp (Ed.), *Reinforcement and behavior*. New York and London: Academic Press, 1969, pp. 285–325.

Carlton, P. L., & Wolgin, D. L. Contingent tolerance to the anorexigenic effects of amphetamine. *Physiology and Behavior*, 1971, *7*, 221–223.

Cazala, P. Y., & Guenet, J. L. The role of genetic factors in the determination of self-stimulation behavior in the mouse: Backcross analysis. *Behavioral Processes*, 1976, *1*, 93–99.

Chalmers, B. M., & Holdstock, T. L. Effects of atropine on heart rate and hippocampal EEG following septal stimulation in rats. *Psychonomic Science*, 1969, *16*, 145–147.

Cherry, C. T. Variability and discrimination reversal learning in the open field following septal lesions in rats. *Physiology and Behavior*, 1975, *15*, 641–646.

Chi, C. C., & Flynn, J. P. Neural pathways associated with hypothalamically elicited attack behavior in cats. *Science*, 1971, *171*, 703–706.

Chin, J. H., Pribram, K. H., Drake, K., & Greene, L. O., Jr. Disruption of temperature discrimination during limbic forebrain stimulation in monkeys. *Neuropsychologia*, 1976, *14*, 293–310.

Chin, T., Donovick, P. J., & Burright, R. G. Septal lesions in rats produce reversal deficits in a simultaneous visual discrimination. *Journal of Comparative and Physiological Psychology*, 1976, *90*, 1133–1143.

Clark, C. V. H., & Isaacson, R. L. Effect of bilateral hippocampal ablation on DRL performance. *Journal of Comparative and Physiological Psychology*, 1965, *59*, 137–140.

Clavier, R. M., & Fibiger, T. C. On the role of ascending catecholamine projections in intracranial self-stimulation of the substantia nigra. *Brain Research*, 1977, *131*, 271–286.

Clody, D. E., & Carlton, P. L. Behavioral effects of lesions of the medial septum of rats. *Journal of Comparative and Physiological Psychology*, 1969, *67*, 344–356.

Cogan, D. C., & Reeves, J. L. Passive avoidance learning in hippocampectomized rats under different shock and intertrial interval conditions. *Physiology and Behavior*, 1979, 22, 1115–1121.

Coindet, J., Chouvet, G., & Mouret, J. Effects of lesions of the suprachiasmatic nuclei on paradoxical sleep and slow wave sleep circadian rhythms in the rat. *Neuroscience Letters*, 1975, 1, 243–247.

Coover, G. D., & Levine, S. Auditory startle response of hippocampectomized rats. *Physiology and Behavior*, 1972, 9, 75–77.

Coover, G. D., Goldman, L., & Levine, S. Plasma corticosterone levels during extinction of a lever-press response in hippocampectomized rats. *Physiology and Behavior*, 1971, 7, 727–732.

Corman, D. C., Meyer, P. M., & Meyer, D. R. Open-field activity and exploration in rats with septal and amygdaloid lesions. *Brain Research*, 1967, 5, 469–476.

Coulombe, D., & White, N. Effects of lesions of the amygdala, pyriform cortex, and stria terminalis on two types of exploration by rats. *Physiological Psychology*, 1978, 6, 319–324.

Cox, V. C., & Valenstein, E. S. Attenuation of aversive properties of peripheral shock by brain stimulation. *Science*, 1965, 149, 323–325.

Cox, V. C., & Valenstein, E. S. Distribution of hypothalamic sites yielding stimulus-bound behavior. *Brain, Behavior, and Evolution*, 1969, 2, 359–376.

Crawford, F. T., & Langdon, J. W. Escape and avoidance responding in the toad. *Psychonomic Science*, 1966, 6, 115–116.

Crosby, E. C., Humphrey, T., & Lauer, E. W. *Correlative anatomy of the nervous system*. New York: Macmillan, 1962.

Crow, T. J. A map of the rat mesencephalon for electrical self-stimulation. *Brain Research*, 1972, 36, 275–287.

Crowne, D. P., & Riddell, W. I. Hippocampal lesions and the cardiac component of the orienting response in the rat. *Journal of Comparative and Physiological Psychology*, 1969, 69, 748–755.

Cummings, J. P., & Felten, P. L. A raphe dendrite bundle in the rabbit medulla. *Journal of Comparative Neurology*, 1979, 183, 1–24.

Curtis, S. D., & Nonneman, A. J. Effects of successive bilateral hippocampectomy on DRL 20 performance in rats. *Physiology and Behavior*, 1977, 19, 707–712.

Dabrowska, J., & Pluta, R. Facilitatory effect of darkness upon spatial reversal learning in septal rats. *Acta Neurobiologiae Experimentalis* (Warsaw), 1978, 38, 223–226.

Dacey, D. M., & Grossman, S. P. Aphagia, adipsia, and sensory-motor deficits produced by amygdala lesions: A function of extra-amygdaloid damage. *Physiology and Behavior*, 1977, 19, 389–398.

Dalby, D. A. Effect of septal lesions on the acquisition of two types of active avoidance behavior in rats. *Journal of Comparative and Physiological Psychology*, 1970, 73, 278–283.

Dalland, T. Response and stimulus perseveration in rats with septal and dorsal hippocampal lesions. *Journal of Comparative and Physiological Psychology*, 1970, 71, 114–118.

Dalland, T. Response perseveration of rats with dorsal hippocampal lesions. *Behavioral Biology*, 1976, 17, 473–484.

Dark, J. G., Chiodo, L. A., Papich, P. S., Yori, J. G., & Asdourian, D. Impairment in a T-maze task following unilateral lateral hypothalamic lesions. *Physiology and Behavior*, 1977, 19, 365–370.

Davis, J. R., & Keesey, R. E. Norepinephrine-induced eating—its hypothalamic locus and an alternate interpretion of action. *Journal of Comparative and Physiological Psychology*, 1971, *77*, 394–402.

Davis, R. E., & Kent, E. W. Transection of direct anterior thalamic afferents from the hippocampus: Effects on activity and active avoidance in rats. *Journal of Comparative and Physiological Psychology*, 1979, *93*, 1182–1192.

Deadwyler, S. A., West, M., & Lynch, G. Activity of dentate granule cells during learning: Differentiation of perforant path input. *Brain Research*, 1979, *169*, 29–43.

Deadwyler, S. A., West, M. O., & Robinson, J. H. Entorhinal and septal inputs differentially control sensory-evoked responses in the rat dentate gyrus. *Science*, 1981, *211*, 1181–1183.

Deagle, J. H., & Lubar, J. F. Effect of septal lesions in two strains of rats on one-way and shuttle avoidance acquisition. *Journal of Comparative and Physiological Psychology*, 1971, *77*, 277–281.

Defendini, R., & Zimmerman, E. A. The magnocellular neurosecretory system of the mammalian hypothalamus. *Research Publications Association for Research in Nervous and Mental Diseases*, 1978, *56*, 137–154.

DeFries, J. C., & Hegmann, J. P. Genetic analysis of open-field behavior. In G. Lindzey & D. D. Thiessen (Eds.), *Contributions to behavior-genetic analysis: The mouse as a prototype*. New York: Appleton-Century-Crofts, 1970, pp. 23–56.

de Groot, J. *The rat forebrain in stereotaxic co-ordinates*. Amsterdam: North-Holland Publishers, 1959.

Delgado, J. M. R., Roberts, W. W., & Miller, N. E. Learning motivated by electrical stimulation of the brain. *American Journal of Physiology*, 1954, *179*, 587.

DeOlmos, J. S. The amygdaloid projection field in the rat as studied by the cupric-silver method. In B. E. Eleftheriou (Ed.), *The neurobiology of the amygdala*. New York: Plenum Press, 1972.

De Ryck, M., & Teitelbaum, P. Neocortical and hippocampal EEG in normal and lateral hypothalamic-damaged rats. *Physiology and Behavior*, 1978, *20*, 403–409.

Deutsch, J. A., & Howarth, C. I. Some tests of a theory of intracranial self-stimulation. *Psychological Review*, 1963, *70*, 444–460.

DeVito, J. L. Subcortical projections to the hippocampal formation in squirrel monkey. *Brain Research Bulletin*, 1980, *5*, 285–289.

de Wied, D. Pituitary-adrenal system hormones and behavior. In F. O. Schmitt & G. F. Worden (Eds.), *The neurosciences: Third study program*. Cambridge, Mass.: MIT Press, 1974, pp. 653–666.

de Wied, D., Bohus, B., van Ree, J. M., & Urban, I. Behavioral and electrophysiological effects of peptides related to lipotropin (β-LPH). *The Journal of Pharmacology and Experimental Therapeutics*, 1978, *204*, 570–580.

Diamond, I. T., & Neff, W. D. Ablation of temporal cortex and discrimination of auditory patterns. *Journal of Neurophysiology*, 1957, *20*, 300–315.

DiCara, L. V. Effect of amygdaloid lesions on avoidance learning in the rat. *Psychonomic Science*, 1966, *4*, 279–280.

Dickinson, A. Septal damage and response output under frustrative nonreward. In R. A. Boakes & M. S. Halliday (Eds.), *Inhibition and learning*. London: Academic Press, 1972, pp. 461–496.

Dicks, D., Myers, R. E., & Kling, A. Uncus and amygdala lesions: Effects on social behavior in the free-ranging rhesus monkey. *Science*, 1979, *165*, 69–71.

Disterhoft, J. F., & Segal, M. Neuron activity in rat hippocampus and motor cortex during discrimination reversal. *Brain Research Bulletin*, 1978, *3*, 583–588.

Dokla, C. P. J., Kasprow, W. J., Sideleau, M. M., & Boitano, J. J. Effects of electro-convulsive shock on open-field behavior and spontaneous alternation in rats. *Behavioral and Neural Biology*, 1980, *28*, 266–284.

Domesick, V. B. Projections from the cingulate cortex in the rat. *Brain Research*, 1969, *12*, 296–320.

Domesick, V. B. The fasciculus cinguli in the rat. *Brain Research*, 1970, *20*, 19–32.

Domesick, V. B. Thalamic relationships of the medial cortex in the rat. *Brain, Behavior, and Evolution*, 1972, *6*, 457–483.

Dominguez, M., & Longo, V. Taming effects of parachlorophenylalanine on septal rats. *Physiology and Behavior*, 1969, *4*, 1031–1033.

Donovick, P. J. Effects of localized septal lesions on hippocampal EEG activity in behavior in rats. *Journal of Comparative and Physiological Psychology*, 1968, *66*, 569–578.

Donovick, P. J., & Burright, R. G. Water consumption in rats with septal lesions following two days of water deprivation. *Physiology and Behavior*, 1968, *3*, 285–288.

Donovick, P. J., & Schwartzbaum, J. S. Effects of low level stimulation of the septal area on two types of discrimination reversal in the rat. *Psychonomic Science*, 1966, *6*, 3–4.

Donovick, P. J., & Wakeman, K. A. Open-field luminance and "septal hyperemotion-ality." *Animal Behavior*, 1969, *17*, 186–190.

Donovick, P. J., Burright, R. G., & Lustbader, S. Isotonic and hypertonic saline inges-tion following septal lesions. *Communications in Behavioral Biology*, 1969, *4*, 17–22.

Donovick, P. J., Burright, R. G., & Zuromski, E. Localization of quinine aversion within the septum, habenula, and interpeduncular nucleus. *Journal of Comparative and Physiological Psychology*, 1970, *17*, 376–383.

Donovick, P. J., Burright, R. G., & Swidler, M. A. Presurgical rearing environment alters exploration, fluid consumption, and learning of septal lesioned and control rats. *Physiology and Behavior*, 1973, *11*, 543–553.

Donovick, P. J., Burright, R. G., & Bentsen, E. O. Presurgical dietary history differ-entially alters the behavior of control and septal lesioned rats. *Developmental Psychobiology*, 1975, *8*, 13–25.

Donovick, P. J., Burright, R. G., Fuller, J. L., & Branson, P. R. Septal lesions and behavior: Effects of presurgical rearing and strain of mouse. *Journal of Comparative and Physiological Psychology*, 1975, *89*, 859–867.

Donovick, P. J., Burright, R. G., Sikorszky, R. D., Stamato, N. J., & MacLaughlin, W. W. Cue elimination effects on discrimination behavior of rats with septal lesions. *Physiology and Behavior*, 1978, *20*, 71–78.

Donovick, P. J., Burright, R. G., Fanelli, R. J., & Engellenner, W. J. Septal lesions and avoidance behavior: Genetic, neurochemical and behavioral considerations. *Physiology and Behavior*, 1981, *26*, 495–507.

Dorsa, D. M., Van Ree, J. M., & De Wied, D. Effects of [des-tyr^1]-γ-endorphin and α-endorphin on substantia nigra self-stimulation. *Pharmacology, Biochemistry and Behavior*, 1979, *10*, 899–905.

Douglas, R. J. Transposition, novelty, and limbic lesions. *Journal of Comparative and Physiological Psychology*, 1966, *62*, 354–357.

Douglas, R. J. The hippocampus and behavior. *Psychological Bulletin*, 1967, *67*, 416–422.

Douglas, R. J. The development of hippocampal function. In R. L. Isaacson & K. H. Pribram (Eds.), *The hippocampus*. New York: Plenum Press, 1975.

Douglas, R. J., & Isaacson, R. L. Hippocampal lesions and activity. *Psychonomic Science*, 1964, *1*, 187–188.

Douglas, R. J., & Isaacson, R. L. Spontaneous alternation and scopolamine. *Psychonomic Science*, 1966, 4, 283–284.

Douglas, R. J., & Marcellus, D. The ascent of man: Deductions based on a multivariate analysis of the brain. *Brain, Behavior and Evolution*, 1975, 11, 179–213.

Douglas, R. J., & Pribram, K. H. Distraction and habituation in monkeys with limbic lesions. *Journal of Comparative and Physiological Psychology*, 1969, 69, 473–480.

Douglas, R. J., & Truncer, P. C. Parallel but independent effects of pentobarbital and scopolamine on hippocampus-related behavior. *Behavioral Biology*, 1976, 18, 359–367.

Dudar, J. D., Whishaw, I. Q., & Szerb, J. C. Release of acetylcholine from the hippocampus of freely moving rats during sensory stimulation and running. *Neuropharmacology*, 1979, 18, 673–678.

Duncan, P. M. The effect of temporary septal dysfunction on conditioning and performance of fear responses. *Journal of Comparative and Physiological Psychology*, 1971, 74, 340–348.

Duncan, P. M., & Duncan, N. C. Free-operant and T-maze avoidance performance by septal and hippocampal-damaged rats. *Physiology and Behavior*, 1971, 7, 687–693.

Dunsmore, R., & Lennox, R. Stimulation and strychninization of supracallosal anterior cingulate gyrus. *Journal of Neurophysiology*, 1950, 13, 207–214.

Dunwiddie, T., & Lynch, G. Long-term potentiation and depression of synaptic responses in the rat hippocampus: Localization and frequency dependency. *Journal of Physiology*, 1978, 276, 353–367.

Eclancher, F. S., & Karli, P. Compartement d'agression interspécifique et comportement alimentaire du rat: Effets de lésions des noyaux ventromédians de l'hypothalamus. *Brain Research*, 1971, 26, 71–79.

Eclancher, F., & Karli, P. Effects of early amygdaloid lesions on the development of reactivity in the rat. *Physiology and Behavior*, 1979, 22, 1123–1134.

Eclancher, F., & Karli, P. Effects of infant and adult amygdaloid lesions upon acquisition of two-way active avoidance by the adult rat: Influence of rearing conditions. *Physiology and Behavior*, 1980, 24, 887–893.

Egger, M. D., & Flynn, J. P. Amygdaloid suppression of hypothalamically elicited attack behavior. *Science*, 1962, 136, 43–44.

Eichelman, B. S., Jr. Effect of subcortical lesions on shock-induced aggression in the rat. *Journal of Comparative and Physiological Psychology*, 1971, 7, 331–339.

Elazar, Z., & Adey, W. R. Spectral analysis of low frequency components in the electrical activity of the hippocampus during learning. *Electroencephalography and Clinical Neurophysiology*, 1967, 23, 225–240.

Elazar, Z., Motles, E., Ely, Y., & Simantov, R. Acute tolerance to the excitatory effect of enkephalin microinjections into hippocampus. *Life Sciences*, 1979, 24, 541–548.

Elde, R., Hökfeldt, T., Johansson, O., & Terenius, L. Immunohistochemical studies using antibodies to leucine-enkephalin: Initial observations on the nervous system of the rat. *Neuroscience*, 1976, 1, 349–351.

Eleftheriou, B. E., Elias, M. F., & Norman, R. L. Effects of amygdaloid lesions on reversal learning in the deermouse. *Physiology and Behavior*, 1972, 9, 69–73.

Elias, M. F., Dupree, M., & Eleftheriou, B. E. Differences in spatial discrimination reversal learning between two inbred mouse strains following specific amygdaloid lesions. *Journal of Comparative and Physiological Psychology*, 1973, 83, 149–156.

Ellen, P., & Aitken, W. C., Jr. Absence of overresponding on a DRL schedule by hippocampally-lesioned rats. *Physiology and Behavior*, 1970, 5, 489–495.

Ellen, P., & Deloache, J. Hippocampal lesions and spontaneous alternation behavior in the rat. *Physiology and Behavior*, 1968, 3, 857–860.

Ellen, P., & Powell, E. W. Effects of septal lesions on behavior generated by positive reinforcement. *Experimental Neurology*, 1962, 6, 1–11. (a)

Ellen, P., & Powell, E. W. Temporal discrimination in rats with rhinencephalic lesions. *Experimental Neurology*, 1962, 6, 538–547. (b)

Ellen, P., Wilson, A. S., & Powell, E. W. Septal inhibition and timing behavior in the rat. *Experimental Neurology*, 1964, 10, 120–132.

Ellen, P., Aitken, W. C., Jr., & Stahl, J. M. Pretraining effects on the DRL performance of rats with septal lesions. *Physiological Psychology*, 1973, 1, 380–384.

Ellen, P., Aitken, W. C., Jr., & Walker, R. Pretraining effects on performance of rats with hippocampal lesions. *Journal of Comparative and Physiological Psychology*, 1973, 84, 622–628.

Ellen, P., Dorsett, P. G., & Richardson, W. K. The effect of cue-fading on the DRL performance of septal and normal rats. *Physiological Psychology*, 1977, 5, 469–476.

Ellen, P., Gillenwater, G., & Richardson, W. K. Extinction responding by septal and normal rats following acquisition under four schedules of reinforcement. *Physiology and Behavior*, 1977, 18, 609–615.

Elliot Smith, G. Some problems relating to the evolution of the brain. *Lancet*, 1910, 1, 1–6, 147–153, 221–227.

Ellison, G. D. Appetite behavior in rats after circumsection of the hypothalamus. *Physiology and Behavior*, 1968, 3, 221–226.

Ellison, G., & Flynn, J. P. Organized aggressive behavior in cats after surgical isolation of the hypothalamus. *Archieves Italienne de Biologie*, 1968, 106, 1–20.

Ellison, G. D., Sorenson, C. A., & Jacobs, B. L. Two feeding syndromes following surgical isolation of the hypothalamus in rats. *Journal of Comparative and Physiological Psychology*, 1970, 70, 173–188.

Elstein, K., Hannigan, J. H., Jr., & Isaacson, R. L. Repeated intracerebroventricular injections of $ACTH_{1-24}$ in rats with hippocampal lesions. *Behavioral and Neural Biology*, 1981, 32, 248–254.

Ely, D. L., Greene, E. G., & Henry, J. P. Effects of hippocampal lesion on cardiovascular, adrenocortical and behavioral responses patterns in mice. *Physiology and Behavior*, 1977, 18, 1075–1083.

Endröczi, E. *Limbic system, learning and pituitary-adrenal function*. Budapest: Akadémia Kiadó, 1972.

Engelhardt, F., & Steward, O. Entorhinal cortical lesions in rats and runway alternation performance: Changes in patterns of response initiation. *Behavioral and Neural Biology*, 1980, 29, 91–104.

Entingh, D. Perseverative responding and hyperphagia following entorhinal lesions in cats. *Journal of Comparative and Physiological Psychology*, 1971, 75, 50–58.

Epstein, A. N. Reciprocal changes in feeding behavior produced by intrahypothalamic chemical injections. *American Journal of Physiology*, 1966, 199, 969–974.

Epstein, A. N. The lateral hypothalamic syndrome: Its implications for the physiological psychology of hunger and thirst. In E. Stellar & J. M. Sprague (Eds.), *Progress in physiological psychology* (Vol. 4). New York: Academic Press, 1971.

Etgen, A. M., Lee, K. S., & Lynch, G. Glucocorticoid modulations of specific protein metabolism in hippocampal slices maintained in vitro. *Brain Research*, 1979, 165, 37–45.

Faillace, L. A., Allen, R. P., McQueen, J. D., & Northrup, B. Cognitive deficits from bilateral cingulotomy for intractable pain in man. *Diseases of the Nervous System*, 1971, *32*, 171–175.

Fallon, D., & Donovick, P. J. Septal lesions, motivation, and secondary reinforcement. Lesion induced somatomotor inhibition. *Journal of Comparative and Physiological Psychology*, 1970, *73*, 155–156.

Fallon, J. H., & Moore, R. Y. Superior colliculus efferents to the hypothalamus. *Neuroscience Letters*, 1979, *14*, 265–270.

Fedio, P., & Ommaya, A. K. Bilateral cingulum lesions and stimulation in man with lateralized impairment in short-term verbal memory. *Experimental Neurology*, 1970, *29*, 84–91.

Feeney, D. M., & Wier, C. S. Sensory neglect after lesions of substantia nigra or lateral hypothalamus: Differential severity and recovery of function. *Brain Research*, 1979, *178*, 329–346.

Feindel, W., & Gloor, P. Comparison of the electrographic effects of stimulation of the amygdala and brain stem reticular formation in cats. *Electroencephalography and Clinical Neurophysiology*, 1954, *6*, 389–402.

Feldman, S., Wajsbort, J., & Birnbaum, D. Effect of combined brain stimulation on gastric secretion, acidity and potassium concentration in cats. *Brain Research*, 1967, *4*, 103–106.

Feldon, J., & Gray, J. A. Effects of medial and lateral septal lesions on the partial reinforcement extinction effect at one trial a day. *Quarterly Journal of Experimental Psychology*, 1979, *31*, 653–674. (a)

Feldon, J., & Gray, J. A. Effects of medial and lateral septal lesions on the partial reinforcement extinction effect at shorter inter-trial intervals. *Quarterly Journal of Experimental Psychology*, 1979, *31*, 675–690. (b)

Felten, D. L., Harrigan, P., Burnett, B. T., & Cummings, J. P. Fourth ventricular tanycytes: A possible relationship with monoaminergic nuclei. *Brain Research Bulletin*, 1981, *6*, 427–436.

Fibiger, H. C., Carter, D. A., & Phillips, A. G. Decreased intracranial self-stimulation after neuroleptics or 6-hydroxydopamine: Evidence for mediation by motor deficits rather than by reduced reward. *Psychopharmacology*, 1976, *47*, 21–27.

File, S., & Wardill, A. Validity of head-dipping as a measure of exploration in a modified hole board. *Psychopharmacology*, 1975, *44*, 53–59.

Filho, L. S. C., Moschovakis, A., & Izquierdo, I. Effect of hippocampal lesions on rat shuttle responses in four different behavioral tests. *Physiology and Behavior*, 1977, *19*, 569–572.

Fisher, A. E. The role of limbic structures on the central regulation of feeding and drinking behavior. *Annals of the New York Academy of Sciences*, 1969, *157*, 894–901.

Flaherty, C. F., & Hamilton, L. W. Responsivity to decreasing sucrose concentrations following septal lesions in the rat. *Physiology and Behavior*, 1971, *6*, 431–437.

Flaherty, C. F., Capobianco, S., & Hamilton, L. W. Effect of septal lesions on retention of negative contrast. *Physiology and Behavior*, 1973, *11*, 625–631.

Flynn, J. The neural basis of aggression in cats. In D. H. Glass (Ed.), *Neurophysiology and emotion*. New York: Rockefeller University Press, 1967, pp. 40–60.

Flynn, J. P. Neural basis of threat and attack. In R. G. Grenell & S. Gabey (Eds.), *Biological foundations of psychiatry*. New York: Raven Press, 1976, pp. 273–295.

Flynn, J. P., Vanegas, H., Foote, W., & Edwards, S. Neural mechanisms involved in a cat's attack on a rat. In R. E. Whalen, R. F. Thompson, M. Verzeano, & N. M. Weinberger (Eds.), *The neural control of behavior*. New York: Academic Press, 1970.

Foltz, E. L. Modification of morphine withdrawal by frontal lobe cingulum lesions. In L. von Bogaert & J. Radermeker (Eds.), *First International Congress of Neurological Sciences*. London: Pergamon, 1959.

Foltz, E. L., & White, L. E., Jr. Experimental cingulumotomy and modification of morphine withdrawal. *Journal of Neurosurgery*, 1957, *14*, 655–673.

Foltz, E. L., & White, L. E., Jr. Pain "relief" by frontal cingulumotomy. *Journal of Neurosurgery*, 1962, *19*, 89–100.

Fonberg, E. The normalizing effect of lateral amygdalar lesions upon the dorsomedial amygdalar syndrome in dogs. *Acta Neurobiologiae Experimentalis*, 1973, *33*, 449–466.

Fonberg, E., & Delgado, J. M. R. Avoidance and alimentary reactions during amygdalar stimulation. *Journal of Neurophysiology*, 1961, *24*, 651–664.

Fonberg, E., Brutkowski, S., & Mempel, E. Defensive conditioned reflexes and neurotic motor reactions following amygdalectomy in dogs. *Acta Biologiae Experimentalis*, 1962, *12*, 51–57.

Fox, C. A. Certain basal telencephalic centers in the cat. *Journal of Comparative Neurology*, 1940, *72*, 1–62.

Franchina, J. J., & Brown, T. S. Reward magnitude shift effects in rats with hippocampal lesions. *Journal of Comparative and Physiological Psychology*, 1971, *76*, 365–370.

Frank, L. H., & Beatty, W. W. Effects of septal lesions on passive avoidance behavior using ice water as the aversive stimulus. *Physiology and Behavior*, 1974, *12*, 321–323.

Frederickson, C. J., & Frederickson, M. H. Emergence of spontaneous alternation in the kitten. *Developmental Psychobiology*, 1979, *12*, 615–621.

Freeman, F. G. Cue utilization and hippocampal lesions in rats. *Physiological Psychology*, 1978, *6*, 275–278.

Freeman, F. G., Mikulka, P. J., Phillips, J., Megarr, M., & Meisel, L. Generalization of conditioned aversion and limbic lesions in rats. *Behavioral Biology*, 1978, *24*, 520–526.

French, J. D., Hernandez-Peon, R., & Livingston, R. B. Projections from cortex to cephalic brain stem (reticular formation) in monkey. *Journal of Neurophysiology*, 1955, *18*, 74–95.

Fried, P. A. The effect of differential hippocampal lesions and pre- and post-operative training on extinction. *Revue Canadienne de Psychologie*, 1972, *26*, 61–70.

Froloff, J. Bedingte Reflexe bei Fischen. *Pflügers Archives Gesamte Physiologie*, 1925, *220*, 339–349.

Fry, J. P., Zieglgänsberger, W., & Herz, A. Specific versus non-specific actions of opioids on hippocampal neurones in the rat brain. *Brain Research*, 1979, *163*, 295–305.

Fuller, J. L., Rosvold, H. E., & Pribram, K. H. The effect on affective and cognitive behavior in the dog of lesions of the pyriform–amygdala–hippocampal complex. *Journal of Comparative and Physiological Psychology*, 1957, *50*, 89–96.

Fuxe, K. Distribution of monoamine nerve terminals in the central nervous system. *Acta Physiologica Scandinavica* (Sweden), 1965, *64*, Suppl. 247.

Fuxe, K., Hökfelt, T., & Ungerstedt, U. Morphological and functional aspects of central monoamine neurons. *International Review of Neurobiology*, 1970, *13*, 93–126.

Gabriel, M., & Saltwick, S. E. Rhythmic, theta-like unit activity of the hippocampal formation during acquisition and performance of avoidance behavior in rabbits. *Physiology and Behavior*, 1980, *24*, 303–312.

Gabriel, M., Foster, K., & Orona, E. Unit activity in cingulate cortex and anteroventral thalamus during acquisition and overtraining of discriminative avoidance behavior in rabbits. In R. F. Thompson, L. H. Hicks, & V. B. Shvyrkov (Eds.), *Neural mechanisms of goal-directed behavior*. New York: Academic Press, 1980, pp. 303–315.

Gabriel, M., Foster, K., Orona, E., Saltwick, S. E., & Stanton, M. Neuronal activity of cingulate cortex, anteroventral thalamus, and hippocampal formation in discriminative conditioning: Encoding and extraction of the significance of conditional stimuli. *Progress in Psychobiology and Physiological Psychology*, 1980, *9*, 125–231.

Gage, F. H., & Olton, D. S. Hippocampal influence on hyperreactivity induced by septal lesions. *Brain Research*, 1975, *98*, 311–325.

Gage, F. H., & Olton, D. S. L-Dopa reduces hyperreactivity induced by septal lesions in rats. *Behavioral Biology*, 1976, *17*, 213–218.

Gage, F. H., Olton, D. S., & Bolanowski, D. Activity, reactivity, and dominance following septal lesions in rats. *Behavioral Biology*, 1978, *22*, 203–210.

Gage, F. H., Armstrong, D. R., & Thompson, R. G. Behavioral kinetics: A method for deriving qualitative and quantitative changes in sensory responsiveness following septal nuclei damage. *Physiology and Behavior*, 1980, *24*, 479–484.

Galef, B. G. Aggression and timidity: Responses to novelty in feral Norway rats. *Journal of Comparative and Physiological Psychology*, 1970, *70*, 370–381.

Galey, D., Simon, H., & Le Moal, M. Behavioral effects of lesions in the A10 dopaminergic area of the rat. *Brain Research*, 1977, *124*, 83–97.

Gallistel, C. R. Electrical self-stimulation and its theoretical implications. *Psychological Bulletin*, 1964, *61*, 23–24.

Gallistel, C. R. Self-stimulation: Failure of pretrial stimulation to affect rats' electrode preference. *Journal of Comparative Physiological Psychology*, 1969, *69*, 722–729.

Gardner, L., & Malmo, R. B. Effects of low-level septal stimulation on escape: Significance for limbic–midbrain interactions in pain. *Journal of Comparative and Physiological Psychology*, 1969, *68*, 65–73.

Gellhorn, E. The emotions and the ergotropic and trophotropic systems. *Psychologische Forschung*, 1970, *34*, 48–94.

Gerbrandt, L. K., Spinelli, D. N., & Pribram, K. H. The interaction of visual attention and temporal cortex stimulation on electrical activity evoked in striate cortex. *Electroencephalography and Clinical Neurophysiology*, 1970, *19*, 146–155.

German, D. L., & Bowden, D. M. Catecholamine systems as the neural substrate for intracranial self-stimulation: A hypothesis. *Brain Research*, 1974, *73*, 381–419.

Gispen, W. H., & Isaacson, R. L. ACTH-induced excessive grooming in the rat. *Pharmacology and Therapeutics*, 1981, *12*, 209–246.

Gittelson, P. L., & Donovick, P. J. The effects of septal lesions on the learning and reversal of a kinesthetic discrimination. *Psychonomic Science*, 1968, *13*, 137–138.

Gittelson, P. L., Donovick, P. J., & Burright, R. G. Facilitation of passive avoidance in rats with septal lesions. *Psychonomic Science*, 1969, *17*, 292–293.

Glass, D. H., Ison, J. R., & Thomas, G. J. Anterior limbic cortex and partial reinforcement effects on acquisition and extinction of a runway response in rats. *Journal of Comparative and Physiological Psychology*, 1969, *69*, 17–24.

Glendenning, K. K. Effects of septal and amygdaloid lesions on social behavior of the cat. *Journal of Comparative and Physiological Psychology*, 1972, *80*, 199–207.

Glickman, S. E., Higgins, T., & Isaacson, R. L. Some effects of hippocampal lesions on the behavior of Mongolian gerbils. *Physiology and Behavior*, 1970, *5*, 931–938.

Goddard, G. V. Amygdaloid stimulation and learning in the rat. *Journal of Comparative and Physiological Psychology*, 1964, *58*, 23–30. (a)

Goddard, G. V. Functions of the amygdala. *Psychological Bulletin*, 1964, *62*, 89–109. (b)

Goddard, G. V. Analysis of avoidance conditioning following cholinergic stimulation of amygdala in rats. *Journal of Comparative and Physiological Psychology*, 1969, *68*, 1–18.

Goddard, G. V., McIntyre, D. C., & Leech, C. K. A permanent change in brain function resulting from daily electrical stimulation. *Experimental Neurology*, 1969, *25*, 295–330.

Gold, P. E., & Van Buskirk, R. B. Enhancement and impairment of memory processes with post-trial injections of adrenocorticotrophic hormone. *Behavioral Biology*, 1976, *16*, 387–400.

Gold, P. E., Macri, J., & McGaugh, J. L. Retrograde amnesia produced by subseizure amygdala stimulation. *Behavioral Biology*, 1973, *9*, 671–680.

Gold, P. E., Edwards, R. M., & McGaugh, J. L. Amnesia produced by unilateral, subseizure, electrical stimulation of the amygdala in rats. *Behavioral Biology*, 1975, *15*, 95–105.

Gold, P. E., Rose, R. P., Hankins, L. L., & Spanis, C. Imparied retention of visual discriminated escape training produced by subseizure amygdala stimulation. *Brain Research*, 1976, *118*, 73–85.

Gold, P. E., Hankins, L. L., & Rose, R. P. Time-dependent post-trial changes in the localization of amnestic electrical sites within the amygdala in rats. *Behavioral Biology*, 1977, *20*, 32–40.

Gold, R. M., & Proulx, D. M. Bait-shyness acquisition is impaired by VMH lesions that produce obesity. *Journal of Comparative and Physiological Psychology*, 1972, *79*, 201–209.

Goldman, P. S. An alternative to developmental plasticity: Heterology of CNS structures in infants and adults. In D. G. Stein & J. J. Rosen (Eds.), *Plasticity and recovery of function in the central nervous system*. New York: Academic Press, 1974.

Gollender, M. Eosinophil and avoidance correlates of stress in anterior cingulate cortex lesioned rat. *Journal of Comparative and Physiological Psychology*, 1967, *64*, 40–48.

Gollender, M., Law, O. T., & Isaacson, R. L. Changes in the circulating eosinophil level associated with learned fear. Conditioned eosinopenia. *Journal of Comparative and Physiological Psychology*, 1960, *53*, 520–523.

Gomer, F. E., & Goldstein, R. Attentional rigidity during exploratory and simultaneous discrimination behavior in septal lesioned rats. *Physiology and Behavior*, 1974, *12*, 19–28.

Gonsiorek, J., Donovick, P., Burright, R. G., & Fuller, J. Aggression in low and high brainweight mice following septal lesions. *Physiology and Behavior*, 1974, *12*, 813–818.

Gonzales, R. C., & Bitterman, M. E. Partial reinforcement effect in the goldfish as a function of amount of reward. *Journal of Comparative and Physiological Psychology*, 1967, *64*, 163–167.

Gotsick, J. E., & Marshall, R. C. Time course of the septal rage syndrome. *Physiology and Behavior*, 1972, *9*, 685–687.

Gottesfeld, Z., & Jacobowitz, D. M. Cholinergic projections from the septal-diagonal band area to the habenular nuclei. *Brain Research*, 1979, *176*, 391–394.

Grastyán, E. Commentary. In E. Gellhorn (Ed.), *Biological foundations of emotion*. Evanston, Ill.: Scott-Foresman, 1968, pp. 114–127.

Grastyán, E., & Buzsáki, G. The orienting-exploratory response hypothesis of discriminative conditioning. *Acta Neurobiologiae Experimentalis* (Warsaw), 1979, *39*, 491–501.

Grastyán, E., Lissák, K., Madarász, I., & Donhoffer, H. Hippocampal electrical activity during the development of conditioned reflexes. *Electroencephalography and Clinical Neurophysiology*, 1959, *11*, 409–429.

Gray, J. A. Sodium amobarbital, the hippocampal theta rhythm, and the partial reinforcement extinction effect. *Psychological Review*, 1970, *77*, 465–480.

Gray, J. A., Feldon, J., Rawlins, J. N. P., Owen, S., & McNaughton, N. The role of the septo-hippocampal system and its noradrenergic afferents in behavioural responses to nonreward. In J. Whelan (Ed.), *Functions of the septo-hippocampal system*. Ciba Foundation Symposium 58 (new series). Amsterdam: Associated Scientific Publishers, 1978.

Green, J. D., & Arduini, A. A. Hippocampal electrical activity in arousal. *Journal of Neurophysiology*, 1954, *17*, 533–557.

Green, J. D., & Petsche, H. Hippocampal electrical activity: II. Virtual generators. *Electroencephalography and Clinical Neurophysiology*, 1961, *13*, 847–853.

Green, J. D., Maxwell, D. S., Schindler, W. J., & Stumpf, C. Rabbit EEG "Theta" rhythm: Its anatomical source and relation to activity in single neurones. *Journal of Neurophysiology*, 1960, *23*, 403–420.

Green, R. H., & Schwartzbaum, J. S. Effects of unilateral septal lesions on avoidance behavior discrimination reversal and hippocampal EEG. *Journal of Comparative and Physiological Psychology*, 1968, *65*, 388–396.

Greene, E. G. Cholinergic stimulation of the medial septum. *Psychonomic Science*, 1968, *10*, 157–158.

Grijalva, C. V., Lindholm, E., & Schallert, T. Gastric pathology and aphagia following lateral hypothalamic lesions in rats: Effects of preoperative weight reduction. *Journal of Comparative and Physiological Psychology*, 1976, *90*, 505–519.

Grossman, S. P. Eating or drinking elicited by direct adrenergic or cholinergic stimulation of the hypothalamus. *Science*, 1960, *132*, 301–302.

Grossman, S. P. The VMH: A center for affective reactions, satiety or both. *Physiology and Behavior*, 1966, *1*, 1–10.

Grossman, S. P. A neuropharmacological analysis of hypothalamic and extrahypothalamic mechanisms concerned with the regulation of food and water intake. *Annals of the New York Academy of Sciences*, 1969, *157*, 902–917.

Grossman, S. P. Aggression, avoidance and reaction to novel environments in female rats with ventromedial hypothalamic lesions. *Journal of Comparative and Physiological Psychology*, 1972, *78*, 274–283.

Grossman, S. P. An experimental "dissection" of the septal syndrome. *Functions of the Septo-Hippocampal System*. Ciba Foundation Symposium 58 (new series). Amsterdam: Elsevier/Excerpta Medica and Elsevier/North Holland, July 1978, pp. 227–273.

Grossman, S. P., & Grossman, L. Surgical interruption of the anterior or posterior connections of the hypothalamus: Effects on aggressive and avoidance behavior. *Physiology and Behavior*, 1970, *5*, 1313–1317.

Grossman, S. P., & Grossman, L. Food and water intake in rats with parasagittal knife cuts medial or lateral to the lateral hypothalamus. *Journal of Comparative and Physiological Psychology*, 1971, *74*, 148–156.

Grossman, S. P., Grossman, L., & Walsh, L. Functional organization of the rat amygdala with respect to avoidance behavior. *Journal of Comparative and Physiological Psychology*, 1975, *88*, 829–850.

Grossman, S. P., Dacey, D., Halaris, A. E., Collier, T., & Routtenberg, A. Aphagia and adipsia after preferential destruction of nerve cell bodies in hypothalamus. *Science*, 1978, *202*, 537–539.

Gurdjian, E. A. The corpus striatum of the rat: Studies on the brain of the rat. No. 3. *Journal of Comparative Neurology*, 1928, *45*, 249–281.

Hahn, M., Haber, S., & Fuller, J. L. Differential agonistic behavior in mice selected for brain weight. *Physiology and Behavior*, 1973, *10*, 759–762.

Hamilton, G., & Isaacson, R. L. Changes in avoidance behavior following epileptogenic lesions on the mesencephalon. *Physiology and Behavior*, 1970, *5*, 1165–1167.

Hamilton, L. W. Behavioral effects of unilateral and bilateral septal lesions in rats. *Physiology and Behavior*, 1970, *5*, 855–859.

Hamilton, L. W. Intrabox and extrabox cues in avoidance responding: Effect of septal lesions. *Journal of Comparative and Physiological Psychology*, 1972, *78*, 268–273.

Hamilton, L. W., McCleary, R. A., & Grossman, S. P. Behavioral effects of cholinergic septal blockade in the cat. *Journal of Comparative and Physiological Psychology*, 1968, *66*, 563–568.

Hamilton, L. W., Kelsey, J. E., & Grossman, S. P. Variation in behavioral inhibition following different septal leions in rats. *Journal of Comparative and Physiological Psychology*, 1970, *70*, 79–86.

Hamilton, L. W., Capobianco, S., & Worsham, E. Lowered response to postingestional cues following septal lesions in rats. *Journal of Comparative and Physiological Psychology*, 1974, *87*, 134–141.

Han, M. F., & Livesey, P. J. Brightness discrimination learning under conditions of cue enhancement by rats with lesions in the amygdala or hippocampus. *Brain Research*, 1977, *125*, 277–292.

Handwerker, M. J., Gold, P. E., & McGaugh, J. L. Impairment of active avoidance learning with posttraining amygdala stimulation. *Brain Research*, 1975, *75*, 324–327.

Harley, C. W. Nonreversal and reversal shifts in the hippocampectomized rat. *Physiology and Behavior*, 1979, *22*, 1135–1139.

Harrell, L. E., de Castro, J. M., & Balagura, S. A critical evaluation of body weight loss following lateral hypothalamic lesions. *Physiology and Behavior*, 1975, *15*, 133–136.

Harris, E. W., Lasher, S., & Steward, O. V. Analysis of the habituation-like changes in transmission in temporo-dentate pathway of the rat. *Brain Research*, 1979, *162*, 21–32.

Harvey, J., & Hunt, H. F. Effect of septal lesions on thirst in the rat as indicated by water consumption and operant responding for water reward. *Journal of Comparative and Physiological Psychology*, 1965, *59*, 49–56.

Heath, R. G., & Mickle, W. A. Evaluation of seven years' experience with depth electrode studies in human patients. In E. R. Ramey & D. S. O'Doherty (Eds.), *Electrical studies of the unanesthetized brain*. New York: Hoeber, 1960, pp. 214–242.

Heatherington, A. W., & Ranson, S. W. Hypothalamic lesions and adiposity in the rat. *Anatomical Record*, 1942, *78*, 149–172.

Hecht, K., Hai, N.-V., Garibyan, A. A., Hecht, T., & Treptow, K. The role of the hippocampus and nucleus caudatus structures in the formation of pathogenetic emotional states of excitation. In K. Lissák (Ed.), *Neural and neurohumoral organization of motivated behaviour*. Proceedings of the Fourth Conference of Interbrain, held in Pécs, Hungary, May 19–23, 1975, pp. 191–203.

Heilman, K. M., & Valenstein, E. *Clinical neuropsychology*. New York: Oxford, 1979.

Heilman, K. M., & Watson, R. T. The neglect syndrome—A unilateral defect of the orienting response. In S. Harnad, R. Doty, L. Goldstein, J. Jaynes, & G. Krauthamer (Eds.), *Lateralization in the nervous system*. New York: Academic Press, 1976, pp. 285–302.

Heilman, K. M., & Watson, R. T. Mechanisms underlying the unilateral neglect syndrome. In E. A. Weinstein & R. P. Friedland (Eds.), *Advances in neurology* (Vol. 18). New York: Raven Press, 1977, pp. 93–106. (a)

Heilman, K. M., & Watson, R. T. The neglect syndrome—A unilateral defect of the orienting response. In S. Harnad, R. W. Doty, L. Goldstein, J. Jaynes, & G. Krauthamer (Eds.), *Lateralization in the nervous system*. New York: Academic Press, 1977. (b)

Heimer, L., & Larsson, K. Drastic changes in the mating behavior of male rats following lesions in the junction of the diencephalon and mesencephalon. *Experientia*, 1964, *20*, 1–4.

Heimer, L., & Larsson, K. Impairment of mating behavior in male rats following lesions in the preoptic-anterior hypothalamic continuum. *Brain Research*, 1966–1967, *3*, 248–263.

Heller, A. Neuronal control of brain serotonin. *Federation Proceedings*, 1972, *31*, 81–90.

Hendrickson, C. W., Kimble, R. J., & Kimble, D. P. Hippocampal lesions and the orienting response. *Journal of Comparative and Physiological Psychology*, 1969, *67*, 220–227.

Henke, P. G. Lesions in the ventromedial hypothalamus and response to frustrative nonreward. *Physiology and Behavior*, 1974, *13*, 143–146.

Henke, P. G. Limbic lesions and the energizing, aversive, and inhibitory effects of nonreward in rats. *Canadian Journal of Psychology/Revue Canadienne de Psychologie*, 1979, *33*, 133–140.

Henke, P. G., Allen, J. D., & Davison, C. Effect of lesions in the amygdala on behavioral contrast. *Physiology and Behavior*, 1972, *8*, 173–176.

Herkenham, M., & Nauta, W. J. H. Efferent connections of the habenular nuclei in the rat. *Journal of Comparative Neurology*, 1979, *187*, 19–47.

Hernandez, L., & Hoebel, B. G. Hypothalamic reward and aversion: A link between metabolism and behavior. *Current Studies of Hypothalamic Function*, 1978, *2*, 72–92.

Herrick, C. J. *Brains of rats and men*. Chicago: University of Chicago Press, 1926.

Herrick, C. J. *The brain of the tiger salamander, Ambystoma tigrinum*. Chicago: University of Chicago Press, 1948.

Hess, W. R. *Das Zwischenhirn*. Basel: Schwabe, 1949.

Hirsh, R. Lack of variability or perseveration: Describing the effect of hippocampal ablation. *Physiology and Behavior*, 1970, *5*, 1249–1254.

Hirsh, R. The hippocampus and contextual retrieval of information from memory: A theory. *Behavioral Biology*, 1974, *12*, 421–444.

Hirsh, R. The hippocampus, conditioned operations, and cognition. *Physiological Psychology*, 1980, *8*, 175–182.

Hirsh, R., & Krajden, J. The hippocampus and the expression of knowledge. In R. L. Isaacson & N. E. Spear (Eds.), *The expression of knowledge*. New York: Plenum Press, in press.

Hirsh, R., Holt, L., & Mosseri, A. Hippocampal mossy fibers, motivational states, and contextual retrieval. *Experimental Neurology*, 1978, *62*, 68–79.

Hirsh, R., Davis, R. E., & Holt, L. Fornix-thalamus fibers, motivational states, and contextual retrieval. *Experimental Neurology*, 1979, *65*, 373–390.

Hjorth-Simonsen, A. Hippocampal efferents to the ipsilateral entorhinal area: An experimental study in the rat. *Journal of Comparative Neurology*, 1971, *142*, 417–438.

Hjorth-Simonsen, A. Projection of the lateral part of the entorhinal area to the hippocampus and fascia dentata. *Journal of Comparative Neurology*, 1972, *147*, 219–232.

Hjorth-Simonsen, A. Some intrinsic connections of the hippocampus in the rat: An experimental analysis. *Journal of Comparative Neurology*, 1973, *147*, 145–162.

Hjorth-Simonsen, A., & Jeune, B. Origin and termination of the hippocampal perforant path in the rat studied by silver impregnation. *Journal of Comparative Neurology*, 1972, *144*, 215–231.

Hodge, G. K., & Butcher, L. L. Pars compacta of the substantia nigra modulates motor activity but is not involved importantly in regulating food and water intake. *Naunyn-Schmiedeberg's Archives of Pharmacology*, 1980, *313*, 51–67.

Hoebel, B. G. The psychopharmacology of feeding. In L. L. Iversen, S. D. Iversen, & S. H. Snyder (Eds.), *Handbook of psychopharmacology* (Vol. 8). New York: Plenum Press, 1977, pp. 55–129.

Hoebel, B. G., & Teitelbaum, P. Weight regulation in normal and hypothalamic hyperphagic rats. *Journal of Comparative and Physiological Psychology*, 1966, *61*, 189–193.

Hoebel, B. G., & Thompson, R. D. Aversion to lateral hypothalamic stimulation caused by intragastric feeding or obesity. *Journal of Comparative and Physiological Psychology*, 1969, *68*, 536–543.

Hökfelt, T., Elde, R., Fuxe, K., Johansson, O., Ljungdahl, A., Goldstein, M., Luft, R., Efendic, S., Nilsson, G., Terenius, L., Ganten, K., Jeffcoat, S. L., Rehfield, J., Said, S., Perec de la Mora, M., Possani, L., Tapia, R., Teran, L., & Palacios, R. Aminergic and peptidergic pathways in the nervous system with special reference to the hypothalamus. In S. Reichlin, R. J. Baldessarini, & J. B. Martin (Eds.), *The hypothalamus*. New York: Raven Press, 1978, pp. 69–135.

Holdstock, T. L. Effect of septal stimulation in rats on heart rate and galvanic skin response. *Psychonomic Science*, 1967, *9*, 37–38.

Holdstock, T. L. Plasticity of autonomic functions in rats with septal lesions. *Neuropsychologia*, 1970, *8*, 147–160.

Holloway, F. A. Effects of septal chemical injections on asymptotic avoidance performance in cats. *Physiology and Behavior*, 1972, *8*, 463–469.

Holmes, J. E., & Beckman, J. Hippocampal theta rhythm used in predicting feline behavior. *Physiology and Behavior*, 1969, *4*, 563–565.

Horel, J. A. The neuroanatomy of amnesia: A critique of the hippocampal memory hypothesis. *Brain*, 1978, *101*, 403–445.

Horvath, F. E. Effects of basolateral amygdalectomy on three types of avoidance behavior in cats. *Journal of Comparative and Physiological Psychology*, 1963, *56*, 386–389.

Hothersall, D., Johnson, D. A., & Collen, A. Fixed-ratio responding following septal lesions in the rat. *Journal of Comparative and Physiological Psychology*, 1970, *73*, 470–476.

Hsaio, S., & Isaacson, R. L. Learning of food and water positions by hippocampally damaged rats. *Physiology and Behavior*, 1971, *6*, 81–83.

Hull, C. L. *A behavior system: An introduction to behavior theory concerning the individual organism*. New York: Yale University Press, 1952.

Humphrey, N. K., & Weiskrantz, L. Vision in monkeys after removal of the striate cortex. *Nature*, 1967, *215*, 595–597.

Huston, J. P. Relationship between motivating and rewarding stimulation of the lateral hypothalamus. *Physiology and Behavior*, 1971, *6*, 711–716.

Huston, J. P., & Borbély, A. A. Operant conditioning in forebrain ablated rats by use of rewarding hypothalamic stimulation. *Brain Research*, 1973, *50*, 467–472.

Ireland, L., & Isaacson, R. L. Reactivity in the hippocampectomized gerbil. *Psychonomic Science*, 1968, *12*, 163–164.

Ireland, L. C., Hayes, W. N., & Schaub, R. E. The effects of bilateral hippocampal lesions on two-way active avoidance in the guinea pig. *Psychonomic Science*, 1969, *14*, 249–250.

Isaacson, R. L. Comment. *Psychonomic Science*, 1967, *7*, 8.

Isaacson, R. L. Hippocampal destruction in man and other animals. *Neuropsychologia*, 1972, *10*, 47–64. (a)

Isaacson, R. L. Neural systems of the limbic brain and behavioral inhibition. In R. Boakes & J. Halliday (Eds.), *Inhibition and learning*. New York: Academic Press, 1972. (b)

Isaacson, R. L. Experimental brain lesions and memory. In M. Rosenzweig & E. L. Bennett (Eds.), *Neural mechanisms of learning and memory*. Cambridge, Mass.: MIT Press, 1976, pp. 521–543.

Isaacson, R. L. Limbic system contributions to goal-directed behavior. In R. F. Thompson, L. H. Hicks, & V. B. Shvyrkov (Eds.), *Neural mechanisms of goal-directed behavior and learning*. New York: Academic Press, 1980, pp. 409–423. (a)

Isaacson, R. L. A perspective for the interpretation of limbic system function. *Physiological Psychology*, 1980, *8*, 183–188. (b)

Isaacson, R. L. The hippocampal formation and its regulation of attention and behavior. In E. Grastyán & P. Molnar (Eds.), *Sensory functions: Advances in physiological sciences* (Vol. 16). New York: Pergamon Press, 1982.

Isaacson, R. L., & Kimble, D. P. Lesions of the limbic system: Their effects upon hypotheses and frustration. *Behavioral Biology*, 1972, *7*, 767–793.

Isaacson, R. L., & McClearn, G. E. The influence of hippocampal damage on locomotor behavior of mice selectively bred for high or low activity in the open field. *Brain Research*, 1978, *150*, 559–567.

Isaacson, R. L., & Pribram, K. H. (Eds.). *The hippocampus: A comprehensive treatise* (2 vols.). New York: Plenum Press, 1975.

Isaacson, R. L., & Spear, N. E. (Eds.). *The expression of knowledge*. New York: Plenum Press, in press.

Isaacson, R. L., & Spear, N. E. Neural and mental capacities. In R. L. Isaacson & N. E. Spear (Eds.), *The expression of knowledge*. New York: Plenum Press, in press.

Isaascon, R. L., & Wickelgren, W. O. Hippocampal ablation and passive avoidance. *Science*, 1962, *138*, 1104–1106.

Isaacson, R. L., Douglas, R. J., & Moore, R. Y. The effect of radical hippocampal ablation on acquisition of avoidance response. *Journal of Comparative and Physiological Psychology*, 1961, *54*, 625–628.

Isaacson, R. L., Olton, D. S., Bauer, B., & Swart, P. The effect of training trials on passive avoidance deficits in the hippocampectomized rat. *Psychonomic Science*, 1966, *5*, 419–420.

Isseroff, A. Limited recovery of spontaneous alternation after extensive hippocampal damage: Evidence for a memory impairment. *Experimental Neurology*, 1979, *64*, 1–11.

Isseroff, A., & Isseroff, R. G. Experience aids recovery of spontaneous alternation following hippocampal damage. *Physiology and Behavior*, 1978, *21*, 469–472.

Ito, M., & Olds, J. Unit activity during self-stimulation behavior. *Journal of Neurophysiology*, 1971, *34*, 263–273.

Iuvone, P. M., & Van Hartesveldt, C. Locomotor activity and plasma corticosterone in rats with hippocampal lesions. *Behavioral Biology*, 1976, *16*, 515–520.

Jackson, F. B., & Gergen, J. A. Acquisition of operant schedules by squirrel monkeys lesioned in the hippocampal area. *Physiology and Behavior*, 1970, *5*, 543–547.

Jackson, W. J., & Strong, P. M. Differential effects of hippocampal lesions upon sequential tasks and maze learning by the rat. *Journal of Comparative and Physiological Psychology*, 1969, *68*, 442–450.

Jacquet, Y. F., & Lajtha, A. Morphine action at central nervous system sites in rat: Analgesia or hyperalgesia depending on site and dose. *Science*, 1973, *182*, 490–492.

Jarrard, L. E. Hippocampal ablation and operant behavior in the rat. *Psychonomic Science*, 1965, *2*, 115–116.

Jarrard, L. E. Behavior of hippocampal lesioned rats in home cage and novel situations. *Physiology and Behavior*, 1968, *3*, 65–70.

Jarrard, L. E. Role of interference and retention by rats with hippocampal lesions. *Journal of Comparative and Physiological Psychology*, 1975, *89*, 400–408.

Jarrard, L. E. Anatomical and behavioral analysis of hippocampal cell fields in rats. *Journal of Comparative and Physiological Psychology*, 1976, *90*, 1035–1050.

Jarrard, L. E. Selective hippocampal lesions and spatial discrimination in the rat. *Society for Neuroscience Abstracts*, 1978, *4*, 222.

Jarrard, L. E. Selective hippocampal lesions and behavior. *Physiological Psychology*, 1980, *8*, 198–206.

Jarrard, L. E., & Becker, J. T. The effects of selective hippocampal lesions on DRL behavior in rats. *Behavioral Biology*, 1977, *21*, 393–404.

Jarrard, L. E., & Bunnell, G. N. Open-field behavior of hippocampal-lesioned rats and hamsters. *Journal of Comparative and Physiological Psychology*, 1968, *66*, 500–502.

Jarrard, L. E., & Korn, J. H. Effects of hippocampal lesions on heart rate during hatituation and passive avoidance. *Communications and Behavioral Biology*, 1969, *3*, 141–150.

Johnson, C. T., Olton, D. S., Gage, F. H., III, & Jenko, P. G. Damage to hippocampus and hippocampal connections: Effects on DRL and spontaneous alternation. *Journal of Comparative and Physiological Psychology*, 1977, *91*, 508–522.

Johnson, D. A., & Thatcher, K. Differential effects of food deprivation on the fixed ratio behavior of normal rats and rats with septal lesions. *Psychonomic Science*, 1972, *26*, 45–46.

Johnson, D. A., Poplawsky, A., & Bieliauskas, L. Alterations of social behavior in rats and hamsters following lesions of the septal forebrain. *Psychonomic Science*, 1972, *26*, 19–20.

Johnston, J. B. Further contributions to the study of the evolution of the forebrain. *Journal of Comparative Neurology*, 1923, *36*, 143–192.

Jonason, K. R., & Enloe, L. J. Alterations in social behavior following septal and amygdaloid lesions in the rat. *Journal of Comparative and Physiological Psychology*, 1971, *75*, 286–301.

Jones, A. B., Barchas, J. D., & Eichelman, B. Taming effects of p-cholrophenylalanine on the aggressive behavior of septal rats. *Pharmacology, Biochemistry and Behavior*, 1976, *4*, 397–400.

Jung, R., & Kornmüller, A. E. Eine Methodik der Ableitung der lokalisierter Potentialschwankungen aus subcorticalen Hirngebieten. *Archiv für Psychiatrie und Nervenkrankheiten*, 1938, *109*, 1–30.

Kaada, B. R. Somatomotor, autonomic and electrocorticographic responses to electrical stimulation of rhinencephalic and other structures in primates, cat and dog. *Acta Physiologica Scandinavica*, 1951, *24*, 83 (Suppl.).

Kaada, B. R. Stimulation and regional ablation of the amygdaloid complex with reference to functional representation. In B. F. Eleftheriou (Ed.), *The neurobiology of the amygdala*. New York: Plenum Press, 1972.

Kaada, B. R., Rasmussen, E. W., & Kveim, O. Impaired acquisition of passive avoidance behavior by subcallosal, septal, hypothalamic and insular lesions in rats. *Journal of Comparative and Physiological Psychology*, 1962, *55*, 661–670.

Kamin, L. J. Attention-like processes in classical conditioning. In M. R. Jones (Ed.), *Miami Symposium on the Prediction of Behavior*. Miami: University of Miami Press, 1968.

Kamin, L. J. Predictability, surprise, attention, and conditioning. In B. Campbell & R. Church (Eds.), *Punishment and aversive behavior*. New York: Appleton-Century-Crofts, 1969.

Kamp, A., Lopes Da Silva, F. H., & Storm Van Leeuwen, W. Hippocampal frequency shifts in different behavioural situations. *Brain Research*, 1971, *31*, 287–294.

Kant, J. J. Influences of amygdala and medial forebrain bundle on self-stimulation in the septum. *Physiology and Behavior*, 1969, *4*, 777–784.

Kaplan, J. Approach and inhibitory reactions in rats after bilateral hippocampal damage. *Journal of Comparative and Physiological Psychology*, 1968, *65*, 274–281.

Kawakami, M., Koshino, T., & Hattori, Y. Changes in the EEG of the hypothalamus and limbic system after administration of ACTH, SU-4885 and Ach in rabbits with special reference to neurohumoral feedback regulation of pituitary-adrenal system. *Japanese Journal of Physiology*, 1966, *16*, 551–569.

Kawakami, M., Seto, K., Terasawa, E., & Yoshida, K. Mechanisms in the limbic system controlling reproductive function of the ovary with special reference to the positive feedback. *Progress in Brain Research*, 1967, *27*, 69–102.

Kawakami, M., Seto, K., Terasawa, E., Yoshida, K., Miyamoto, T., Sekiguchi, M., & Hattori, Y. Influence of electrical stimulation of lesion in the limbic structure upon biosynthesis of adrenocorticoid in the rabbit. *Neuroendocrinology*, 1968, *3*, 337–348.

Kawamura, H., Nakamura, T., & Tokizane, T. Effect of acute brain stem lesions on the electrical activities of the limbic system and neocortex. *Japanese Journal of Physiology*, 1961, *11*, 565–575.

Kearley, R. C., Van Hartesveldt, C., & Woodruff, M. L. Behavioral and hormonal effects of hippocampal lesions on male and female rats. *Physiological Psychology*, 1974, *2*, 187–196.

Keene, J. J., & Casey, K. L. Excitatory connection from lateral hypothalamic self-stimulation sites to escape sites in medullary reticular formation. *Experimental Neurology*, 1970, *28*, 155–166.

Kelsey, J. E., & Grossman, S. P. Cholinergic blockade and lesions in the ventro-medial septum of the rat. *Physiology and Behavior*, 1969, *4*, 837–845.

Kelsey, J. E., & Grossman, S. P. Nonperseverative disruption of behavioral inhibition following septal lesions in rats. *Journal of Comparative and Physiological Psychology*, 1971, *75*, 305–311.

Kelsey, J. E., & Grossman, S. P. Influence of central cholinergic pathways on performance on free-operant avoidance and DRL schedules. *Pharmacology, Biochemistry and Behavior*, 1975, *3*, 1043–1050.

Kemble, E. D., & Beckman, G. J. Escape latencies at three levels of electric shock in rats with amygdaloid lesions. *Psychonomic Science*, 1969, *14*, 205–206.

Kemble, E. D., & Beckman, G. J. Vicarious trial and error following amygdaloid lesions in rats. *Neuropsychologia*, 1970, *8*, 161–169.

Kemble, E. D., & Nagel, J. A. Failure to form a learned taste aversion in rats with amygdaloid lesions. *Bulletin of the Psychonomic Society*, 1973, *2*, 155–156.

Kemble, E. D., & Nagel, J. A. Persistent depression of rearing behavior in rats after extensive septal lesions. *Journal of Comparative and Physiological Psychology*, 1975, *89*, 747–758.

Kemble, E. D., & Strand, M. H. Effect of septal lesions on the acquisition of three tasks requiring jumping or rearing responses. *Behavioral Biology*, 1977, *20*, 387–397.

Kemble, E. D., Levine, M. S., Gregoire, K., Koepp, K., & Thomas, T. T. Reactivity to saccharin and quinine solutions following amygdaloid or septal lesions in rats. *Behavioral Biology*, 1972, *7*, 503–512.

Kemble, E. D., Studelska, D. R., & Nagel, J. A. Rearing behavior of rats after amygdaloid, hippocampal, olfactory bulb, cortical, or striatal lesions. *Bulletin of the Psychonomic Society*, 1976, *8*, 163–166.

Kemp, I. R., & Kaada, B. R. The relation of hippocampal theta activity to arousal, attentive behaviour and somato-motor movements in unrestrained cats. *Brain Research*, 1975, *95*, 323–342.

Kent, M. A., & Peters, R. H. Effects of ventromedial hypothalamic lesions on hunger-motivated behavior in rats. *Journal of Comparative and Physiological Psychology*, 1973, *83*, 92–97.

Kenyon, J., & Krieckhaus, E. E. Decrements in one-way avoidance learning following septal lesions in rats. *Psychonomic Science*, 1965, *3*, 113–114.

Kesner, R. P. An attribute analysis of memory: The role of the hippocampus. *Physiological Psychology*, 1980, *8*, 189–197.

Kesner, R. P., & Berman, R. F. Effects of midbrain reticular formation, hippocampal, and lateral hypothalamic stimulation upon recovery from neophobia and taste aversion learning. *Physiology and Behavior*, 1977, *18*, 763–768.

Kesner, R. P., & Conner, H. S. Effects of electrical stimulation of rat limbic system and mid-brain reticular formation upon short- and long-term memory. *Physiological Behavior*, 1974, *12*, 5–12.

Killeffer, F. A., & Stern, W. E. Chronic effects of hypothalamic injury—Report of a case of near total hypothalamic destruction resulting from removal of a craniopharyngioma. *Archives of Neurology*, 1970, *22*, 419–429.

Kim, C., Choi, H., Kim, J. K., Chang, H. K., Park, R. S., & Kang, G. General behavioral activity and its component patterns in hippocampectomized rats. *Brain Research*, 1970, *19*, 379–394.

Kim, C., Choi, H., Kim, J. K., Kim, M. S., Huh, M. K., & Moon, Y. B. Sleep pattern of hippocampectomized cat. *Brain Research*, 1971, *29*, 223–236.

Kim, C., Kim, C. C., Kim, J. K., Kim, M. S., Chang, H. K., Kim, J. Y., & Lee, I. G. Fear response and aggressive behavior of hippocampectomized house rats. *Brain Research*, 1971, *29*, 237–251.

Kim, C., Choi, H., Kim, J. K., Kim, M. S., Park, H. J., Ahn, B. T., & Kang, S. H. Influence of hippocampectomy on gastric ulcer in rats. *Brain Research*, 1976, *109*, 245–254.

Kimble, D. P. *The effect of bilateral hippocampal damage on cognitive and emotional behavior in the rat.* Unpublished doctoral dissertation, University of Michigan, 1961.

Kimble, D. P. The effects of bilateral hippocampal lesions in rats. *Journal of Comparative and Physiological Psychology*, 1963, *56*, 273–283.

Kimble, D. P. Hippocampus and internal inhibition. *Psychological Bulletin*, 1968, *70*, 285–295.

Kimble, D. P. Changes in behavior of hippocampal-lesioned rats across a 6-week postoperative period. *Physiological Psychology*, 1976, *4*, 289–293.

Kimble, D. P., & Dannen, E. Persistent spatial maze-learning deficits in hippocampal-lesioned rats across a 7-week postoperative period. *Physiological Psychology*, 1977, *5*, 409–413.

Kimble, D. P., & Gostnell, D. Role of cingulate cortex in shock avoidance behavior of rats. *Journal of Comparative and Physiological Psychology*, 1968, *65*, 290–294.

Kimble, D. P., & Greene, E. G. Absence of latent learning in rats with hippocampal lesions. *Psychonomic Science*, 1968, *11*, 99–100.

Kimble, D. P., & Kimble, R. J. The effect of hippocampal lesions on extinction and "hypothesis" behavior in rats. *Physiology and Behavior*, 1970, *5*, 735–738.

Kimble, D. P., Kirkby, R. J., & Stein, D. G. Response perseveration interpretation of passive avoidance deficits in hippocampectomized rats. *Journal of Comparative and Physiological Psychology*, 1966, *61*, 141–143.

Kimble, D. P., Anderson, S., Bremiller, R., & Dannen, E. Hippocampal lesions, superior cervical ganglia removal, and behavior in rats. *Physiology and Behavior*, 1979, *22*, 461–466.

Kimble, D. P., Bremiller, R., Stickrod, G., & Smotherman, W. P. Failure to find a behavioral role for anomalous sympathetic innervation of the hippocampus in male rats. *Physiology and Behavior*, 1980, *25*, 675–681.

Kimura, D. Effects of selective hippocampal damage on avoidance behavior in the rat. *Canadian Journal of Psychology*, 1958, *12*, 213–218.

King, B. M. A re-examination of the ventromedial hypothalamic paradox. *Neuroscience and Biobehavioral Reviews*, 1980, *4*, 151–160.

King, B. M., & Gaston, M. G. Factors influencing the hunger and thirst motivated behavior of hypothalamic hyperphagic rats. *Physiological Behavior*, 1976, *16*, 33–41. (a)

King, B. M., & Gaston, M. G. Impaired free-operant avoidance behavior following ventromedial hypothalamic lesions in rats. *Physiological Behavior*, 1976, *16*, 719–726. (b)

King, B. M., Alheid, G. F., & Grossman, S. P. Factors influencing active avoidance behaviors in rats with ventromedial hypothalamic lesions. *Physiology and Behavior*, 1977, *18*, 901–913.

King, F. A. Effects of septal and amygdala lesions on emotional behavior and conditioned avoidance responses in the rat. *Journal of Nervous and Mental Diseases*, 1958, *126*, 57–63.

King, F. A., & Meyer, P. M. Effects of amygdaloid lesions upon septal hyperemotionality in the rat. *Science*, 1958, *128*, 655–656.

King, R. B., & Grossman, S. P. Impaired and enhanced shuttle box avoidance behavior following ventromedial hypothalamic lesions. *Physiology and Behavior*, 1978, *20*, 51–56.

King, R. B., Schricker, J. L., & O'Leary, J. L. An experimental study of the transition from normal to convulsoid cortical activity. *Journal of Neurophysiology*, 1953, *16*, 286–298.

Kirkby, R. J., Stein, D. G., Kimble, R. J., & Kimble, D. P. Effects of hippocampal lesions and duration of sensory input on spontaneous alternation. *Journal of Comparative and Physiological Psychology*, 1967, *64*, 342–345.

Kiser, R. S., & German, D. C. Opiate effects on aversive midbrain stimulation in rats. *Neuroscience Letters*, 1978, *10*, 197–202.

Klemm, W. R. Correlation of hippocampal theta rhythm, muscle activity, and brain stem reticular formation activity. *Communications in Behavioral Biology*, 1970, *3*, 147–156.

Klemm, W. R., & Dreyfus, L. R. Septal- and caudate-induced behavioral inhibition in relation to hippocampal EEG of rabbits. *Physiology and Behavior*, 1975, *15*, 561–567.

Kling, A. Effects of amygdalectomy on social affiliative behavior in non-human primates. In B. E. Eleftheriou (Ed.), *The neurobiology of the amygdala*. New York: Plenum Press, 1972, pp. 511–536.

Kling, A., & Steklis, H. D. A neural substrate for affiliative behavior in nonhuman primates. *Brain, Behavior, and Evolution*, 1976, *13*, 216–238.

Kling, A. J., Orbach, J., Schwarz, N., & Towne, J. Injury to the limbic system and associated structures in cats. *Archives of General Psychiatry*, 1960, *3*, 391–420.

Kling, A., Steklis, H. D., & Deutsch, S. Radiotelemetered activity from the amygdala during social interactions in the monkey. *Experimental Neurology*, 1979, *66*, 88–96.

Klüver, H., & Bucy, P. C. Preliminary analysis of the temporal lobes in monkeys. *Archives of Neurology and Psychiatry*, 1939, *42*, 979–1000.

Knigge, K. M. Adrenocortical response to immobilization in rats with lesion in hippocampus and amygdala. *Federation Proceedings*, 1961, *20*, 185.

Knigge, K. M., Joseph, S. A., & Hoffman, G. E. Organization of LRF and SRIF-neurons in the endocrine hypothalamus. In S. Reichlin, R. J. Baldessarini, & J. B. Martin (Eds.), *The hypothalamus*. New York: Raven Press, 1978, pp. 49–67.

Köhler, C. Habituation of the orienting response after medial and lateral septal lesions in the albino rat. *Behavioral Biology*, 1976, *16*, 63–72.

Köhler, C., & Srebro, B. Effects of lateral and medial septal lesions on exploratory behavior in the albino rat. *Brain Research*, 1980, *182*, 423–440.

Koikegami, H., & Fuse, S. Studies on the functions and fiber connections of the amygdaloid nuclei and periamygdaloid cortex: Experiment on the respiratory movements. *Folia Psychiatrica et Neurologica Japonica*, 1952, *5*, 188–197.

Koikegami, H., Dodo, T., Mochida, Y., & Takahashi, H. Stimulation experiments on the amygdaloid nuclear complex and related structures: Effects upon the renal volume, urinary secretion, movements of the urinary bladder, blood pressure and respiratory movements. *Folia Psychiatrica et Neurologica Japonica*, 1957, *11*, 157–206.

Kolb, B., & Whishaw, I. Q. Effects of brain lesions and atropine on hippocampal and neocortical EEG in the rat. *Experimental Neurology*, 1977, *56*, 1–22.

Komisaruk, B. R. Phasic synchrony of EEG theta rhythm: EKG and certain oscillatory EMG patterns in awake rats. *Proceedings of the International Union of the Physiological Sciences, 24th International Congress*, 1968, *7*, 244.

Komisaruk, B. R. Synchrony between limbic system theta activity and rhythmical behavior in rats. *Journal of Comparative and Physiological Psychology*, 1970, *70*, 482–492.

Komisaruk, B. R. The role of rhythmical brain activity in sensorimotor integration. In J. M. Sprague & A. N Epstein (Eds.), *Progress in psychobiology and physiological psychobiology* (Vol. 7). New York: Academic Press, 1977, pp. 55–90.

Kramis, R. C., & Routtenberg, A. Dissociation of hippocampal EEG from its behavioral correlates by septal and hippocampal electrical stimulation. *Brain Research*, 1977, *125*, 37–49.

Kramis, R., Vanderwolf, C. H., & Bland, B. H. Two types of hippocampal rhythmical slow activity in both the rabbit and the rat: Relations to behavior and effects of atropine, diethyl ether, urethane and pentobarbital. *Experimental Neurology*, 1975, *49*, 58–85.

Kratz, K. E., & Mitchell, J. C. Internal and external cue use following septal ablation in the rat. *Physiological Psychology*, 1977, *5*, 177–180.

Krayniak, P. F., Siegel, A., Meibach, R. C., Fruchtman, D., & Scrimenti, M. Origin of the fornix system in the squirrel monkey. *Brain Research*, 1979, *160*, 401–411.

Krayniak, P. F., Weiner, S., & Siegel, A. An analysis of the efferent connections of the septal area in the cat. *Brain Research*, 1980, *189*, 15–29.

Krayniak, P. F., Meibach, R. C., & Siegel, A. A projection from the entorhinal cortex to the nucleus accumbens in the rat. *Brain Research*, 1981, *209*, 427–431.

Krechevsky, I. Brain mechanisms and "hypotheses." *Journal of Comparative Psychology*, 1935, *19*, 425–462.

Kreindler, A., & Steriade, M. Functional differentiation within the amygdaloid complex inferred from peculiarities of epileptic afterdischarges. *Electroencephalography and Clinical Neurophysiology*, 1963, *15*, 811–826.

Kreindler, A., & Steriade, M. EEG patterns of arousal and sleep induced by stimulating various amygdaloid levels in the cat. *Archieves Italienne de Biologie*, 1964, *102*, 576–586.

Krettek, J. E., & Price, J. L. The cortical projections of the mediocortical nucleus and adjacent thalamic nuclei in the rat. *Journal of Comparative Neurology*, 1977, *171*, 157–192. (a)

Krettek, J. E., & Price, J. L. Projections from the amygdaloid complex and adjacent olfactory structures to the entorhinal cortex and to the subiculum in the rat and cat. *Journal of Comparative Neurology*, 1977, *172*, 723–752. (b)

Krettek, J. E., & Price, J. L. Projections from the amygdaloid complex to the cerebral cortex and thalamus in the rat and cat. *Journal of Comparative Neurology*, 1977, *172*, 687–722. (c)

Krettek, J. E., & Price, J. L. Amygdaloid projections to subcortical structures within the basal forebrain and brainstem in the rat and cat. *Journal of Comparative Neurology*, 1978, *178*, 225–254. (a)

Krettek, J. E., & Price, J. L. A description of the amygdaloid complex in the rat and cat with observations on intra-amygdaloid axonal connections. *Journal of Comparative Neurology*, 1978, *178*, 255–280. (b)

Krieckhaus, E. E. *Behavioral changes in cats following lesions of the mammillothalamic tracts.* Unpublished doctoral dissertation, University of Illinois, 1962.

Krieckhaus, E. E. Decrements in avoidance behavior following mammillothalamic tractotomy in cats. *Journal of Neurophysiology*, 1964, *27*, 753–767.

Krieckhaus. E. E. Decrements in avoidance behavior following mammillothalamic tractotomy in rats and subsequent recovery with *d*-amphetamine. *Journal of Comparative and Physiological Psychology*, 1965, *60*, 31–35.

Krieckhaus, E. E. Role of freezing and fear in avoidance decrements following mammillothalamic tractotomy in cat: I. Two-way avoidance behavior. *Psychonomic Science*, 1966, *4*, 263–264.

Krieckhaus, E. E., & Chi, C. C. Role of freezing and fear in avoidance decrements following mammillothalamic tractotomy in cat. *Psychonomic Science*, 1966, *4*, 264–266.

Krieckhaus, E. E., & Lorenz, R. Retention and relearning of lever-press avoidance following mammillothalamic tractotomy. *Physiology and Behavior*, 1968, *3*, 433–438.

Krieckhaus, E. E., & Randall, D. Lesions of mammillothalamic tract in rat produce no decrements in recent memory. *Brain*, 1968, *91*, 369–378.

Krieckhaus, E. E., Coons, E. E., Greenspon, T., Weiss, J., & Lorenz, R. L. Retention of choice behavior in rats following mammillothalamic tractotomy. *Physiology and Behavior*, 1968, *3*, 125–131.

Krieger, D. T., Hauser, H., & Krey, L. C. Suprachiasmatic nuclear lesions do not abolish food-shifted circadian adrenal and temperature rhythmicity. *Science*, 1977, *197*, 398–399.

Lammers, H. J., & Lohman, A. H. M. Experimental anatomisch onderzoek naar de verbindingen van piriforme cortex en amygdalakernen bij de kat. *Nederlands Tijdschrift voor Geneeskunde*, 1957, *101*, 1–2.

Lang, H., Tourinen, T., & Valleala, P. Amygdaloid afterdischarge and galvanic skin response. *Electroencephalography and Clinical Neurophysiology*, 1964, *16*, 366–374.

Lanier, L. P., & Isaacson, R. L. Activity changes related to the location of lesions in the hippocampus. *Behavioral Biology*, 1975, *13*, 59–69.

Lash, L. Response discriminability and the hippocampus. *Journal of Comparative and Physiological Psychology*, 1964, *57*, 251–256.

Lasher, S. S., & Stewart, O. The time course of changes in open field activity following bilateral entorhinal lesions in rats and cats. *Behavioral and Neural Biology*, 1981, *32*, 1–10.

Lashley, K. S. *Brain mechanisms and intelligence*. Chicago: University of Chicago Press, 1929.

Laughlin, M. E., Donovick, P. J., & Burright, R. G. Septal lesions in meadow voles and mongolian gerbils: Consummatory and investigatory behavior. *Physiology and Behavior*, 1975, *15*, 191–198.

LaVaque, T. J. Conditioned avoidance response perseveration and septal rats during massed extinction trials. *Psychonomic Science*, 1966, *5*, 409–410.

Leibowitz, S. A hypothalamic beta-adrenergic "satiety" system antagonizes an alpha-adrenergic "hunger" system in the rat. *Nature*, 1970, *226*, 963–964.

Leibowitz, S. F. Brain catecholaminergic mechanisms for control of hunger. In D. Novin, W. Wyrwicka, & C. Bray (Eds.), *Hunger: Basic mechanisms and clinical implications*. New York: Raven Press, 1976, pp. 1–18.

Leibowitz, S. F. Paraventricular nucleus: A primary site mediating adrenergic stimulation of feeding and drinking. *Pharmacology, Biochemistry and Behavior*, 1978, *8*, 163–175.

Leibowitz, S. F., & Rossakis, C. Analysis of feeding suppression produced by perifornical hypothalamic injection of catecholamines, amphetamines and mazindol. *European Journal of Pharmacology*, 1978, *53*, 69–81. (a)

Leibowitz, S. F., & Rossakis, C. Pharmacological characterization of perifornical hypothalamic α-adrenergic receptors mediating feeding inhibition in the rat. *Neuropharmacology*, 1978, *17*, 691–702. (b)

Leibowitz, S. F., Chang, K., & Oppenheimer, R. L. Feeding elicited by noradrenergic stimulation of the paraventricular nucleus: Effects of corticosterone and other hormone manipulations. *Neuroscience Abstracts*, 1976, *2*, 292.

Le Motte, C. C., Snowman, A., Pert, C. B., & Snyder, S. H. Opiate receptor binding in rhesus monkey brain: Association with limbic structures. *Brain Research*, 1978, *155*, 374–379.

Lengvári, I., & Halász, B. Evidence for a diurnal fluctuation in plasma corticosterone levels after fornix transections in the rat. *Neuroendocrinology*, 1973, *11*, 191–196.

Leonard, C. M. The prefrontal cortex of the rat: I. Cortical projection of the mediodorsal nucleus. II. Efferent connections. *Brain Research*, 1969, *12*, 321–343.

Leung, L. S. Behavior-dependent evoked potentials in the hippocampal CA1 region of the rat: I. Correlation with behavior and EEG. *Brain Research*, 1980, *198*, 95–117.

Lewellyn, D., Lowes, G., & Isaacson, R. L. Visually mediated behaviors following neocortical destruction in the rat. *Journal of Comparative and Physiological Psychology*, 1969, *69*, 25–32.

Lidsky, T. I., Levine, M. S., Kreinick, C. J., & Schwartzbaum, J. S. Retrograde effects of amygdaloid stimulation on conditioned suppression (CER) in rats. *Journal of Comparative and Physiological Psychology*, 1970, *73*, 135–149.

Liebeskind, J. C. *The effect of cingulate cortex lesions on the development of resistance to stress*. Unpublished doctoral dissertation, University of Michigan, 1962.

Liebeskind, J. C., Giesler, G. J., Jr., & Urca, G. Evidence pertaining to an endogenous mechanism of pain inhibition in the central nervous system. In Y. Zotterman (Ed.), *Sensory functions of the skin in primates*. Oxford: Pergamon Press, 1976, pp. 561–573.

Lieblich, I., & Olds, J. Selection for the readiness to respond to electrical stimulation of the hypothalamus as a reinforcing agent. *Brain Research*, 1971, *27*, 153–161.

Lieblich, I., Gross, R., & Cohen, E. Effects of testosterone replacement on the recovery from increased emotionality, produced by septal lesions in prepubertal castrated male rats. *Physiology and Behavior*, 1977, *18*, 1159–1164.

Lieblich, I., Cohen, E., Ben-Zion, M., & Dymshitz, J. A genetically mediated relationship between the readiness to self-stimulate lateral hypothalamus and the intensity of the septal and ventromedial rage syndromes. *Brain Research*, 1980, *185*, 253–263.

Liebman, J. M., Mayer, D. J., & Liebeskind, J. C. Mesencephalic central gray lesions and fear-motivated behavior in rats. *Brain Research*, 1970, *23*, 353–370.

Lindsley, D. B., & Wilson, C. L. Brain stem-hypothalamic systems influencing hippocampal activity and behavior. In R. L. Isaacson & K. H. Pribram (Eds.), *The hippocampus: A comprehensive treatise*. New York: Plenum Press, 1975, pp. 247–278.

Lipp, H. P. Differential hypothalamic self-stimulation behaviour in Roman high avoidance and low avoidance rats. *Brain Reserrch Bulletin*, 1979, *4*, 553–559.

Livesey, P. J., & Bayliss, J. The effects of electrical (blocking) stimulation to the dentate of the rat on learning of a simultaneous brightness discrimination and reversal. *Neuropsychologia*, 1975, *13*, 395–407.

Livesey, P. J., & Meyer, P. Functional differentiation in the dorsal hippocampus with local electrical stimulation during learning by rats. *Neuropsychologia*, 1975, *13*, 431–438.

Livesey, P. J., Meyer, P., & Smith, J. P. Effects of disruption of hippocampal function on learning of a go–no-go discrimination in the rat. *Brain Research*, 1980, *195*, 197–202.

Lømo, T. Potentiation of monosynaptic EPSPs in the perforant path—Dentate granule cell synapse. *Experimental Brain Research*, 1971, *12*, 46–63.

Lopes Da Silva, F. H., & Arnolds, D. E. A. T. Physiology of the hippocampus and related structures. *Annual Review of Physiology*, 1979, *36*, 291–301.

Lopes Da Silva, F. H., & Kamp, A. Hippocampal theta frequency shifts and operant behaviour. *Electroencephalography and Clinical Neurophysiology*, 1969, *26*, 133–143.

Lorens, S. A., & Kondo, C. Y. Effects of septal lesions on food and water intake and operant responding for food. *Physiology and Behavior*, 1969, *4*, 729–732.

Lorens, S. A., & Sainati, S. M. Naloxone blocks the excitatory effect of ethanol and chlordiazepoxide on lateral hypothalamic self-stimulation behavior. *Life Sciences*, 1978, *23*, 1359–1364. (a)

Lorens, S. A., & Sainati, S. M. Opiate receptors mediate the excitatory (euphorigenic) effect of ethanol, chordiazepoxide, and morphine on brain stimulation reward. *Neuroscience Abstracts*, 1978, *4*, 35. (b)

Lovely, R. H. Hormonal dissociation of limbic lesion effects on shuttle box avoidance in rats. *Journal of Comparative and Physiological Psychology*, 1975, *89*, 224–230.

Lown, B. A., Hayes, W. N., & Schaub, R. E. The effects of bilateral septal lesions on two-way active avoidance in the guinea pig. *Psychonomic Science*, 1969, *16*, 13–14.

Lubar, J. F. Effect of medial cortical lesions on the avoidance behavior of the cat. *Journal of Comparative and Physiological Psychology*, 1964, *58*, 38–46.

Lubar, J. F., & Perachio, A. A. One-way and two-way learning and transfer of an active avoidance response in normal and cingulectomized cats. *Journal of Comparative and Physiological Psychology*, 1965, *60*, 46–52.

Lubar, J. F., Perachio, A. A., & Kavanagh, A. J. Deficits in active avoidance behavior following lesions of the lateral and posterolateral gyrus of the cat. *Journal of Comparative and Physiological Psychology*, 1966, *62*, 263–269.

Lubar, J. F., Boyce, B. A., & Shaefer, C. S. Etiology of polydipsia and polyuria in rats with septal lesions. *Physiology and Behavior,* 1968, *3,* 289–292.

Lubar, J. F., Shaefer, C. S., & Wells, D. G. The role of the septal area in the regulation of water intake and associated motivational behavior. *Annals of the New York Academy of Sciences,* 1969, *157,* 875–893.

Macadar, A. W., Chalupa, L. M., & Lindsley, D. B. Differentiation of brain stem loci which affect hippocampal and neocortical electrical activity. *Experimental Neurology,* 1974, *43,* 449–514.

MacDougall, J. M., & Bevan, W. Influence of pretest shock upon rate of electrical self-stimulation of the brain. *Journal of Comparative and Physiological Psychology,* 1968, *65,* 261–264.

MacDougall, J. M., Van Hoesen, G. W., & Mitchell, J. C. Development of post S^r and post non S^r DRL performance and its retention following septal lesions in rats. *Psychonomic Science,* 1969, *16,* 45–46.

MacDougall, J. M., Pennebaker, J. W., & Stevenson, M. Effects of septal lesions on the social behavior of two subspecies of deer mice. *Physiology and Behavior,* Unpublished manuscript, 1973.

MacKintosh, N. J. A theory of attention: Variations in the associability of stimuli with reinforcement. *Psychological Review,* 1975, *82,* 276–298.

MacLean, P. D. Psychosomatic disease and the "visceral brain": Recent developments bearing on the Papez theory of emotion. *Psychosomatic Medicine,* 1949, *11,* 338–353.

MacLean, P. D. The triune brain, emotion, and scientific bias. In F. O. Schmitt (Ed.), *The neurosciences; Second study program.* New York: Rockefeller University Press, 1970, pp. 336–349.

MacLean, P. D. Cerebral evolution and emotional processes. *Annals of the New York Academy of Sciences,* 1972, *193,* 137–149.

MacLean, P. D. Role of pallidal projections in species-typical display behavior of squirrel monkey. *Transactions of the American Neurological Association,* 1975, *100,* 25–28.

MacLean, P. D. A mind of three minds: Educating the triune brain. *Seventy-seventh Yearbook of the National Society for the Study of Education.* Chicago: University of Chicago Press, 1978, pp. 308–342. (a)

MacLean, P. D. Effects of lesions of globus pallidus on species-typical display behavior of squirrel monkeys. *Brain Research,* 1978, *149,* 175–196. (b)

Maeda, H., & Hirata, K. Two-stage amygdaloid lesions and hypothalamic rage: A method useful for detecting functional localization. *Physiology and Behavior,* 1978, *21,* 529–530.

Maier, N. R. F. Cortical destruction of the posterior part of the brain and its effects on reasoning in rats. *Journal of Comparative Neurology,* 1932, *56,* 179–214. (a)

Maier, N. R. F. The effect of cerebral destruction on reasoning and learning in rats. *Journal of Comparative Neurology,* 1932, *54,* 45–75. (b)

Maier, N. R. F. *Frustration: The study of behavior without a goal.* New York: McGraw-Hill, 1949.

Maier, N. R. F. Frustration theory: Restatement of extension. In N. R. F. Maier & T. C. Schneirla (Eds.), *Principles of animal psychology* (enlarged ed.). New York: Dover, 1964, pp. 595–620.

Mair, W. G. P. Warrington, E. K., & Weiskrantz, L. Memory disorders in Korsakoff's psychosis: A neuropathological and neuropsychological investigation of two cases. *Brain,* 1979, *102,* 749–783.

Malmo, R. Classical and instrumental conditioning with special stimulation as reinforcement. *Journal of Comparative and Physiological Psychology,* 1965, *60,* 1–8.

Mandell, A. J. Toward a psychobiology of transcendence: God in the brain. In J. M. Davidson & R. J. Davidson (Eds.), *The psychobiology of consciousness*. New York: Plenum Press, 1980, pp. 379–464.

Margalit, D., & Segal, M. A pharmacologic study of analgesia produced by stimulation of the nucleus locus coeruleus. *Psychopharmacology*, 1979, *62*, 169–173.

Margules, D. L. Noradrenergic basis of inhibition between reward and punishment in amygdala. *Journal of Comparative and Physiological Psychology*, 1968, *66*, 329–334.

Margules, D. L. Alpha-adrenergic receptors in hypothalamus for the suppression of feeding behavior by satiety. *Journal of Comparative and Physiological Psychology*, 1970, *73*, 1–12. (a)

Margules, D. L. Beta-adrenergic receptors in hypothalamus for learned and unlearned taste-aversions. *Journal of Comparative and Physiological Psychology*, 1970, *73*, 13–21. (b)

Margules, D. L., & Stein, L. Neuroleptics vs. tranquilizers: Evidence from animals of mode and site of action. In H. Brill (Ed.), *Neuropsychopharmacology*. Amsterdam: Excerpta Medica Foundation, 1967.

Margules, D. L., Lewis, M. J., Dragovich, J. A., & Margules, A. S. Hypothalamic norepinephrine: Circadian rhythms and the control of feeding behavior. *Science*, 1972, *178*, 640–642.

Marotta, R. F., Logan, N., Potegal, M., Glusman, M., & Gardner, E. L. Dopamine agonists induce recovery from surgically-induced septal rage. *Nature*, 1977, *269*, 513–515.

Marshall, J. F. Comparison of the sensorimotor dysfunctions produced by damage to lateral hypothalamus or superior colliculus in the rat. *Experimental Neurology*, 1978, *58*, 203–217.

Marshall, J. F., Turner, B. H., & Teitelbaum, P. Sensory neglect produced by lateral hypothalamic damage. *Science*, 1971, *174*, 523–525.

Martin, J. R. Motivated behaviors elicited from hypothalamus, midbrain, and pons of the guinea pig *(Cavia porcellus)*. *Journal of Comparative and Physiological Psychology*, 1976, *90*, 1011–1034.

Martinez, J. L., Jr., Jensen, R. A., Creager, R., Veliquette, J., Messing, R. B., McGaugh, J. L., & Lynch, G. Selective effects of enkephalin on electrical activity of the *in vitro* hippocampal slice. *Behavioral and Neural Biology*, 1979, *26*, 128–131.

Maru, E., Takahashi, L. K., & Iwahara, S. Effects of median raphe nucleus lesions on hippocampal EEG in the freely moving rat. *Brain Research*, 1979, *163*, 223–234.

Mason, C. A., & Lincoln, D. W. Visualization of the retino-hypothalamic projections in the rat by cobalt precipitation. *Cell Tissue Research*, 1976, *168*, 117–131.

Masserman, J. H., Levitt, M., McAvoy, T., Kling, A., & Pechtel, C. The amygdalae and behavior. *American Journal of Psychiatry*, 1958, *115*, 14–17.

Matheson, G. K., Branch, B. J., & Taylor, N. Effects of amygdaloid stimulation on pituitary-adrenal activity in conscious cats. *Brain Research*, 1971, *32*, 151–168.

Max, D. M., Cohen, E., & Lieblich, I. Effects of capture procedures on emotionality scores in rats with septal lesions. *Physiology and Behavior*, 1974, *13*, 617–620.

Mayer, D. J., & Liebeskind, J. C. Pain reduction by focal electrical stimulation of the brain: An anatomical and behavior analysis. *Brain Research*, 1974, *68*, 73–93.

McBride, R. L., & Sutin, J. Amygdaloid and pontine projections to the ventromedial nucleus of the hypothalamus. *The Journal of Comparative Neurology*, 1977, *174*, 377–396.

McCaughran, J. A., Jr., Corcoran, M. E., & Wada, J. A. Role of the forebrain commissures in amygdaloid kindling in rats. *Epilepsia*, 1978, *19*, 19–33.

McCleary, R. A. Response specificity in the behavioral effects of limbic system lesions in the cat. *Journal of Comparative and Physiological Psychology*, 1961, *54*, 605–613.

McCleary, R. A. Response-modulating functions of the limbic system: Initiation and suppression. In E. Stellar & J. M. Sprague (Eds.), *Progress in physiological psychology* (Vol 1). New York: Academic Press, 1966.

McConnell, J. V., & Jacobson, A. L. Learning in invertebrates. In D. A. Dewsbury & D. A. Rethlingshafer (Eds.), *Comparative psychology: A modern survey*. New York: McGraw-Hill, 1973.

McDaniel, J. R., Donovick, P. J., Burright, R. G., & Fanelli, R. J. Genetics, septal lesions, and avoidance behavior in mice. *Behavioral and Neural Biology*, 1980, *28*, 285–299.

McDermott, L. J., Alheid, G. F., Kelly, J., Halaris, A. E., & Grossman, S. P. Regulatory deficits after surgical transections of three components of the MFB: Correlation with regional amine depletions. *Pharmacology, Biochemistry and Behavior*, 1977, *6*, 397–407.

McEwen, B. S., Weiss, J. M., & Schwartz, L. S. Uptake of corticosterone by rat brain and its concentration by certain limbic structures. *Brain Research*, 1969, *16*, 227–241.

McEwen, B. S., Gerlach, J. L., & Micco, D. J., Jr., Putative glucocorticoid receptors in hippocampus and other regions of the rat brain. In R. L. Isaacson & K. H. Pribram (Eds.), *The hippocampus. Vol. 1: Structure and Development*. New York: Plenum Press, 1975, pp. 285–322.

McGinty, D., Epstein, A. N., & Teitelbaum, P. The contribution of oropharyngeal sensations to hypothalamic hyperphagia. *Animal Behavior*, 1965, *13*, 413–418.

McGowan, B., Hankins, W., & Garcia, J. Limbic lesions and control of the internal and external environment. *Behavioral Biology*, 1972, *7*, 841–852.

McGowan, B. K., Garcia, J., Ervin, F. R., & Schwartz, J. Effects of septal lesions on bait shyness in the rat. *Physiology and Behavior*, 1969, *4*, 907–909.

McGowan-Sass, B. K., & Timiras, P. S. The hippocampus and hormonal cyclicity. In R. L. Isaacson & K. H. Pribram (Eds.), *The hippocampus. Vol. 1: Structure and development*. New York: Plenum Press, 1975, pp. 355–374.

McIntyre, D. C. Split-brain rat: Transfer and interference of kindled amygdala convulsions. *Canadian Journal of Neurological Science*, 1975, *2*, 429–437.

McIntyre, D. C. Effects of focal vs. generalized kindled convulsions from anterior neocortex or amygdala on CER acquisition in rats. *Physiology and Behavior*, 1979, *23*, 855–859.

McIntyre, D. C., & Goddard, G. V. Transfer, interference and spontaneous recovery of convulsions kindled from rat amygdala. *Electroencephalography and Clinical Neurophysiology*, 1973, *35*, 533–543.

McIntyre, D. C., & Molino, A. Amygdala lesions and CER learning long-term effect of kindling. *Physiology and Behavior*, 1972, *8*, 1055–1058.

McNaughton, B. L. Evidence for two physiologically distinct perforant pathways to the fascia dentata. *Brain Research*, 1980, *199*, 1–19.

McNew, J. J., & Thompson, R. Role of the limbic system in active and passive avoidance conditioning in the rat. *Journal of Comparative and Physiological Psychology*, 1966, *61*, 173–180.

Means, L. W., Walker, D. W., & Isaacson, R. L. Facilitated single alternation go, no-go performance following hippocampectomy in the rat. *Journal of Comparative and Physiological Psychology*, 1970, *22*, 278–285.

Mendelson, J. Ecological modulation of brain stimulation effects. *International Journal of Psychobiology*, 1972, *2*, 285–304.

Meyer, P. M., & Meyer, D. R. Memory, remembering and amnesia. In R. L. Isaacson & N. E. Spear (Eds.), *The expression of knowledge.* New York: Plenum Press, in press.

Meyer, P. M., Johnson, D. A., & Vaughn, D. W. The consequences of septal and neocortical ablations upon learning a two-way conditioned avoidance response. *Brain Research,* 1970, *22,* 113–120.

Meyer, J. S., Luine, V. N., Khylchevskaya, R. I., & McEwen, B. S. Glucocorticoids and hippocampal enzyme activity. *Brain Research,* 1979, *166,* 172–175.

Meyers, B., & Domino, E. F. The effect of cholinergic blocking drugs on spontaneous alternation in rats. *Archives Internationales de Pharmacodynamie,* 1964, *150,* 525–529.

Micco, D. J., Jr., McEwen, B. S., & Shein, W. Modulation of behavioral inhibition in appetitive extinction following manipulation of adrenal steroids in rats: Implications for involvement of the hippocampus. *Journal of Comparative and Physiological Psychology,* 1979, *93,* 323–329.

Miczek, K. A., & Grossman, S. P. Effects of septal lesions in inter- and intraspecies aggression in rats. *Journal of Comparative and Physiological Psychology,* 1972, *79,* 318–327.

Mikulka, P. J., Freeman, F. G., & Lidstrom, P. The effect of training technique and amygdala lesions on the acquisition and retention of a taste aversion. *Behavioral Biology,* 1977, *19,* 509–517.

Mikulka, P. J., Freeman, F., & Hughes, J. The effect of lesions of the amygdala and hippocampus on behavioral contrast in the rat. *Behavioral and Neural Biology,* in press.

Milgram, N. W. Effect of hippocampal stimulation on feeding in the rat. *Physiology and Behavior,* 1969, *4,* 665–670.

Miller, J. J., & Mogenson, G. J. Effect of septal stimulation on lateral hypothalamic unit activity in the rat. *Brain Research,* 1971, *32,* 125–142. (a)

Miller, J. J., & Mogenson, G. J. Modulatory influences of the septum on lateral hypothalamic self stimulation. *Experimental Neurology,* 1971, *33,* 671–683. (b)

Miller, N. E., Bailey, C. J., & Stevenson, J. A. F. Decreased "hunger" but increased food intake resulting from hypothalamic lesions. *Science,* 1950, *112,* 256–259.

Miller, V. M., & Best, P. J. Spatial correlates of hippocampal unit activity are altered by lesions of the fornix and entorhinal cortex. *Brain Research,* 1980, *194,* 311–323.

Millhouse, O. E. Optic chiasm collaterals afferent to the suprachiasmatic nucleus. *Brain Research,* 1977, *137,* 351–355.

Milner, B., Corkin, S., & Teuber, H. L. Further analysis of the hippocampal amnesic syndrome: 14-year follow-up study of H.M. *Neuropsychology,* 1968, *6,* 215–234.

Mishkin, M. Memory in monkeys severely impaired by combined but not by separate removal of amygdala and hippocampus. *Nature,* 1978, *273,* 297–298.

Mogenson, G. J., & Calaresu, F. R. Cardiovascular responses to electrical stimulation of the amygdala in the rat. *Experimental Neurology,* 1973, *39,* 166–180.

Mogenson, G. J., Jones, D. L., & Yim, C. Y. From motivation to action: functional interface between the limbic system and the motor system. In G. A. Kerkut & J. W. Phillis (Eds.), *Progress in neurobiology* (Vol. 14). New York: Karger, 1980, pp. 69–97.

Mok, A. C. S., & Mogenson, G. J. An evoked potential study of the projections to the lateral habenular nucleus from the septum and the lateral preoptic area in the rat. *Brain Research,* 1972, *43,* 343–360.

Montgomery, R. L., & Christian, E. L. Norepinephrine concentrations in brains and hearts of hyperactive septally lesioned rats. *Pharmacology, Biochemistry and Behavior,* 1973, *1,* 491.

Moore, J. W. Brain processes and conditioning. In A. Dickinson & R. A. Boakes (Eds.), *Mechanisms of learning and motivation: A memorial volume to Jerzy Konorski.* Hillsdale, N. J.: Erlbaum, 1979.

Moore, J. W., & Stickney, K. J. Formation of attentional-associative networks in real time: Role of the hippocampus and implications for conditioning. *Physiological Psychology* 1980, *8*, 207–217.

Moore, R. Y. Effects of some rhinencephalic lesions on retention of conditioned avoidance behavior in cats. *Journal of Comparative and Physiological Psychology*, 1964, *53*, 540–548.

Moore, R. Y. Retinohypothalamic projection in mammals: A comparative study. *Brain Research*, 1973, *49*, 403–409.

Moore, R. Y. Suprachiasmatic nucleus, secondary synchronizing stimuli and the central neural control of circadian rhythms. *Brain Research*, 1980, *183*, 13–28.

Moore, R. Y., & Eichler, V. B. Loss of circadian adrenal corticosterone rhythm following suprachiasmatic lesions. *Brain Research*, 1972, *42*, 201–206.

Moore, R. Y., & Lenn, N. J. A retino-hypothalamic projection in the rat. *Journal of Comparative Neurology*, 1972, *146*, 1–14.

Moore, R. Y., Björklund, A., & Stenevi, U. Plastic changes in the adrenergic innervation of the rat septal area in response to denervation. *Brain Research*, 1971, *33*, 13–35.

Morgan, J. M., & Mitchell, J. C. Septal lesions enhance delay of responding on a free operant avoidance schedule. *Psychonomic Science*, 1969, *16*, 10–11.

Morrison, J. H., Molliver, M. E., Grzanna, R., & Coyle, J. T. Noradrenergic innervation patterns in the regions of medial cortex: An immunofluorescence characterization. *Brain Research Bulletin*, 1979, *4*, 849–857.

Morrow, J. E., & Smithson, B. L. Learning sets in an invertebrate. *Science*, 1969, *164*, 850–851.

Mountcastle, V. B. Brain mechanisms for directed attention. *Journal of the Royal Society of Medicine*, 1978, *71*, 14–28.

Munn, N. L. *Handbook of psychological research on the rat.* Boston: Houghton-Miffin, 1950.

Munñoz, C., & Grossman, S. P. Some behavioral effects of selective neuronal depletion by kainic acid in the dorsal hippocampus of rats. *Physiology and Behavior*, 1980, *25*, 581–587.

Murphy, L. R., & Brown, T. S. Hippocampal lesions and learned taste aversion. *Physiological Psychology*, 1974, *2*, 60–64.

Myers, R. E., & Swett, C., Jr. Social behavior deficits of free-ranging monkeys after anterior temporal cortex removal: A preliminary report. *Brain Research*, 1970, *18*, 551–556.

Myhrer, T. Locomotor and avoidance behavior in rats with partial or total hippocampal perforant paths sections. *Physiology and Behavior*, 1975, *15*, 217–224.

Myhrer, T. Shuttle-box performance in rats with disruption of hippocampal CA1 output. *Brain Research*, 1976, *110*, 376–380.

Nachman, M., & Ashe, J. H. Effects of basolateral amygdala lesions on neophobia, learned taste aversions, and sodium appetite in rats. *Journal of Comparative and Physiological Psychology*, 1974, *87*, 622–643.

Nadel, L. Dorsal and ventral hippocampal lesions and behavior. *Physiology and Behavior*, 1968, *3*, 891–900.

Nagel, J. A., & Kemble, E. D. Effects of amygdaloid lesions on the performance of rats in four passive avoidance tasks. *Physiology and Behavior*, 1976, *17*, 245–250.

Nakajima, S. Interference with relearning in the rat after hippocampal injection of actinomycin D. *Journal of Comparative and Physiological Psychology*, 1969, *67*, 457–461.

Nauta, W. J. H. Fiber degeneration following lesions of the amygdaloid complex in the monkey. *Journal of Anatomy*, 1961, *95*, 515–531.

Nauta, W. J. H. In C. H. Hockman (Ed.), *Limbic system mechanisms and autonomic function*. Springfield, Ill.: Charles C Thomas, 1972.

Nicoll, R. A., Alger, B. E., & Jahr, C. E. Peptides as putative excitatory neurotransmitters: Carnosine, enkephalin, substance P and TRH. *Proceedings of the Royal Society of London B*, 1980, *210*, 133–149. (a)

Nicoll, R. A., Alger, B. E., & Jahr, C. E. Enkephalin blocks inhibitory pathways in the vertebrate CNS. *Nature*, 1980, *287*, 22–25. (b)

Nielson, H., McIver, H., & Boswell, R. Effect of septal lesions on learning, emotionality, activity, and exploratory behavior in rats. *Experimental Neurology*, 1965, *11*, 147–157.

Nonneman, A. J., & Isaacson, R. L. Task dependent recovery after early brain damage. *Behavioral Biology*, 1973, *8*, 143–172.

Novick, I., and Pihl, R. Effect of amphetamine on the septal syndrome in rats. *Journal of Comparative and Physiological Psychology*, 1969, *68*, 220–225.

Nyakas, C., de Kloet, E. R., & Bohus, B. Hippocampal function and putative corticosterone receptors: Effect of septal lesions. *Neuroendocrinology*, 1979, *29*, 301–312.

O'Keefe, J. Place units in the hippocampus of the freely moving rat. *Experimental Neurology*, 1976, *51*, 78–109.

O'Keefe, J., & Conway, D. H. Hippocampal place units in the freely moving rat: Why they fire where they fire. *Experimental Brain Research*, 1978, *31*, 573–590.

O'Keefe, J., & Dostrovsky, J. The hippocampus as a spatial map: Preliminary evidence from unit activity in the freely-moving rat. *Brain Research*, 1971, *34*, 171–175.

O'Keefe, J., & Nadal, L. *The hippocampus as a cognitive map*. Oxford: Clarendon Press, 1978.

O'Keefe, J., & Nadel, L. Precis of O'Keefe and Nadel's *The Hippocampus as a Cognitive Map*. *The Behavioral and Brain Sciences*, 1979, *2*, 487–533.

Olds, J., & Milner P. Positive reinforcement produced by electrical stimulation of septal area and other regions of rat brain. *Journal of Comparative and Physiological Psychology*, 1954, *47*, 419–427.

Olds, J., & Peretz, E. A motivational analysis of the reticular activating system. *Electroencephalography and Clinical Neurophysiology*, 1960, *12*, 445–454.

Olds, M. E. Comparative effects of amphetamine, scopolamine, chlordiazepoxide, and diphenylhydantoin on operant and extinction behavior with brain stimulation and food reward. *Neuropharmacology*, 1970, *9*, 519–532.

Olds, M. E., & Frey, J. H. Effects of hypothalamic lesions on escape behavior produced by midbrain electrical stimulation. *American Journal of Physiology*, 1971, *221*, 8–18.

Olds, M. E., & Olds, J. Approach–escape interactions in the rat brain. *American Journal of Physiology*, 1962, *203*, 803–810.

Olds, M. E., & Olds, J. Approach–avoidance analysis of rat diencephalon. *Journal of Comparative Neurology*, 1963, *120*, 259–295.

Olton, D. S. Specific deficits in active avoidance behavior following penicillin injection into the hippocampus. *Physiology and Behavior*, 1970, *5*, 957–963.

Olton, D. S. Behavioral and neuroanatomical differentiation of response suppression and response-shift mechanisms in the rat. *Journal of Comparative and Physiological Psychology*, 1972, *78*, 450–456.

Olton, D. S. (1973). Shock-motivated avoidance and the analysis of behavior. *Psychological Bulletin 79*, 243–251.

Olton, D. S. Characteristics of spatial memory. In S. H. Hulse, H. F. Fowler, & W. K. Honig (Eds.), *Cognitive aspects of animal behavior*. Hillsdale, N.J.: Erlbaum, 1978.

Olton, D. W., & Feustle, W. A. Hippocampal function required for nonspatial working memory. *Experimental Brain Research*, 1981, *41*, 380–389.

Olton, D. S., & Gage, F. H. Role of the fornix in the septal syndrome. *Physiology and Behavior*, 1974, *13*, 269–279.

Olton, D. S., & Isaacson, R. L. Fear, hippocampal lesions, and avoidance behavior. *Communications in Behavioral Biology*, 1969, *3*, 1–4.

Olton, D. S., & Papas, B. Spatial memory and hippocampal function. *Neuropsychologia*, 1979, *17*, 669–682.

Olton, D. S., & Samuelson, R. J. Remembrance of places passed: Spatial memory in rats. *Journal of Experimental Psychology: Animal Behavior Processes*, 1976, *2*, 97–116.

Olton, D. S., Becker, J. T., & Handelmann, G. E. Hippocampus, space and memory. *The Behavioral and Brain Sciences*, 1979, *2*, 313–365.

Olton, D. S., Becker, J. T., & Handelmann, G. E. Hippocampal function: Working memory or cognitive map. *Physiological Psychology*, 1980, *8*, 239–246.

Opsahl, C. A., & Powley, T. L. Body weight and gastric acid secretion in rats with subdiaphragmatic vagotomy and lateral hypothalamic lesions. *Journal of Comparative and Physiological Psychology*, 1977, *91*, 1284–1296.

Osborne, B., & Black, A. A detailed analysis of behaviour during the transition from acquisition to extinction in rats with fornix lesions. *Behavioral Biology*, 1978, *23*, 271–290.

Osborne, B., Sivakumaran, T., & Black, A. H. Effects of fornix lesions on adrenocortical responses to changes in environmental stimulation. *Behavioral Biology*, 1979, *25*, 227–241.

Pampiglione, G., & Falconer, M. A. Some observations upon stimulation of the hippocampus in man. *Electroencephalography and Clinical Neurophysiology*, 1956, *8*, 718.

Papez, J. W. A proposed mechanism of emotion. *Archives of Neurology and Psychiatry*, 1937, *38*, 725–744.

Papsdorf, J. D., & Woodruff, M. L. Effects of bilateral hippocampectomy on the rabbit's acquisition of shuttle-box and passive-avoidance responses. *Journal of Comparative and Physiological Psychology*, 1970, *73*, 486–489.

Pasquier, D. A., & Reinoso-Suarez, F. The topographic organization of hypothalamic and brain stem projections to the hippocampus. *Brain Research Bulletin*, 1978, *3*, 373–389.

Pellegrino, L. The effects of amygdaloid stimulation on passive avoidance. *Psychonomic Science*, 1965, *2*, 189–190.

Pellegrino, L. Amygdaloid lesions and behavioral inhibition in the rat. *Journal of Comparative and Physiological Psychology*, 1968, *65*, 483–491.

Pellegrino, L. J., & Clapp, D. F. Limbic lesions and externally cued DRL performance. *Physiology and Behavior*, 1971, *7*, 863–868.

Penfield, W., & Milner, B. Memory deficit produced by bilateral lesions in the hippocampal zone. *AMA Archives of Neurology and Psychiatry*, 1958, *79*, 475–497.

Pepeu, G., Mulas, A., Ruffi, A., & Sotgiu, P. Brain acetylcholine levels in rats with septal lesions. *Life Sciences*, 1971, *10*, 181–184.

Peretz, E. The effects of lesions of the anterior cingulate cortex on the behavior of the rat. *Journal of Comparative and Physiological Psychology*, 1960, *53*, 540–548.

Pfaff, D. W., Silva, M. T. A., & Weiss, J. M. Telemetered recording of hormone effects on hippocampal neurons. *Science*, 1971, *172*, 394–395.

Phillips, A. G., & LePiane, F. G. Disruption of conditioned taste aversion in the rat by stimulation of amygdala: A conditioning effect, not amnesia. *Journal of Comparative and Physiological Psychology*, 1980, *94*, 664–674.

Phillips, A. G., & LePiane, F. G. Differential effects of electrical stimulation of amygdala or caudate on inhibitory shock avoidance: A role for state-dependent learning. *Behavioural Brain Research*, 1981, *2*, 103–111.

Phillips, A. G., & Lieblich, I. Developmental and hormonal aspects of hyperemotionality produced by septal lesions in male rats. *Physiology and Behavior*, 1972, *9*, 237–242.

Phillips, A. G., Brooke, S. M., & Fibiger, H. C. Effect of amphetamine isomers and neuroleptics on self-stimulation from the nucleus accumbens and dorsal noradrenergic bundle. *Brain Research*, 1975, *85*, 13–22.

Phillips, A. G., Carter, D. A., & Fibiger, H. C. Dopaminergic substrates of intracranial self-stimulation in the caudate-putamen. *Brain Research*, 1976, *104*, 221–232.

Pigareva, M. L. Elaboration of conditioned alimentary reflexes having different probabilities of reinforcement in rats with hippocampal lesions. *Acta Neurobiological Experimentalis* (Warsaw), 1974, *34*, 423–433.

Pinel, J. P. J., Treit, D., & Rovner, L. I. Temporal lobe aggression in rats. *Science*, 1977, *197*, 1088–1089.

Pittendrigh, C. A. Circadian oscillations in cells and the circadian organization of multicellular systems. In F. O. Schmitt & F. G. Worden (Eds.), *The neurosciences: Third study program*. Cambridge, Mass.: MIT Press, 1974, pp. 437–458.

Ploog, D. W., & MacLean, P. D. On functions of the mammillary bodies in the squirrel monkey. *Experimental Neurology*, 1963, *7*, 76–85.

Plunkett, R. P. Effect of bilateral hippocampal lesions on cue utilization in the rat. *Psychological Reports*, 1978, *43*, 863–866.

Plunkett, R. P., & Faulds, B. D. The effect of cue distinctiveness on successive discrimination performance in hippocampal lesioned rats. *Physiological Psychology*, 1979, *7*, 49–52.

Pond, F. J., & Schwartzbaum, J. S. Hippocampal electrical activity evoked by rewarding and aversive brain stimulation in rats. *Communications in Behavioral Biology*, 1970, *5*, 89–103.

Pond, F. J., Lidsky, T. I., Levine, M. S., & Schwartzbaum, J. S. Hippocampal electrical activity during hypothalamic-evoked consummatory behavior in rats. *Psychonomic Science*, 1970, **21**, 21–23.

Poplawsky, A. Long-term maintenance of shuttlebox avoidance behavior before and after septal lesions. *Physiological Psychology*, 1978, *6*, 294–299.

Poplawsky, A., & Cohen, S. L. Septal lesions and the reinforcer-omission effect. *Physiology and Behavior*, 1977, *18*, 983–985.

Poplawsky, A., & Johnson, D. A. Open-field social behavior of rats following lesions of medial or lateral septal nuclei or cingulate cortex. *American Zoologist*, 1972, *12*, 83.

Poplawsky, A., & Johnson, D. A. Open-field social behavior of rats following lateral or medial septal lesions. *Physiology and Behavior*, 1973, *11*, 845–854.

Powley, T. L. The ventromedial hypothalamic syndrome, satiety, and a cephalic phase hypothesis. *Psychological Review*, 1977, *84*, 89–126.

Powley, T. L., & Keesey, R. E. Relationship of body weight to the lateral hypothalamic feeding syndrome. *Journal of Comparative and Physiological Psychology*, 1970, *70*, 25–36.

Powley, T. L., & Opsahl, C. A. Ventromedial hypothalamic obesity abolished by subdiaphragmatic vagotomy. *American Journal of Physiology*, 1974, *226*, 25–33.

Pribram, K. H. *Languages of the brain: Experimental paradoxes and principles in neuropsychology*. Englewood Cliffs, N.J.: Prentice-Hall, 1971.

Pribram, K. H., & Bagshaw, M. Further analysis of the temporal lobe syndrome utilizing frontotemporal ablations. *Journal of Comparative Neurology*, 1953, *99*, 347–375.

Pribram, K. H., & Fulton, J. F. An experimental critique of the effects of anterior cingulate ablations in monkey. *Brain*, 1954, *77*, 34–44.

Pribram, K. H., & MacLean, P. D. Neuronographic analysis of medial and basal cortex: II. Monkey. *Journal of Neurophysiology*, 1953, *16*, 323–340.

Pribram, K. H., & Weiskrantz, L. A comparison of the effects of medial and lateral cerebral resections on conditioned avoidance behavior of monkeys. *Journal of Comparative and Physiological Psychology*, 1957, *50*, 74–80.

Pribram, K. H., Douglas, R. J., & Pribram, B. J. The nature of nonlimbic learning. *Journal of Comparative and Physiological Psychology*, 1969, *69*, 765–772.

Price, J. L. An autoradiographic study of complementary laminar patterns of termination of afferent fibers to the olfactory cortex. *Journal of Comparative Neurology*, 1973, *150*, 87–108.

Pubols, L. M. Changes in food motivated behavior of rats as a function of septal and amygdaloid lesions. *Experimental Neurology*, 1966, *15*, 240–254.

Rabe, A., & Haddad, R. K. Effect of selective hippocampal lesions in the rat on acquisition, performance, and extinction of bar pressing on a fixed ratio schedule. *Experimental Brain Research*, 1968, *5*, 159–266.

Rabe, A., & Haddad, R. K. Integrative deficit after hippocampal lesions. *Proceedings of the 77th Annual Convention of the American Psychological Association*, 1969, *4*, 213–214.

Rabin, B. M. Ventromedial hypothalamic control of food intake and satiety: A reappraisal. *Brain Research*, 1972, *43*, 317–342.

Ramon y Cajal, S. *The structure of Ammon's horn*. Springfield, Ill.: Charles C Thomas, 1968.

Ranck, J. B., Jr. Studies on single neurons in dorsal hippocampal formation and septum in unrestrained rats. *Experimental Neurology*, 1973, *41*, 461–555.

Ranck, J. B., Jr. Behavioral correlates and fixing repertoires of neurons in the dorsal hippocampal formation and septum of unrestrained cats. In R. L. Isaacson & K. H. Pribram (Eds.), *The hippocampus (Vol. 2)*. New York: Plenum Press, 1975, pp. 207–244.

Ransom, W. B. On tumors of the corpus callosum with account of a case. *Brain*, 1895, *18*, 531–550.

Raphelson, A. C., Isaacson, R. L., & Douglas, R. J. The effect of distracting stimuli on the runway performance of the limbic damaged rats. *Psychonomic Science*, 1965, *3*, 483–484.

Reeves, A. G., & Plum, F. Hyperphagia, rage, and dementia accompanying a ventromedial hypothalamic neoplasm. *Archives of Neurology, Chicago*, 1969, *20*, 616–624.

Reeves, C. D. Discrimination of light of different wave lengths by fish. *Behavioral Monographs*, 1919, *4*, 1–106.

Reinberg, A., & Halberg, F. Circadian chronopharmacology. *Annual Review of Pharmacology*, 1971, *11*, 455–492.

Reinstein, D. K. *Behavioral and biochemical changes after hippocampal damage*. Unpublished Ph.D. dissertation, State University of New York at Binghamton, 1981.

Reinstein, D. K., Hannigan, J. H., Jr., & Isaacson, R. L. Behavioral and biochemical changes after hippocampal destruction involve forebrain dopaminergic systems. *Pharmacology, Biochemistry and Behavior*, in press.

Reis, D. J., & Gunne, L. M. Brain catecholamines: Relation to the defense reaction evoked by amygdaloid stimulation in cat. *Science*, 1965, *149*. 450–451.

Reis, D. J., & McHugh, P. R. Hypoxia as a cause of bradycardia during amygdala stimulation in monkey. *American Journal of Physiology*, 1968, *214*, 601–610.

Reis, D. J., & Oliphant, M. C. Bradycardia and tachycardia following electrical stimulation of the amygdaloid region in monkey. *Journal of Neurophysiology*, 1964, *27*, 893–912.

Reynolds, D. V. Surgery in the rat during electrical analgesia induced by focal brain stimulation. *Science*, 1969, *164*, 444–445.

Reynolds, R. W. Equivalence of radio frequency and electrolytic lesions in producing septal rage. *Psychonomic Science*, 1965, *2*, 35–36.

Rhodes, D. L., & Liebeskind, J. C. Analgesia from rostral brain stem stimulation in the rat. *Brain Research*, 1978, *143*, 521–532.

Richardson, D. E., & Akil, H. Pain reduction by electrical brain stimulation in man: I. Acute administration in periaqueductal and periventricular sites. *Journal of Neurosurgery*, 1977, *47*, 178–183. (a)

Richardson, D. E., & Akil, H. Pain reduction by electrical brain stimulation in man: II. Chronic self-administration in the periventricular gray matter. *Journal of Neurosurgery*, 1977, *47*, 184–194. (b)

Rickert, E. J., Bennett, T. L., Lane, P. L., & French, J. Hippocampectomy and the attenuation of blocking. *Behavioral Biology*, 1978, *22*, 147–160.

Rickert, E. J., Lorden, J. F., Dawson, R., Jr., Smyly, E., & Callahan, M. F. Stimulus processing and stimulus selection in rats with hippocampal lesions. *Behavioral and Neural Biology*, 1979, *27*, 454–465.

Riopelle, A. J., Alper, R. G., Strong, P. N., & Ades, H. W. Multiple discrimination and patterned string performance of normal and temporal-lobectomized monkey. *Journal of Comparative and Physiological Psychology*, 1953, *46*, 145–149.

Roberts, W. W. Both rewarding and punishing effects from stimulation of posterior hypothalamus of cat with same electrode at same intensity. *Journal of Comparative and Physiological Psychology*, 1958, *51*, 400–407.

Roberts, W. W., Dember, W. N., & Brodwick, M. Alternation and exploration in rats with hippocampal lesions. *Journal of Comparative and Physiological Psychology*, 1962, *55*, 695–700.

Roberts, W. W., Steinberg, M. L., & Means, L. W. Hypothalamic mechanisms for sexual, aggressive, and other motivational behaviors in the opossum, *Didelphis virginiana*. *Journal of Comparative and Physiological Psychology*, 1967, *64*, 1–15.

Robinson, E. Effects of amygdalectomy on fear-motivated behavior in rats. *Journal of Comparative and Physiological Psychology*, 1963, *56*, 814–820.

Robinson, T. E. Hippocampal rhythmic slow activity (RSA; theta): A critical analysis of selected studies and discussion of possible species-differences. *Brain Research Reviews*, 1980, *2*, 69–101.

Robinson, T. E., & Vanderwolf, C. H. Electrical stimulation of the brain stem in freely moving rats: II. Effects on hippocampal and neocortical electrical activity, and relations to behavior. *Experimental Neurology*, 1978, *61*, 485–515.

Robinson, T. E., & Whishaw, I. Q. Effects of posterior hypothalamic lesions on voluntary behaviour and hippocampal electroencelphalogramms in the rat. *Journal of Comparative and Physiological Psychology*, 1974, *86*, 768–786.

Rolls, B. J., & Rolls, E. T. Effects of lesions in the basolateral amygdala on fluid intake in the rat. *Journal of Comparative and Physiological Psychology*, 1973, *83*, 240–247.

Rolls, E. T. Contrasting effects of hypothalamic and nucleus accumbens septi self-stimulation on brain stem single unit activity and cortical arousal. *Brain Research*, 1971, *31*, 275–285.

Rolls, E. T. *The brain and reward.* New York; Pergamon Press, 1975.

Rolls, E. T., & Kelly, P. H. Neural basis of stimulus-bound locomotor activity in the rat. *Journal of Comparative and Physiological Psychology,* 1972, *81,* 173–182.

Rose, M. Cytoarchitektonischer Atlas der Grosshirnrinde der Maus. *Journal of Psychology and Neurology,* 1929, *40,* 1–51.

Rosene, D. L., & Van Hoesen, G. W. Hippocampal efferents reach widespread areas of cerebral cortex and amygdala in the rhesus monkey. *Science,* 1977, *198,* 315–317.

Ross, J. F., & Grossman, S. P. Transections of stria medullaris or stria terminalis in the rat: Effects on aversively controlled behavior. *Journal of Comparative and Physiological Psychology, 91,* 907–917.

Ross, J. F., Walsh, L. L., & Grossman, S. P. Some behavioral effects of entorhinal cortex lesions in the albino rat. *Journal of Comparative Physiological Psychology,* 1973, *85,* 70–81.

Ross, J. F., Grossman, L., & Grossman, S. P. Some behavioral effects of transecting ventral or dorsal fiber connections of the septum in the rat. *Journal of Comparative and Physiological Psychology,* 1975, *89,* 5–18.

Rosvold, H. E., Fuller, J. L., & Pribram, K. H. Ablation of the pyriform, amygdala, hippocampal complex in genetically pure strain cocker spaniels. In J. F. Fulton (Ed.), *Frontal lobotomy and affective behavior: A neurophysiological analysis.* New York: Norton, 1951, pp. 80–82.

Rosvold, H. E., Mirsky, A. F., & Pribram, K. H. Influence of amygdalectomy on social behavior in monkeys. *Journal of Comparative and Physiological Psychology,* 1954, *47,* 173–178.

Routtenberg, A. Forebrain pathways of reward in *Rattus norvegicus. Journal of Comparative and Physiological Psychology,* 1971, *75,* 269–276.

Routtenberg, A., & Olds, J. Attenuation of response to an aversive brain stimulus by concurrent rewarding septal stimulation. *Federation Proceedings,* 1963, *22,* 515 (abst.).

Routtenberg, A., & Sloan, M. Self-stimulation in the frontal cortex of *Rattus norvegicus. Behavioral Biology,* 1972, *7,* 567–572.

Rowland, N., Marshall, F. J., Antelman, S. M., & Edwards, D. J. Hypothalamic hyperphagia prevented by damage to brain dopamine-containing neurons. *Physiology and Behavior,* 1979, *22,* 635–640.

Roźkowska, E., & Fonberg, E. The effects of ventromedial hypothalamic lesions on food intake and alimentary instrumental conditioned reflexes in dogs. *Acta Neurobiologiae Experimentalis,* 1971, *31,* 354–364.

Rudell, A. P., Fox, S. E., & Ranck, J. B., Jr. Hippocampal excitability phase-locked to the theta rhythm in walking rats. *Experimental Neurology,* 1980, *68,* 87–96.

Rusak, B., & Zucker, I. Neural regulation of circadian rhythms. *Physiology Reviews,* 1979, *59,* 449–526.

Sagvolden, T. Acquisition of two-way active avoidance behavior following septal lesions in the rat: Effect of intensity of discontinuous shock. *Behavioral Biology,* 1975, *14,* 59–74. (a)

Sagvolden, T. Operant responding for water in rats with septal lesions: Effect of deprivation level. *Behavioral Biology,* 1975, *13,* 323–330. (b)

Sagvolden, T. Behavior of rats with septal lesions during low levels of water deprivation. *Behavioral and Neural Biology,* 1979, *26,* 431–441.

Saleh, M. A., & Winget, C. M. Effect of suprachiasmatic lesions on diurnal heart rate rhythm in the rat. *Physiology and Behavior,* 1977, *19,* 561–564.

Saltwick, S. E., & Gabriel, M. Relationships of non-bursting neuronal activity of the hippocampal formation to acquisition and performance of discriminative avoidance behavior in rabbits. Manuscript in preparation, 1982.

Sanders, F. K. Second-order olfactory and visual learning in the optic tectum of goldfish. *Journal of Experimental Biology*, 1940, *30*, 412–415.

Sanwald, J. C., Porzio, N. R., Deane, G. E., & Donovick, P. J. The effects of septal and dorsal hippocampal lesions on the cardiac component of the orienting response. *Physiology and Behavior*, 1970, *5*, 883–888.

Saper, C. B., Loewy, A. D., Swanson, L. W., & Cowan, W. M. Direct hypothalamo-autonomic connections. *Brain Research*, 1976, *117*, 305–312.

Saper, C. B., Swanson, L. W., & Cowan, W. M. The efferent connections of the ventromedial nucleus of the hypothalamus of the rat. *Journal of Comparative Neurology*, 1976, *169*, 409–442.

Saper, C. B., Swanson, L. W., & Cowan, W. M. The efferent connections of the anterior hypothalamic area of the rat, cat and monkey. *Journal of Comparative Neurology*, 1978, *182*, 575–600.

Saper, C. B., Swanson, L. W., & Cowan, W. M. An autoradiographic study of the efferent connections of the lateral hypothalamic area in the rat. *Journal of Comparative Neurology*, 1979, *183*, 689–706.

Sar, M., Stumpf, W. E., Miller, R. J., Chang, K.-H., & Cuatrecasas, P. Immunohistochemical localization of enkephalin in rat brain and spinal cord. *Journal of Comparative Neurology*, 1978, *182*, 17–38.

Scalia, F., & Winans, S. The differential projections of the olfactory bulb in mammals. *Journal of Comparative Neurology*, 1975, *161*, 31–56.

Scheff, S. W., & Cotman, C. W. Recovery of spontaneous alternation following lesions of the entorhinal cortex in adult rats: Possible correlation to axon sprouting. *Behavioral Biology*, 1977, *21*, 286–293.

Schmaltz, L. W. Deficit in active avoidance learning in rats following penicillin injection into hippocampus. *Physiology and Behavior*, 1971, *6*, 667–674.

Schmaltz, L. W., & Isaacson, R. L. The effects of preliminary training conditions upon DRL 20 performance in the hippocampectomized rat. *Physiology and Behavior*, 1966, *1*, 175–182.

Schmaltz, L. W., & Isaacson, R. L. Effects of caudate and frontal lesions on retention and relearning of a DRL schedule. *Journal of Comparative and Physiological Psychology*, 1968, *65*, 343–348.

Schmaltz, L. W., & Theios, J. Acquisition and extinction of a classically conditioned response in hippocampectomized rabbits *(oryctolagus cuniculus) Journal of Comparative and Physiological Psychology*, 1972, *79*, 328–333.

Schnurr, R. Localization of the septal rage syndrome in Long-Evans rats. *Journal of Comparative and Physiological Psychology*, 1972, *81*, 291–296.

Schreiner, L., & Kling, A. Behavioral changes following rhinencephalic injury in cat. *Journal of Neurophysiology*, 1953, *16*, 643–659.

Schwaber, J. S., Kapp, B. S., & Higgins, G. The origin and extent of direct amygdala projections to the region of the dorsal motor nucleus of the vagus and the nucleus of the solitary tract. *Neuroscience Letters*, 1980, *20*, 15–20.

Schwartz, W. J., & Gainer, H. Suprachiasmatic nucleus: Use of ^{14}C-labeled deoxyglucose uptake as a functional marker. *Science*, 1977, *197*, 1089–1091.

Schwartzbaum, J. S. Changes in reinforcing properties of stimuli following ablation of the amygdaloid complex in monkeys. *Journal of Comparative and Physiological Psychology*, 1960, *53*, 388–395.

Schwartzbaum, J. S. Some characteristics of "amygdaloid hyperphagia" in monkeys. *American Journal of Psychology*, 1961, 74, 252–259.

Schwartzbaum, J. S., & Donovick, P. J. Discrimination reversal and spatial alternation associated with septal and caudate dysfunction in rats. *Journal of Comparative and Physiological Psychology*, 1968, 65, 83–92.

Schwartzbaum, J. S., & Gay, P. E. Interacting behavioral effects of septal and amygdaloid lesions in the rat. *Journal of Comparative and Physiological Psychology*, 1966, 61, 59–65.

Schwartzbaum, J. S., & Gustafson, J. W. Peripheral shock, implanted electrodes and artifactual interactions: A renewed warning. *Psychonomic Science*, 1970, 20, 49–50.

Schwartzbaum, J. S., & Poulos, D. A. Discrimination behavior after amygdalectomy in monkeys: Learning set and discrimination reversals. *Journal of Comparative and Physiological Psychology*, 1965, 60, 320–328.

Schwartzbaum, J. S., & Pribram, K. H. The effects of amygdalectomy in monkeys on transportation along a brightness continuum. *Journal of Comparative and Physiological Psychology*, 1960, 53, 396–399.

Schwartzbaum, J. S., Wilson, W. A., Jr., & Morrissette, J. R. The effect of amygdalectomy on locomotor activity in monkeys. *Journal of Comparative and Physiological Psychology*, 1961, 54, 334–336.

Schwartzbaum, J. S., Kellicutt, M. H., Spieth, L. M., & Thompson, J. D. Effects of septal lesions in rats on response inhibition associated with food reinforced behavior. *Journal of Comparative and Physiological Psychology*, 1964, 58, 217–224.

Schwartzbaum, J. S., Thompson, J. D., & Kellicutt, M. H. Auditory frequency discrimination and generalization following lesions of the amygdaloid area in rats. *Journal of Comparative and Physiological Psychology*, 1964, 57, 257–266.

Schwartzbaum, J., Green, R., Beatty, W., & Thompson, J. D. Acquisition of avoidance behavior following septal lesions in the rat. *Journal of Comparative and Physiological Psychology*, 1967, 63, 95–104.

Schwartzbaum, J. S., DiLorenzo, P. M., Mello, W. F., & Kreinick, C. J. Further evidence of dissociation between reactivity and visual evoked response following septal lesions in rats. *Journal of Comparative and Physiological Psychology*, 1972, 80, 143–149.

Schwartzbaum, J. S., Kreinick, C. J., & Levine, M. S. Behavioral reactivity and visual evoked potentials to photic stimuli following septal lesions in rats. *Journal of Comparative and Physiological Psychology*, 1972, 80, 123–142.

Schwartzkroin, P. A., & Wester, K. Long-lasting facilitation of a synaptic potential following tetanization in the *in vitro* hippocampal slice. *Brain Research*, 1975, 89, 107–119.

Sclafani, A., & Grossman, S. P. Reactivity of hyperphagic and normal rats to quinine and electric shock. *Journal of Comparative and Physiological Psychology*, 1971, 74, 157–166.

Scoville, W. B., The limbic lobe in man. *Journal of Neurosurgery*, 1954, 11, 64–66.

Scoville, W. B., & Milner, B. Loss or recent memory after bilateral hippocampal lesions. *Journal of Neurology, Neurosurgery and Psychiatry*, 1957, 20, 11–21.

Sears, R. Effect of optic lobe ablation on the visuomotor behavior of the goldfish. *Journal of Comparative Psychology*, 1934, 17, 233–265.

Segal, M. Flow of conditioned responses in limbic telencephalic system of the rat. *Journal of Neurophysiology*, 1973, 36, 840–854.

Segal, M. Excitability changes in rat hippocampus during conditioning. *Experimental Neurology*, 1977, 55, 67–73.

Segal, M., & Bloom, F. E. The action of nor-epinephrine in the rat hippocampus: IV. The effect of locus coeruleus stimulation on evoked hippocampal unit activity. *Brain Research*, 1976, *107*, 513–525. (a)

Segal, M., & Bloom, F. E. The action of norepinephrine in the rat hippocampus: III. Hippocampal cellular responses to locus coeruleus stimulation in the awake rat. *Brain Research*, 1976, *107*, 499–511. (b)

Segal, M. E., Disterhoft, J., & Olds, J. Hippocampal unit activity during aversive and appetitive conditioning. *Science*, 1972, *175*, 791–794.

Seggie, J. Endocrine and circadian variables in manifestation of affective behavior following septal ablation in rats. *Proceedings of the 78th Annual Convention of the American Psychological Association*, 1970, *5*, 199–200.

Sen, R. N., & Anand, B. K. Effects of electrical stimulation of the limbic system of brain ("visceral brain") on gastric secretory activity and ulceration. *Indian Journal of Medical Research*, 1957, *45*, 515–521.

Sherrick, M. F., Brunner, R. L., Roth, T. G., & Dember, W. N. Rats' sensitivity to their direction of movement and spontaneous alternation. *Quarterly Journal of Experimental Psychology*, 1979, *31*, 83–93.

Showers, M. J. C. The cingulate gyrus: Additional motor area and cortical autonomic regulator. *Journal of Comparative Neurology*, 1959, *112*, 231–301.

Sibole, W., Miller, J. J., & Mogenson, G. J. Effects of septal stimulation on drinking elicited by electrical stimulation of the lateral hypothalamus. *Experimental Neurology*, 1971, *32*, 466–477.

Sideroff, S., Schneiderman, N., & Powell, D. A. Motivational properties of septal stimulation as the US in classical conditioning of heart rate in rabbits. *Journal of Comparative and Physiological Psychology*, 1971, *74*, 1–10.

Siegel, A., & Tassoni, J. P. Differential efferent projections from the ventral and dorsal hippocampus of the cat. *Brain, Behavior, and Evolution*, 1971, *4*, 185–200. (a)

Siegel, A., & Tassoni, J. P. Differential efferent projections of the lateral and medial septal nuclei to the hippocampus in the cat. *Brain, Behavior, and Evolution*, 1971, *4*, 201–219. (b)

Sikorzsky, R. D., Donovick, P. J., Burright, R. G., & Chin, T. Experiential effects on acquisition and reversal of discrimination tasks by albino rats with septal lesions. *Physiology and Behavior*, 1977, *18*, 231–236.

Simantov, R., Kuhar, M. J., Uhl, G. R., & Snyder, S. H. Opioid peptide enkephalin: Immunohistichemical mapping in the rat central nervous system. *Proceedings of the National Academy of Sciences*, 1977, *74*, 2167–2171.

Singh, D. Comparison of hyperemotionality caused by lesions in the septal and ventromedial hypothalamic areas in the rat. *Psychonomic Science*, 1969, *16*, 3–4.

Slangen, J. L., & Miller, N. E. Pharmacological tests for the function of hypothalamic norepinephrine in eating behavior. *Physiology and Behavior*, 1969, *4*, 543–552.

Slonaker, R. L., & Hothersall, D. Collateral behaviors and the DRL deficit of rats with septal lesions. *Journal of Comparative Physiological Psychology*, 1972, *80*, 91–96.

Slotnick, B. M. Disturbance of maternal behaviour in the rat following lesions in the cingulate cortex. *Behaviour*, 1967, *29*, 204–236.

Slotnick, B. M., & McMullen, M. F. Intraspecific fighting in albino mice with septal forebrain lesions. *Physiology and Behavior*, 1972, *8*, 333–337.

Slusher, M. A. Effects of cortisol implants in the brainstem and ventral hippocampus on diurnal corticosteroid levels. *Experimental Brain Research*, 1966, *1*, 184–194.

Smith, G. P., Levin, B. E., & Ervin, G. N. Loss of active avoidance responding after lateral hypothalamic injections of 6-hydroxydopamine. *Brain Research*, 1975, *88*, 483–498.

Smith, R. F., & Schmaltz, L. W. Acquisition of appetitively and aversively motivated lesions on two types of passive avoidance tasks. *Psychological Reports*, 1965, *16*, 1277–1290.

Snapir, N., Yaakobi, M., Robinzon, B., Ravona, H., & Perek, M. Involvement of the medial hypothalamus and the septal area in the control of food intake and body weight in geese. *Pharmacology, Biochemistry and Behavior*, 1976, *5*, 609–615.

Snyder, D. R., & Isaacson, R. L. Effects of large and small bilateral hippocampal lesions on two types of passive-avoidance responses. *Psychological Reports*, 1965, *16*, 1277–1290.

Sodetz, F. J. Septal ablation and free-operant avoidance behavior in the rat. *Physiology and Behavior*, 1970, *5*, 773–777.

Sodetz, F. J., & Bunnell, B. N. Septal ablation and the social behavior of the golden hamster. *Physiology and Behavior*, 1970, *6*, 79–88.

Sodetz, F. J., Matalka, E. S., & Bunnell, B. N. Septal ablation and affective behavior in the golden hamster. *Psychonomic Science*, 1967, *7*, 189–190.

Solomon, P. R. Role of the hippocampus in blocking and conditioned inhibition of the rabbit's nictitating membrane response. *Journal of Comparative and Physiological Psychology*, 1977, *91*, 407–417.

Solomon, P. R. Temporal versus spatial information processing theories of hippocampal function. *Psychological Bulletin*, 1979, *86*, 1272–1279.

Solomon, P. R. A time and a place for everything? Temporal processing views of hippocampal function with sepcial reference to attention. *Physiological Psychology*, 1980, *8*, 254–261.

Solomon, P. R., & Moore, J. W. Latent inhibition and stimulus generalization of the classically conditioned nictitating membrane response in rabbits (*Oryctolagus cuniculus*) following dorsal hippocampal ablation. *Journal of Comparative and Physiological Psychology*, 1975, *89*, 1192–1203.

Solomon, P. R., Nichols, G. L., Kiernan, J. M., III, Kamer, R. S., & Kaplan, L. J. Differential effects of lesions in medial and dorsal raphe of the rat: Latent inhibition and septohippocampal serotonin levels. *Journal of Comparative and Physiological Psychology*, 1980, *94*, 145–154.

Sorensen, J. P., Jr., & Harvey, J. A. Decreased brain acetylcholine after septal lesions in rats: Correlation with thirst. *Physiology and Behavior*, 1971, *6*, 723–725.

Springer, J., Hannigan, J. H., Jr., & Isaacson, R. L. Changes in dopamine and DOPAC following systemic administration of apomorphine and DPI in rats. *Brain Research*, 1981, *220*, 226–230.

Srebro, B. Retention of successive position eversals in rats with septal and fronto-polar lesions. *Physiology and Behavior*, 1973, *11*, 103–105.

Stahl, J. M., & Ellen, P. Septal lesions and reasoning performance in the rat. *Journal of Comparative and Physiological Psychology*, 1973, *84*, 629–638.

Stahl, J. M., & Ellen, P. Performance of rats on the Maiere three-table task following septal lesions occurring 24 hours after birth. *Journal of Comparative and Physiological Psychology*, 1979, *93*, 1145–1153.

Stamm, J. S. The function of the median cerebral cortex in maternal behavior of rats. *Journal of Comparative and Physiological Psychology*, 1955, *48*, 347–356.

Stein, D. G., & Kirkby, R. J. The effects of training on passive avoidance deficits in rats with hippocampal lesions: A reply to Isaacson, Olton, Bauer, and Swart. *Psychonomic Science*, 1967, *7*, 7–8.

Stein, L. Chemistry of purposive behavior. In J. T. Tapp (Ed.), *Reinforcement and behavior*. New York and London: Academic Press, 1969, pp. 329–352.

Stein, L., & Belluzzi, J. D. Brain endorphins: Possible role in reward and memory formation. *Federation Proceedings*, 1979, *38*, 2468–2472.

Stein, L., Wise, C. D., & Berger, B. D. Noradrenergic reward mechanisms, recovery of function, and schizophrenia. In J. L. McGaugh (Ed.), *The chemistry of mood, motivation, and memory*. New York: Plenum Press, 1972, pp. 81–103.

Stephan, F. K., & Zucker, I. Circadian rhythms in drinking behavior and locomotor activity of rats are eliminated by hypothalamic lesions. *Proceedings of the National Academy of Science*, 1972, *69*, 1583–1586.

Stephan, F. K., Swann, J. M., & Sisk, C. L. Anticipation of 24-hr. feeding schedules in rats with lesions of the suprachiasmatic nucleus. *Neuroscience Abstracts*, 1978, *4*, 181.

Stern, J. J., & Zwick, G. Effects of intraventricular norepinephrine and estradiol benzoate on weight regulatory behavior in female rats. *Behavioral Biology*, 1973, *9*, 605–612.

Stevens, J. R. Schizophrenia and dopamine regulation in the mesolimbic system. *Trends in Neuroscience*, April 1979, pp. 102–105.

Stevens, R. Effects of duration of sensory input and intertrial interval on spontaneous alternation in rats with hippocampal lesions. *Physiological Psychology*, 1973, *1*, 41–44.

Stevenson, J. A. F., & Montemurro, D. G. Loss of weight and metabolic rate of rats with lesions in the medial and lateral hypothalamus. *Nature*, 1963, *198*, 92.

Stewart, O., Loesche, J., & Horton, W. C. Behavioral correlates of denervation and reinervation of the hippocampal formation of the rat: Open field activity and cue utilization following bilateral entorhinal cortex lesions. *Brain Research Bulletin*, 1977, *2*, 41–48.

Stiglick, A., & White, N. Effects of lesions of various medial forebrain bundle components on lateral hypothalamic self-stimulation. *Brain Research*, 1977, *133*, 45–63.

Straus, E., & Yalow, R. S. Cholecystokinin in the brains of obese and nonobese mice. *Science*, 1979, *203*, 68–69.

Stricker, E. M. Drinking by rats after lateral hypothalamic lesions: A new look at the lateral hypothalamic syndrome. *Journal of Comparative Physiological Psychology*, 1976, *90*, 127–143.

Stricker, E. M. Excessive drinking by rats with septal lesions during hypovolemia induced by subcutaneous colloid treatment. *Physiology and Behavior*, 1978, *21*, 905–907.

Stricker, E. M., Cooper, P. H., Marshall, J. F., & Zigmond, M. J. Acute homeostatic imbalances reinstate sensorimotor dysfunctions in rats with lateral hypothalamic lesions. *Journal of Comparative and Physiological Psychology*, 1979, *93*, 512–521.

Strong, P. N., Jr. The effect of cul length and hippocampal lesions on maze learning in the rat. *Pavlovian Journal of Biological Sciences*, October–December 1978, *13*, 246–250.

Stumpf, C. H. The fast component in the electrical activity of the rabbit's hippocampus. *Electroencephalography and Clinical Neurophysiology*, 1965, *18*, 477–486.

Stumpf, W. E. Estrogen-neurons and estrogen-neuron systems in the periventricular brain. *American Journal of Anatomy*, 1970, *129*, 207–217.

Suess, W. M., & Berlyne, D. E. Exploratory behavior as a function of hippocampal damage, stimulus complexity, and stimulus novelty in the hooded rat. *Behavioral Biology*, 1978, *23*, 487–499.

Suits, E., & Isaacson, R. L. The effects of scopolamine hydrobromide on one-way and two-way avoidance learning in rats. *International Journal of Neuropharmacology*, 1968, *7*, 441–446.

Swanson, A. M., & Isaacson, R. L. Hippocampal lesions and the frustration effect in rats. *Journal of Comparative and Physiological Psychology,* 1969, *68,* 562–567.

Swanson, L. W. An autoradiographic study of the efferent connections of the preoptic region in the cat. *Journal of Comparative Neurology,* 1976, *167,* 227–256.

Swanson, L. W. Immunohistochemical evidence for a neurophysin-containing autonomic pathway arising in the paraventricular nucleus of the hypothalamus. *Brain Research,* 1977, *128,* 346–353.

Swanson, L. W., & Cowan, W. M. The efferent connections of the suprachiasmatic nucleus of the hypothalamus. *Journal of Comparative Neurology,* 1975, *160,* 1–12. (a)

Swanson, L. W., & Cowan, W. M. Hippocampo-hypothalamic connections: Origin in subicular cortex, not Ammon's horn. *Science,* 1975, *189,* 303–304. (b)

Swanson, L. W., & Cowan, W. M. A note on the connections and development of the nucleus accumbens. *Brain Research,* 1975, *92,* 324–330. (c)

Swanson, L. W., & Cowan, W. M. An autoradiographic study of the organization of the efferent connections of the hippocampal formation in the rat. *Journal of Comparative Neurology,* 1977, *172,* 49–84.

Swanson, L. W., & Cowan, W. M. The connections of the septal area in the rat. *Journal of Comparative Neurology,* 1979, *186,* 621–656.

Swanson, L. W., & Hartman, B. K. The central adrenergic system: An immunofluorescence study of the location cell bodies and their efferent connections in the rat utilizing dopamine-β-hydroxylase as a marker. *Journal of Comparative Neurology,* 1975, *163,* 467–506.

Swanson, L. W., Cowan, W. M., & Jones, E. G. An autoradiographic study of the efferent connections of the ventral lateral geniculate nucleus in the albino rat and cat. *Journal of Comparative Neurology,* 1974, *156,* 143–164.

Swanson, L. W., Wyss, J. M., & Cowan, W. M. An autoradiographic study of the organization of intrahippocampal association pathways in the rat. *Journal of Comparative Neurology,* 1978, *181,* 681–716.

Swanson, L. W., Sawchenko, P. E., & Cowan, W. M. Evidence that the commissural, associational and septal projections of the regio inferior of the hippocampus arise from the same neurons. *Brain Research,* 1980, *197,* 207–212.

Szentagothai, J., Flerko, B., Mess, B., & Halaz, B. *Hypothalamic control of the anterior pituitary.* Budapest: Akademiai Kiado, 1968.

Szerb, J. C. Cortical acetycholine release and electroencephalographic arousal. *Journal of Physiology (London),* 1967, *192,* 329–343.

Tassin, J.-P. Stinus, L., Simon, H., Blanc, G., Thierry, A.-M., Le Moal, M., Cardo, B., & Glowinski, J. Relationship between the locomotor hyperactivity induced by A10 lesions and the destruction of the fronto-cortical dopaminergic innervation in the rat. *Brain Research,* 1978, *141,* 278–281.

Teitelbaum, H., & Milner, P. M. Activity changes following partial hippocampal lesions in rats. *Journal of Comparative and Physiological Psychology,* 1963, *56,* 284–289.

Teitelbaum, P. Sensory control of hypothalamic hyperphagia. *Journal of Comparative and Physiological Psychology,* 1955, *48,* 158–163.

Teitelbaum, P. Random and food-directed activity in hyperphagica and normal rats. *Journal of Comparative and Physiological Psychology,* 1957, *50,* 486–490.

Teitelbaum, P., & Campbell, B. A. Injection patterns in hyperphagic and normal rats. *Journal of Comparative and Physiological Psychology,* 1958, *51,* 135–141.

Teitelbaum, P., & Epstein, A. N. The lateral hypothalamic syndrome. Recovery of feeding and drinking after lateral hypothalamic lesions. *Psychological Review,* 1962, *69,* 74–90.

Teitelbaum, H., & McFarland, W. L. Power spectral shifts in hippocampal EEG associated with conditioned locomotion in the rat. *Physiology and Behavior*, 1971, *7*, 545–549.

Teitelbaum, P., & Wolgin, D. Neurotransmitters and the regulation of food intake. In W. H. Gispen, Tj. B. Van Wimersma Griedanus, B. Bohus, & D. de Wied (Eds.), *Progress in brain research, Vol. 42: Hormones, homeostasis, and the brain*. Amsterdam: Elsevier, 1975, pp. 235–239.

Teitelbaum, P., Cheng, M. F., & Rozin, P. Development of feeding parallels its recovery after hypothalamic damage. *Journal of Comparative and Physiological Psychology*, 1969, *67*, 430–441.

Terasawa, E., & Timiras, P. S. Electrical activity during the estrous cycle of the rat: Cyclic changes in limbic structures. *Endocrinology*, 1968, *83*(2), 207–216.

Teyler, T. J., Vardaris, R. M., Lewis, D., & Rawitch, A. B. Gonadal steroids: Effect on excitability of hippocampal pyramidal cells. *Science*, 1980, *209*, 1017–1019.

Thierry, A. M., Tassin, J. P., Blanc, G., & Glowinski, J. Selective activation of the mesocortical DA system by stress. *Nature*, 1976, *263*, 242–244.

Thomas, G. J. Delayed alternation in rats after pre- or postcommissural fornicotomy. *Journal of Comparative and Physiological Psychology*, 1978, *92*, 1128–1136.

Thomas, G. J., & Slotnick, B. M. Effect of lesions in the cingulum on maze learning and avoidance conditioning in the rat. *Journal of Comparative and Physiological Psychology*, 1962, *55*, 1085–1096.

Thomas, G. J., & Slotnick, B. M. Impairment of avoidance responding by lesions in the cingulate cortex in rats depends on food drive. *Journal of Comparative and Physiological Psychology*, 1963, *56*, 959–964.

Thomas, G. J., Frey, W. J., Slotnick, B. M., & Krieckhaus, E. E. Behavioral effects of mammillothalamic tractotomy in cats. *Journal of Neurophysiology*, 1963, *26*, 857–876.

Thomas, G. J., Hostetter, G., & Barber, D. J. Behavioral functions of the limbic system. In E. Stellar & J. M. Sprague (Eds.), *Progress in physiological psychology (Vol. 2)*. New York: Academic Press, 1968, pp. 229–311.

Thomas, J. B., & McCleary, R. A. One-way avoidance behavior and septal lesions in the rat. *Journal of Comparative and Physiological Psychology*, 1974, *86*, 751–759.

Thomas, J. B., & Thomas, K. A. Square-runway avoidance behavior and septal lesions in the rat. *Physiology and Behavior*, 1974, *13*, 577–582.

Thomas, J. B., & Van Atta, E. L. Hyperirritability, lever press avoidance, and septal lesions in the albino rat. *Physiology and Behavior*, 1972, *8*, 225–232.

Thompson, C. I., Bergland, R. M., & Towfighi, J. T. Social and nonsocial behaviors of adult rhesus monkeys after amygdalectomy in infancy or adulthood. *Journal of Comparative and Physiological Psychology*, 1977, *91*, 533–548.

Thompson, J. D., & Schwartzbaum, J. S. Discrimination behavior and conditioned suppression (CER) following localized lesions in the amygdala and putamen. *Psychological Reports, Monograph Supplement*, No. 4-VI5, 1964.

Thompson, R. In J. M. Warren, & K. Akert (Eds.), *The frontal granular cortex and behavior: A symposium*, New York: McGraw-Hill, 1964.

Thompson, R. Hippocampal and cortical function in a maze devoid of left and right turns. *Physiology and Behavior*, 1979, *23*, 601–603.

Thompson, R., Langer, S. K., & Rich, I. Lesion studies on the functional significance of the posterior thalamomesencephalic tract. *Journal of Comparative Neurology*, 1964, *123*, 29–44.

Thompson, R. F., Berger, T. W., Berry, S. D., Hoehler, F. K., Kettner, R. E., & Weisz, D. J. Hippocampal substrate of classical conditioning. *Physiological Psychology*, 1980, *8*, 262–279.

Tondat, L. M., & Almli, C. R. Hyperdipsia produced by severing ventral septal fiber systems. *Physiology and Behavior*, 1975, *15*, 701–706.

Torii, S. Two types of pattern of hippocampal electrical activity induced by stimulation of hypothalamus and surrounding areas of rabbit's brain. *Japanese Journal of Psychology*, 1961, *11*, 147–157.

Trafton, C. L., & Marques, P. R. Effects of septal area and cingulate cortex lesions on opiate addiction behavior in rats. *Journal of Comparative and Physiological Psychology*, 1971, *75*, 277–285.

Trafton, C. L., Fibley, R. A., & Johnson, R. W. Avoidance behavior in rats as a function of the size and location of anterior cingulate cortex lesions. *Psychonomic Science*, 1969, *14*, 100–102.

Tsou, K., & Jang, C. S. Studies on the site of analgesic action of morphine by intracerebral micro-injection. *Scientia Sinica*, 1964, *13*, 1099–1109.

Turner, B. H. Neural structures involved in the rage syndrome of the rat. *Journal of Comparative and Physiological Psychology*, 1970, *71*, 103–113.

Turner, B. H. Sensorimotor syndrome produced by lesions of the amygdala and lateral hypothalamus. *Journal of Comparative Physiological Psychology*, 1973, *82*, 37–47.

Turner, B. H., Mishkin, M., & Knapp, M. Organization of the amygdalopetal projections from modality-specific cortical association areas in the monkey. *Journal of Comparative Neurology*, 1980, *191*, 515–543.

Ungerstedt, U. Stereotaxic mapping of the monoamine pathways in the rat brain. *Acta Physiologica Scandinavica*, 1971, *367* (Suppl.), 1–48.

Urban, I., & de Wied, D. Changes in excitability of the theta activity generating substrate by $ACTH_{4-10}$ in the rat. *Experimental Brain Research*, 1976, *24*, 325–344.

Urban, I., Lopes Da Silva, F. H., Storm van Leeuwen, W., & de Wied, D. A frequency shift in the hippocampal theta activity: An electrical correlate of central action of ACTH analogues in the dog? *Brain Research*, 1974, *69*, 361–365.

Ursin, H. The effect of amygdaloid lesions on flight and defense behavior in cats. *Experimental Neurology*, 1965, *11*, 61–79.

Ursin, H., & Kaada, B. R. Functional localization within the amygdaloid complex in the cat. *Electroencephalography and Clinical Neurophysiology*, 1960, *12*, 1–20.

Ursin, H., Wester, K., & Ursin, R. Habituation to electrical stimulation of the brain in unanesthetized cats. *Electroencephalography and Clinical Neurophysiology*, 1967, *23*, 41–49.

Ursin, H., Sundberg, H., & Menaker, S. I. Habituation of the orienting response elicited by stimulation of the caudate nucleus in the cat. *Neuropsychologia*, 1969, *7*, 313–318.

Usui, S., & Iwahara, S. Effects of atropine upon the hippocampal electrical activity in rats with special reference to paradoxical sleep. *Electroencephalography and Clinical Neurophysiology*, 1977, *42*, 510–517.

Valdes, J. J., Cameron, W. R., Evans, S., & Gage, F. H. Regional brain morphine injections selectively attenuate aspects of septal hyperreactivity: A multivariate assessment. *Pharmacology, Biochemistry and Behavior*, 1980, *12*, 563–572.

Valenstein, E. S., & Campbell, J. F. Medial forebrain bundle–lateral hypothalamic area and reinforcing brain stimulation. *American Journal of Physiology*, 1966, *210*, 270–274.

Valenstein, E. S., & Cox, V. C. The influence of hunger, thirst and previous experience in the test chamber on stimulus-bound eating and drinking. *Journal of Comparative and Physiological Psychology*, 1970, *70*, 189–199.

Valenstein, E. S., Cox, V. C., & Kakolewski, J. Behavior elicited by hypothalamic stimuli. *Brain, Behavior and Evolution*, 1969, *2*, 295–316.

Valenstein, E. S., Cox, V. C., & Kakolewski, J. A reexamination of the role of the hypothalamus in motivation. *Psychological Review*, 1970, *77*, 16–31.

Valverde, F. Amygdaloid projection field. In W. Bargmann & J. P. Schade (Eds.), *Progress in brain research, Vol. 3: The rhinencephalon and related structures,* Amsterdam: Elsevier, 1963.

Vanderwolf, C. H. Effect of combined medial thalamic and septal lesions on active-avoidance behavior. *Journal of Comparative and Physiological Psychology,* 1964, *58,* 31–37.

Vanderwolf, C. H. Hippocampal electrical activity and voluntary movement in the rat. *Electroencephalography and Clinical Neurophysiology,* 1969, *26,* 407–418.

Vanderwolf, C. H. Limbic-diencephalic mechanisms of voluntary movement. *Psychological Reviews,* 1971, *78,* 83–113.

Vanderwolf, C. H., & Robinson, T. E. Reticulo-cortical activity and behavior: A critique of the arousal theory and a new synthesis. *The Behavioral and Brain Sciences,* 1981, *4,* 459–514.

Vanderwolf, C. H., Kolb, B., & Cooley, R. K. Behavior of the rat after removal of the neocortex and hippocampal formation. *Journal of Comparative and Physiological Psychology,* 1978, *92,* 156–175.

Vanderwolf, C. H., Kramis, R., & Robinson, T. E. Hippocampal electrical activity during waking behavior and sleep: Analyses using centrally acting drugs. *Functions of the Septo-hippocampal System.* Ciba Foundation Symposium 58 (new series). Amsterdam: Elsevier, Excerpta Medica, North-Holland, 1978.

Vandesande, F., Dierckx, K., & DeMey, J. Identification of the vasopressin-neurophysin producing neurons in the rat suprachiasmatic nuclei. *Cell Tissue Research,* 1975, *156,* 377–380.

Van Hartesveldt, C. Size of reinforcement and operant responding in hippocampectomized rats. *Behavioral Biology,* 1973, *8,* 347–356.

Van Hartesveldt, C. Effect of drugs on DRL performance by rats with hippocampal lesions. Unpublished manuscript, 1974.

Van Hartesveldt, C. The hippocampus and regulation of the hypothalamic-hypophyseal-adrenal cortical axis. In R. L. Isaacson & K. H. Pribram (Eds.), *The hippocampus. Vol. 1: Structure and development.* New York: Plenum Press, 1975, pp. 375–391.

Van Hartesveldt, C., Petit, T. L., & Isaacson, R. L. Epileptogenic effects of several penicillins and penicillin-related compounds in rat neocortex. *Epilepsia,* 1975, *16,* 449–455.

Van Hoesen, G. W., MacDougall, J. M., & Mitchell, J. C. Anatomical specificity of septal projections in active and passive avoidance behaviour in rats. *Journal of Comparative and Physiological Psychology,* 1969, *68,* 80–89.

Van Hoesen, G. W., MacDougall, J. M., Wilson, J. R., & Mitchell, J. C. Septal lesions and the acquisition and maintenance of a discrete-trial DRL task. *Physiology and Behavior,* 1971, *7,* 471–475.

Van Hoesen, G. W., Pandya, D. N., & Butters, N. Cortical afferents to the entorhinal cortex of the rhesus monkey. *Science,* 1972, *175,* 1471–1473.

Van Hoesen, G. W., Wilson, L. M., McDougall, J. M., & Mitchell, J. C. Selective hippocampal complex deafferentation and deeferentation and avoidance behavior in rats. *Physiolgoical Behavior,* 1972, *8,* 873–897.

Van Wimersma Greidanus, T. B., Croiset, G., Bakker, E., & Bouman, H. Amygdaloid lesions block the effect of neuropeptides (Vasopressin, $ACTH_{4-10}$) on avoidance behavior. *Physiology and Behavior,* 1979, *22,* 291–295.

Velasco, M. E., & Taleisnik, S. Effect of hippocampal stimulation on the release of gonadotropin. *Endocrinology,* 1969, *85*(6), 1154–1159.

Verhoef, J., Witter, A., & de Wied, D. Specific uptake of a behaviorally potent [³H]ACTH₄₋₁₀ analog in the septal area after intraventricular injection in rats. *Brain Research*, 1977, *131*, 117–128.

Victor, M., Adams, R. D., & Collins, G. H. *The Wernicke-Korsakoff syndrome*. Oxford: Blackwell, 1971.

Votaw, C. L. Certain functional and anatomical relations of the cornu ammonis of the macaque monkey: I. Functional relations. *Journal of Comparative Neurology*, 1959, *112*, 353–382.

Votaw, C. L. Study of septal stimulation and ablation in the macaque monkey. *Neurology*, 1960, *10*, 202–209.

Votaw, C. L., & Lauer, E. W. Blood pressure, pulse and respiratory changes produced by stimulation of the hippocampus of the monkey. *Experimental Neurology*, 1963, *7*, 502–517.

Wada, J. A., & Sato, M. The generalized convulsive seizure state induced by daily electrical stimulation of the amygdala in split brain cats. *Epilepsia*, 1975, *16*, 417–430.

Wakefield, C. The intrinsic connections of the basolateral amygdaloid nuclei as visualized with the HRP method. *Neuroscience Letters*, 1979, *12*, 17–21.

Walsh, L. L., Halaris, A. E., Grossman, L., & Grossman, S. P. Some biochemical effects of zona incerta lesions that interfere with the regulation of water intake. *Pharmacology, Biochemistry and Behavior*, 1977, *7*, 351–356.

Warburton, D. M., & Russell, R. W. Some behavioral effects of cholinergic stimulation in the hippocampus. *Life Sciences*, 1969, *8*, 617–627.

Warrington, E. K., & Weiskrantz, L. An analysis of short-term and long-term memory defects in man. In J. A. Deutsch, (Ed.), *Physiological basis of memory*. New York: Academic Press, 1973.

Wayner, M. J., Loullis, C. C., & Barone, F. C. Effects of lateral hypothalamic lesions on schedule dependent and schedule induced behavior. *Physiology and Behavior*, 1977, *18*, 503–511.

Weiskrantz, L. Behavioral change associated with ablation of the amygdaloid complex in monkeys. *Journal of Comparative and Physiological Psychology*, 1956, *49*, 381–391.

Weiskrantz, L. Varieties of residual experience. *Quarterly Journal of Experimental Psychology*, 1980, *32*, 365–386.

Weiskrantz, L., & Warrington, E. K. The problem of the amnesic syndrome in man and animals. In R. L. Isaacson & K. H. Pribram (Eds.), *The hippocampus*. New York: Plenum Press, 1975, pp. 411–428.

Weiskrantz, L., & Wilson, W. A., Jr. The effects of reserpine (serpasil) on emotional behavior of normal and brain-operated monkeys. *Annals of the New York Academy of Sciences*, 1955, *61*, 36–55.

Weiskrantz, L., & Wilson, W. A. The effect of ventral rhinencephalic lesions on avoidance thresholds in monkeys. *Journal of Comparative and Physiological Psychology*, 1958, *51*, 167–171.

Weiss, C. S., & Hertzler, D. R. Facilitation of two-way avoidance of the guinea pig following intrahippocampal injections of procaine hydrochloride. *Physiological Psychology*, 1973, *1*, 305–307.

Weiss, K. R., Friedman, R., & McGregor, S. Effects of septal lesions on latent inhibition and habituation of the orienting response in rats. *Acta Neurobiologica Experimentalis*, 1974, *34*, 491–504.

Werka, T., Skår, J., & Ursin, H. Exploration and avoidance in rats with lesions in amygdala and piriform cortex. *Journal of Comparative and Physiological Psychology*, 1978, *92*, 672–681.

Wetzel, A. B., Conner, R. L., & Levine, S. Shock-induced fighting in septal-lesioned rats. *Psychonomic Science*, 1967, 9, 133–134.

Whishaw, I. Q. Hippocampal electroencephalographic activity in the Mongolian gerbil during natural behaviors and in wheel running and conditioned immobility. *Canadian Journal of Psychology*, 1972, 26, 219–239.

Whishaw, I. Q. The effects of alcohol and atropine on EEG and behavior in the rabbit. *Psychopharmacologica* (Berlin), 1976, 48, 83–90.

Whishaw, I. Q., Bland, B. H., Robinson, T. E., & Vanderwolf, C. H. Neuromuscular blockade: The effects on two hippocampal RSA (theta) systems and neocortical desynchronization. *Brain Research Bulletin*, 1976, 1, 573–581.

White, L. E., Jr. Ipsilateral afferents to the hippocampal formation in the albino rat: I. Cingulum projections. *Journal of Comparative Neurology*, 1959, 113, 1–32.

White, N. Perseveration by rats with amygdaloid lesions. *Journal of Comparative and Physiological Psychology*, 1971, 77, 416–426.

White, N., & Weingarten, H. Effects of amygdaloid lesions on exploration by rats. *Physiology and Behavior*, 1976, 17, 73–79.

Wickelgren, W. O., & Isaacson, R. L. Effect of the introduction of an irrelevant stimulus in runway performance of the hippocampectomized rat. *Nature*, 1963, 200, 48–50.

Wigal, T., Goodlett, C., Eisenberg, S., Spear, N., Hannigan, J. H., Jr., Donovick, P., Burright, R., & Isaacson, R. The effects of home contextual cues on spontaneous alternation and conditional place aversion in rats with septal or hippocampal lesions. *Neuroscience Abstracts*, 1981, 7, 649.

Wigstrom, H., Swann, J. W., & Andersen, P. Calcium dependency of synaptic long-lasting potentiation in the hippocampal slice. *Acta Physiologica Scandinavica*, 1979, 105, 126–128.

Wikler, A., Norrell, H., & Miller, D. Limbic system and opioid addiction in the rat. *Experimental Neurology*, 1972, 34, 545–557.

Wilson, M., Kaufman, H. M., Zieler, R. E., & Lieb, J. P. Visual identification and memory in monkeys with circumscribed inferotemporal lesions. *Journal of Comparative and Physiological Psychology*, 1972, 78, 173–183.

Wilsoncroft, W. E. Effects of medial cortex lesions on the maternal behavior of the rat. *Psychological Reports*, 1963, 13, 835–838.

Wimer, R. E., Wimer, C. C., Chernow, C. R., & Balvanz, B. A. The genetic organization of neuron number in the pyramidal cell layer of hippocampal regio superior in house mice. *Brain Research*, 1980, 196, 59–77.

Winocur, G. The effects of interference on discrimination learning and recall by rats with hippocampal lesions. *Physiology and Behavior*, 1979, 22, 339–345.

Winocur, G., & Mills, J. A. Transfer between related and unrelated problems following hippocampal lesions in rats. *Journal of Comparative and Physiological Psychology*, 1970, 73, 162–169.

Winocur, G., & Olds, J. Effects of context manipulation on memory and reversal learning in rats with hippocampal lesions. *Journal of Comparative and Physiological Psychology*, 1978, 92, 312–321.

Winson, J. Interspecies differences in the occurrence of theta. *Behavioral Biology*, 1972, 7, 479–487.

Winson, J. The theta mode of hippocampal function. In R. L. Isaacson & K. H. Pribram (Eds.), *The hippocampus: A comprehensive treatise*. New York: Plenum Press, 1974.

Winson, J., & Abzug, C. Gating of neuronal transmission in the hippocampus: Efficacy of transmission varies with behavioral state. *Science*, 1977, 196, 1223–1225.

Winson, J., & Abzug, C. Neuronal transmission through hippocampal pathways dependent on behavior. *Journal of Neurophysiology:* 1978, *41,* 716–732.

Wise, R. A. Individual differences in effects of hypothalamic stimulation: The role of stimulation locus. *Physiological Behavior,* 1971, *6,* 569–572.

Wise, R. A. Catecholamine theories of reward: A critical review. *Brain Research,* 1978, *152,* 215–247.

Wishart, T., & Mogenson, G. Effects of lesions of the hippocampus and septum before and after passive avoidance training. *Physiology and Behavior,* 1969, *5,* 31–34.

Wishart, T. B., & Mogenson, G. J. Effects of lesions of the hippocampus and septum before and after passive avoidance training. *Physiology and Behavior,* 1970, *5,* 31–34. (a)

Wishart, T. B., & Mogenson, G. J. Reduction of water intake by electrical stimulation of the septal region of the rat brain. *Physiology and Behavior,* 1970, *5,* 1399–1404. (b)

Wodinsky, J., & Bitterman, M. E. Partial reinforcement in the fish. *American Journal of Psychology,* 1959, *72,* 184–199.

Wodinsky, J., & Bitterman, M. E. Resistance to extinction in the fish after extensive training with partial reinforcement. *American Journal of Psychology,* 1960, *73,* 429–434.

Wolgin, D. L., & Teitelbaum, P. Role of activation and sensory stimuli in recovery from lateral hypothalamic damage in the cat. *Journal of Comparative and Physiological Psychology,* 1978, *92,* 474–500.

Wolgin, D. L., Cytawa, J., & Teitelbaum, P. The role of activation in the regulation of food intake. In D. Novin, W. Wyricka, & G. Bray (Eds.), *Hunger: Basic mechanisms and clinical implications.* New York: Raven Press, 1976, pp. 179–191.

Woodruff, M. L., & Isaacson, R. L. Discrimination learning in animals with lesions of hippocampus. *Behavioral Biology,* 1972, *7,* 489–501.

Woodruff, M. L., & Kantor, H. *Fornix transection eliminates the kamin effect: Possible mediation by ACTH.* Presented at a meeting of the American Psychological Association, Montreal, 1980.

Woodruff, M. L., Schneiderman, B., & Isaacson, R. L. Impaired acquisition of a simultaneous brightness discrimination by cortically and hippocampally lesioned rats. *Psychonomic Science,* 1972, *27,* 269–271.

Woodruff, M. L., Gage, F. H., & Isaacson, R. L. Changes in focal epileptic activity produced by brain stem sections in the rabbit. *Electroencephalography and Clinical Neurophysiology,* 1973, *35,* 475–486. (a)

Woodruff, M. L., Kearley, R. C., & Isaacson, R. L. Deficient brightness discrimination acquisition produced by daily intracranial injections of penicillin in rats. *Behavioral Biology,* 1974, *12,* 445–460.

Woodruff, M. L., Hatton, D. C., & Meyer, M. E. Hippocampal ablation prolongs immobility response in rabbits. *(Oryctolagus cuniculus). Journal of Comparative and Physiological Psychology,* 1975, *88,* 329–334.

Woodruff, M. L., Fish, B. S., & Alderman, A. O. Epileptiform lesions in rat hippocampus and acquisition of two-way avoidance. *Physiology and Behavior,* 1977, *19,* 401–410.

Worsham, E., & Hamilton, L. W. Acquisition and retention of avoidance behaviors following septal lesions or scopolamine injections in rats. *Physiological Psychology,* 1973, *1,* 219–226.

Wurtz, R. H., & Olds, J. Amygdaloid stimulation and operant reenforcement in the rat. *Journal of Comparative and Physiological Psychology,* 1963, *56,* 941–949.

Wyss, J. M., Swanson, L. W., & Cowan, W. M. Evidence for an input to the molecular layer and the *stratum granulosum* of the dentate gyrus from the supramammillary region of the hypothalamus. *Anatomy and Embryology*, 1979, *156*, 165–176. (a)

Wyss, J. M., Swanson, L. W., & Cowan, W. M. A study of subcortical afferents to the hippocampal formation in the rat. *Neuroscience*, 1979, *4*, 463–476. (b)

Yeudall, L. T., & Walley, R. E. Methylphenidate, amygdalectomy, and active performance in the rat. *Journal of Comparative and Physiological Psychology*, 1977, *91*, 1207–1219.

Young, R. C., Ervin, G. N., & Smith, G. P. Abnormal open field behavior after anterolateral hypothalamic injection of 6-hydroxydopamine. *Pharmacology, Biochemistry and Behavior*, 1976, *5*, 565–570.

Yunger, L. M., & Harvey, J. A. Effect of lesions in the medial forebrain bundle on three measures of pain sensitivity and noise-elicited startle. *Journal of Comparative and Physiological Psychology*, 1973, *83*, 173–183.

Zeigler, H. P. Feeding behavior of the pigeon. In J. S. Rosenblatt, R. A. Hinde, E. Shaw & C. Beer (Eds.), *Advances in the Study of Behavior*, (Vol. 7). New York: Academic Press, 1976.

Zeman, W., & King, F. A. Tumors of the septum pellucidum and adjacent structures with abnormal affective behaviour: An anterior midline structure syndrome. *Journal of Nervous and Mental Disease*, 1958, *127*, 490–502.

Zigmond, M. J., & Stricker, E. M. Recovery of feeding and drinking by rats after intraventricular 6-hydroxydopamine or lateral hypothalamic lesions. *Science*, 1973, *182*, 717–720.

Zucker, I., & McCleary, R. A. Perseveration in septal cats. *Psychonomic Science*, 1964, *1*, 387–388.

Zucker, I., Rusak, B., & King, R. G. Neural bases for circadian rhythms in rodent behavior. In A. H. Riesen & R. F. Thompson (Eds.), *Advances in psychobiology* (Vol. 3). New York: Wiley, 1976, pp. 35–76.

Zuromski, E. S., Donovick, P. J., & Burright, R. J. The effect of septal lesions on the albino rat's ability to regulate light. *Journal of Comparative and Physiological Psychology*, 1972, *78*, 83–90.

Author Index

313

Subject Index